Cardiovascular Disease

METHODS IN MOLECULAR MEDICINE™

John M. Walker, SERIES EDITOR

METHODS IN MOLECULAR MEDICINE™

Cardiovascular Disease

Methods and Protocols

Volume 2: Molecular Medicine

Edited by

Qing K. Wang, PhD, MBA

Department of Molecular Medicine
Cleveland Clinic Lerner College of Medicine
Case Western Reserve University, Cleveland, OH

HUMANA PRESS ✹ TOTOWA, NEW JERSEY

Production Editor: Jennifer Hackworth

Cover illustration: Figure 2 from Volume 2, Chapter 13, "Methods for Isolation of Endothelial and Smooth Muscle Cells and In Vitro Proliferation Assays" by Ganapati H. Mahabeleshwar, Payaningal R. Somanath, and Tatiana V. Byzova

Cover design by Patricia F. Cleary

For additional copies, pricing for bulk purchases, and/or information about other Humana titles, contact Humana at the above address or at any of the following numbers: Tel.: 973-256-1699; Fax: 973-256-8341; E-mail: orders@humanapr.com; or visit our Website: www.humanapress.com

Printed in the United States of America. 10 9 8 7 6 5 4 3 2 1
1-59745-213-0 (e-book)

Library of Congress Cataloging in Publication Data
    Cardiovascular disease : methods and protocols / edited by Qing Wang.
        v. ; cm. -- (Methods in molecular medicine ; 128-129)
    Includes bibliographical references and index.
    Contents: v. 1. Genetics -- v. 2. Molecular medicine.
    ISBN 1-58829-572-9 (v. 1 : alk. paper) -- ISBN 1-58829-892-2 (v. 2 : alk. paper)
    1. Cardiovascular system--Diseases--Genetic aspects--Laboratory manuals.   I. Wang, Qing, 1965-   . II. Series.
    [DNLM: 1. Cardiovascular Diseases--genetics--Laboratory Manuals. 2. Cardiovascular Diseases--physiopathology--Laboratory Manuals. 3. Molecular Biology--methods--Laboratory Manuals.   WG 25 C2678 2006]
    RC687.C37 2006
    616.1'042--dc22   2006000450

Preface

Cardiovascular disease is the leading cause of death in developed countries, but is quickly becoming an epidemic in such well-populated countries as China, India, and other developing nations. Cardiovascular research is the key to the prevention, diagnosis, and management of cardiovascular disease. Vigorous and cross-disciplinary approaches are required for successful cardiovascular research. As the boundries between different scientific disciplines, particularly in the life sciences, are weakening and disappearing, a successful investigator needs to be competent in many different areas, including genetics, cell biology, biochemistry, physiology, and structural biology. The newly developed field of molecular medicine is a cross-disciplinary science that seeks to comprehend disease causes and mechanisms at the molecular level, and to apply this basic research to the prevention, diagnosis, and treatment of diseases and disorders. This volume in the *Methods in Molecular Medicine* series, *Cardiovascular Disease,* provides comprehensive coverage of both basic and the most advanced approaches to the study and characterization of cardiovascular disease. These methods will advance knowledge of the mechanisms, diagnoses, and treatments of cardiovascular disease.

Cardiovascular Disease is a timely volume in which the theory and principles of each method are described in the Introduction section, followed by a detailed description of the materials and equipment needed, and step-by-step protocols for successful execution of the method. A notes section provides advice for potential problems, any modifications, and alternative methods.

We have gathered a group of highly experienced cardiovascular researchers to describe in detail the most important techniques in molecular medicine that are employed in genetic, molecular, cellular, structural, and physiological studies of cardiovascular disease. The thirty-seven chapters in the two volumes cover varied methods that include the following:

- Cytogenetic analyses (karyotyping, FISH, array CGH, somatic hybrid analysis).
- Linkage programs for mapping chromosomal locations of disease genes.
- Bioinformatics.
- Human genetics for identifying genes for both monogenic and common complex diseases (positional cloning and genome-wide association study).
- Mouse genetics for identifying genes for complex disease traits (chromosome substitution strains).
- Mutation screening, genetic testing, and high throughput genotyping of single-nucleotide polymorphisms (SNPs).
- Microarray (Genechips) analysis.

- Proteomics.
- Generation of knockout, knock-in, and conditional mutant mice and transgenic overexpression mice for cardiovascular genes.
- Animal models for coronary artery disease, heart failure, hypertension, cardiac arrhythmias, and thrombosis.
- Cardiac physiology (recording techniques for action potentials, sodium and other ionic currents, and optical mapping).
- Cell biology (isolation of adult cardiomyocytes, endothelial cells, smooth muscle cells, angiogenesis, cell proliferation, adhesion, migration, and apoptosis assays).
- Gene transfer and gene therapy (adenovirus vectors, HIV-based retroviral vectors, nucleofection®).
- Structural biology (X-ray crystallography, NMR spectroscopy, and electron cryomicroscopy).
- Stem cells.

Cardiovascular Disease should be particularly useful for inspiring undergraduate students, graduate students, postdoctoral fellows, cardiology fellows, clinicians, basic scientists, and other researchers who are entering a new area of cardiovascular research to experience the new challenges. It will serve as a valuable resource book for active researchers when they design new experiments. Although many techniques are described for studying cardiovascular disease, they should be equally valuable for researchers studying other human diseases.

I especially thank Susan De Stefano for her valuable assistance in preparing, reformatting and compiling all the chapters. I also thank Professor John M. Walker, the Series Editor for his invitation to develop this book and his help in editing this book. Finally, I thank all of the authors for the time-consuming job of preparing their chapters.

Qing K. Wang, PhD, MBA

Contents

CONTENTS OF THE COMPANION VOLUME
Volume 1: Genetics

Contributors

RONALD W. ALFA • *Department of Neurosciences, University of California, San Diego, La Jolla, CA*

ALEXANDRU ALMASAN • *Department of Cancer Biology, Lerner Research Institute, and Department of Radiation Oncology, The Cleveland Clinic Foundation, Cleveland, OH*

ANDREA AMALFITANO • *Department of Pediatrics, Duke University Medical Center, Durham, NC*

STEPHEN R. ARCHACKI • *Center for Molecular Genetics, The Cleveland Clinic Foundation, Cleveland, OH*

MICHAEL BADER • *Max-Delbrück Center for Molecular Medicine, Berlin-Buch, Germany*

JULIE BAGLIONE • *Department of Cell Biology, The Cleveland Clinic Foundation, Cleveland, OH*

MARCOS E. BARBOSA • *Max-Delbrück Center for Molecular Medicine, Berlin-Buch, Germany*

ARMIN BLESCH • *Department of Neurosciences, University of California, San Diego, La Jolla, CA*

TATIANA V. BYZOVA • *Department of Molecular Cardiology, The Cleveland Clinic Foundation, Cleveland, OH*

YUANNA CHENG • *Department of Cardiovascular Medicine, The Cleveland Clinic Foundation, Cleveland, OH*

RONALD A. CONLON • *Department of Genetics, Case Western Reserve University, Cleveland, OH*

MEREDITH E. CROSBY • *Department of Cancer Biology, Lerner Research Institute, and Department of Environmental Health Science, Case Western Reserve University, Cleveland, OH*

MARGARET S. DICE • *Department of Biology, Utah State University, Logan, UT*

SUDHIRANJAN GUPTA • *Department of Molecular Cardiology, The Cleveland Clinic Foundation, Cleveland, OH*

PUDUR JAGADEESWARAN • *Department of Cellular and Structural Biology, The University of Texas Health Science Center at San Antonio, San Antonio, TX*

TYCE KEARL • *Department of Biology, Utah State University, Logan, UT*

ASHRAF KITMITTO • *School of Medicine, University of Manchester, UK*

DAVID F. LEPAGE • *Department of Genetics, Case Western Reserve University, Cleveland, OH*

GANAPATI H. MAHABELESHWAR • *Department of Molecular Cardiology, The Cleveland Clinic Foundation, Cleveland, OH*

NILADRI MAL • *Departments of Cardiovascular Medicine and Cell Biology, The Cleveland Clinic Foundation, Cleveland, OH*

SUPARNA MAZUMDER • *Department of Cancer Biology, Cleveland Clinic Lerner Research Institute, Cleveland, OH*

MICHAEL NIX • *amaxa biosystems, Cologne, Germany*

MARCELA OANCEA • *Department of Cancer Biology, Cleveland Clinic Lerner Research Institute, and Department of Chemistry, Cleveland State University, Cleveland, OH*

RYAN PARIS • *Department of Cellular and Structural Biology, The University of Texas Health Science Center at San Antonio, San Antonio, TX*

XUEJUN PENG • *Department of Quantitative Health Sciences, The Cleveland Clinic Foundation, Cleveland, OH*

MARC S. PENN • *Departments of Cardiovascular Medicine and Cell Biology, The Cleveland Clinic Foundation, Cleveland, OH*

RALPH PLEHM • *Max-Delbrück Center for Molecular Medicine, Berlin-Buch, Germany*

EDWARD F. PLOW • *Joseph J. Jacobs Center for Thrombosis and Vascular Biology and Department of Molecular Cardiology, The Cleveland Clinic Foundation, Cleveland, OH*

ELZBIETA PLUSKOTA • *Joseph J. Jacobs Center for Thrombosis and Vascular Biology and Department of Molecular Cardiology, The Cleveland Clinic Foundation, Cleveland, OH*

JUN QIN • *Structural Biology Program, The Cleveland Clinic Foundation, Cleveland, OH*

PRASHANTH RAO • *Department of Cellular and Structural Biology, The University of Texas Health Science Center at San Antonio, San Antonio, TX*

PETER C. RUBEN • *Department of Biology, Utah State University, Logan, UT*

SUBHA SEN • *Department of Molecular Cardiology, The Cleveland Clinic Foundation, Cleveland, OH*

DELILA SERRA • *Department of Pediatrics, Duke University Medical Center, Durham, NC*

JONATHAN D. SMITH • *Department of Cell Biology, The Cleveland Clinic Foundation, Cleveland, OH*

DMITRY A. SOLOVIEV • *Joseph J. Jacobs Center for Thrombosis and Vascular Biology and Department of Molecular Cardiology, The Cleveland Clinic Foundation, Cleveland, OH*

PAYANINGAL R. SOMANATH • *Department of Molecular Cardiology, The Cleveland Clinic Foundation, Cleveland, OH*

SOICHI TAKEDA • *Department of Cardiac Physiology, National Cardiovascular Research Institute, Japan*

XIAO-LI TIAN • *Department of Molecular Cardiology, The Cleveland Clinic Foundation, Cleveland, OH*

CORINNA THIEL • *amaxa biosystems, Cologne, Germany*

QING K. WANG • *Department of Molecular Cardiology, Center for Cardiovascular Genetics, Department of Cardiovascular Medicine, The Cleveland Clinic Foundation, Cleveland, OH*

FANG XU • *Department of Pediatrics, Duke University Medical Center, Durham, NC*

SANDRO L. YONG • *Department of Molecular Cardiology, The Cleveland Clinic Foundation, Cleveland, OH*

SUN-AH YOU • *Department of Molecular Cardiology, The Cleveland Clinic Foundation, Cleveland, OH*

1

Microarray Analysis of Cardiovascular Diseases

Stephen R. Archacki and Qing K. Wang

Summary

Microarray analysis is a powerful technique for high-throughput, global transcriptonomic profiling of gene expression. It holds great promise for analyzing the genetic and molecular bases of cardiovascular diseases and various other complex diseases and permits the analysis of thousands of genes simultaneously, both in diseased and nondiseased tissues and/or cell lines. Microarrays or microchips are made by depositing spots of DNA or oligonucleotides representing thousands of genes on a solid support such as a coated glass surface, and can allow the comparison of gene expression patterns in any two samples. Total RNA is isolated from the tissue or cells of interest, converted to cDNA and then cRNA labeled with biotin, and hybridized to the chips. Hybridization signals are then quantified and compared among different samples. We used oligonucleotide microarrays to obtain an unbiased assessment of expression levels of thousands of genes simultaneously in normal and diseased coronary arteries. Fifty-six genes showed differential expression in atherosclerotic coronary artery tissues, and 49 of them represent new linked genes for coronary artery disease. These studies can generate novel hypotheses relating to the pathologies of disease and further studies with animal models, molecular biology, cell biology, and biochemistry will validate these hypotheses and provide novel insights into the pathogenesis of disease.

Key Words: Oligonucleotide array; microarray, genechip; expression profiling; coronary artery disease; gene; genetics; atherosclerosis.

1. Introduction

Gene expression is central to the pathogenesis of many disease processes. Microarray analysis is a powerful technique for studying gene expression. Different from other methods, such as Northern blot analysis and reverse-transcription (RT)-PCR, that can study a single gene each time, microarray analysis permits the analysis of thousands of genes simultaneously in both

From: *Methods in Molecular Medicine, vol. 129:*
Cardiovascular Disease: Methods and Protocols, Volume 2: Molecular Medicine
Edited by: Q. K. Wang © Humana Press Inc., Totowa, NJ

diseased and nondiseased tissues as occurs in coronary artery disease, congestive heart failure, and congenital heart disease *(1)*. This technology has identified novel genes and pathways involved in the generation of these diseases at both the organ/tissue level (coronary arteries, cardiac tissues) and cell level (endothelial cells, vascular smooth muscle cells, macrophages). It is important to note that several studies have confirmed the expression of genes previously linked with these disease processes, suggesting that expression profiling with microarrays is a valid approach for identifying gene expression alternations associated with disease *(2)*. Yet, many more novel genes have been identified as well and will serve as a valuable resource to identify novel pathways involved in the generation of disease *(3)*. With the continued use of the technology and its accelerated application to these diseases, we will eventually identify a common group of genes, which can serve as markers for these disease processes on a global scale.

Microarrays or GeneChips are made by depositing spots of cDNA or oligonucleotides on a solid support such as a coated glass surface. A flat glass surface makes it possible to (1) array molecules in a parallel fashion, (2) miniaturize the procedure, and (3) use fluorescent dyes for detection and, thus, avoid radioactivity. This differs from conventional methods such as filter-based supports of charged nylon and nitrocellulose for studying mRNA expression.

Expression profiling begins by harvesting the total RNA from the tissue of interest. The total RNA is then converted to a single-stranded molecule of DNA followed by the synthesis of the complementary strand of DNA, resulting in a doubled-stranded molecule (cDNA). Consequently, the cDNA is then converted back to a complementary, single-stranded RNA (which is labeled with biotin) and can be hybridized to the microarrays or chips for expression profiling. An example of this labeling assay is shown in **Fig. 1**.

The data generated from the microarray contains the raw score values from each spot on the micrroarray representing the gene expression. Several programs are available to analyze the data. A general schematic overview of the process is shown in **Fig 2**. Briefly, the analysis of the data occurs in five main steps: (1) entering the raw data into the program, (2) experimental data normalization (designating groups of replicates and control samples), (3) experimental interpretation (choosing how the raw data is translated into a value [using the raw score or a log ratio]), (4) statistical analysis (using analysis of variance [ANOVA] to determine a statistically significant gene list), and (5) clustering (K means or gene tree).

Microarray analysis can generate novel hypotheses related to the pathology of the disease, and further studies with animal models, molecular biology, cell biology, and biochemistry will validate the hypothesis and provide novel

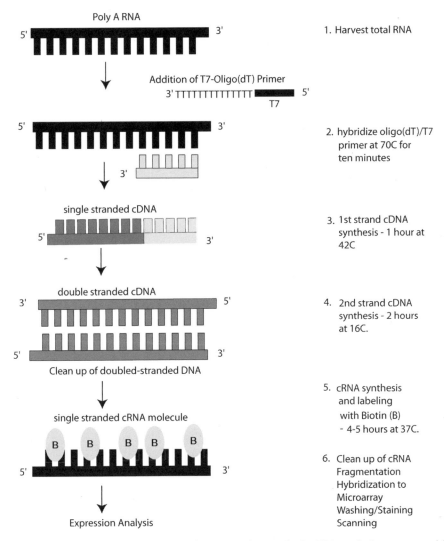

Poly A RNA

1. Harvest total RNA

Addition of T7-Oligo(dT) Primer

2. hybridize oligo(dT)/T7 primer at 70C for ten minutes

single stranded cDNA

3. 1st strand cDNA synthesis - 1 hour at 42C

double stranded cDNA

4. 2nd strand cDNA synthesis - 2 hours at 16C.

Clean up of doubled-stranded DNA

5. cRNA synthesis and labeling with Biotin (B) - 4-5 hours at 37C.

single stranded cRNA molecule

6. Clean up of cRNA Fragmentation Hybridization to Microarray Washing/Staining Scanning

Expression Analysis

Fig. 1. Microarray labeling assays for expression analysis. This technique starts with harvesting intact total RNA from tissue such as coronary artery, its reverse transcription to a single-stranded complementary DNA molecule and double stranded DNA synthesis, and ultimately the final product of a complementary RNA molecule labeled with agents such as bioton (B), which can then be placed on the microarray of gene expression.

insights into the pathogenesis of disease. These studies will eventually generate novel diagnostic and therapeutic markers, and identify potential drug targets for the development of more effective management of cardiovascular disease.

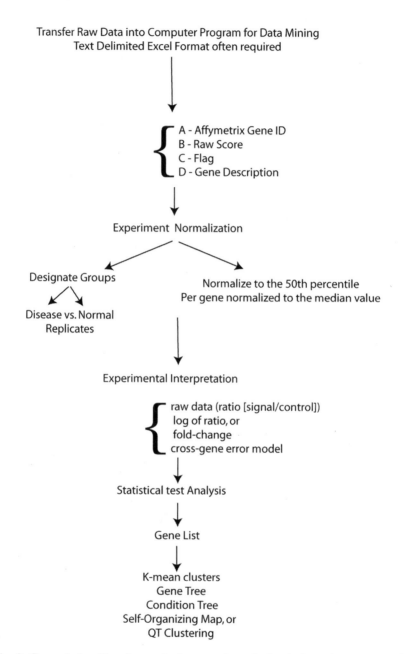

Fig. 2. General algorithm for analyzing raw data obtained after microarray analysis. Many experimental parameters can be modified to selectively filter a statistically significant gene list.

2. Materials

2.1. Microarrays

1. Human Genome U33 Array (Affymetrix) or purchased from existing core facilities providing tailor-made arrays.
2. The Affymetrix gene chip U133 plus 2.0 contains 54,675 probe sets.

2.2. cRNA Synthesis

1. Total RNA isolating kits with TRIZol reagent (Invitrogen).
2. Double-stranded complementary DNA Kit with Superscript Choice System (Invitrogen) with a high-performance liquid chromatography (HPLC)-purified oligo-T primer containing a T7 RNA polymerase promoter (GENSET, La Jolla, CA).
3. In vitro transcription (IVT) kit (ENZO, Diagnostics, Farmingdale, NY).
4. Qiagen total RNA cleanup kit.
5. Glycogen (Ambion).
6. 7.5 M ammonium acetate.
7. Absolute ethanol (EtOH).
8. 25:24:1 phenol:chloroform:isoamyl alcohol (saturated with 10 mM Tris-HCl, pH 8.0/1 mM EDTA).
9. Phase lock gels (PLGs).
10. 1 M dithiothreitol (DTT).
11. 100 mM dNTP.
12. Diethylpyrocarbonate (DEPC)-treated water.

2.3. Tissue Samples

1. Tissue harvested from human subjects should be flash-frozen in liquid nitrogen and stored at –80°C until use for extraction of total RNA.
2. Ideally, approx 0.2 g of tissue is sufficient for total RNA extraction and synthesis of nucleic acids for analysis on the microarray.
3. Tissue should be pulverized (e.g., mortar and pestle) into a fine powder before the addition of TRIZol.
4. It is best to continuously work through the synthesis of the cRNA probe from the start after total RNA extraction. However, when necessary, various steps can be carried out overnight and resumed the next day without altering the integrity of the original RNA.
5. Each of the initial steps does require a conscientious precaution of preventing RNase contamination from the hands or unclean glassware. All efforts should be made to follow the timed algorithm for the synthesis of the cRNA probe to prevent degradation.

3. Methods

3.1. Microarray Probe Synthesis

3.1.1. First-Strand Synthesis

1. Approximately 5–400 µg of total RNA is used (total reaction volume is not to exceed 20 µL). Mix T7 (dt-24) primer: 5′GGCCAGTGAATTGTAATACGACT-

CACTATAGGGAGGCGG(dT)$_{24}$-3′ with target total RNA and DEPC-treated water in 1.5 mL RNAse-free tube. Hybridize probe at 70°C for 10 min, then place on ice.

2. To each tube on ice, add 5X first-strand buffer, 0.1 M DTT, and 10 mM dNTP; mix and incubate at 42°C for 2 min.

3. Proceed immediately to add SSII Reverse Transcriptase enzyme to sample tubes, mix well and incubate at 42°C for 1 h. Place reactions on ice when complete, then quick-spin. The conversion of the mRNA to a single-stranded DNA molecule has now been synthesized. This can be stored at –20°C.

3.1.2. Second-Strand Synthesis

1. Prepare the second-strand synthesis reaction master mixture for all tubes (includes DEPC-treated water, 5X second-strand buffer, dNTPs, 10 U/µL DNA ligase [enzymatically links polynucleotide chains together being synthesized], 10 U/µL DNA polymerase I, and 2 U/µL RNase H [enzymatically degrades original RNA strand]). To each of the tubes (containing 20 µL first-strand synthesis), add the 130 µL of the second-strand reaction mixture. The total volume is now 150 µL. Gently tap the tube to mix and quick-spin. During this reaction, the single-stranded DNA molecule is now being used as a template for the synthesis of a complementary double-stranded molecule.

2. Incubate for 2 h at 16°C.

3. Add 2 µL (10 U) T4 DNA polymerase to each tube (this fills in any gaps in the final polynucleotide strand) and incubate for another 5 min at 16°C.

4. Add 10 µL 0.5 M EDTA and place reaction on ice. Store at –20°C or proceed to cleanup.

3.2. Cleanup of dsDNA

3.2.1. PLG–Phenol/Chloroform Extraction

1. Pellet the PLG at ≥10,000g for 20–30 s.

2. Add 162 µL (equal volume) of 25:24:1 phenol:chloroform:isoamyl alcohol (saturated with 10 mM Tris-HCl, pH 8.0/1 mM EDTA) to the final cDNA synthesis preparation (162 µL) to reach a final volume of 324 µL.

3. Vortex.

4. Transfer cDNA-phenol/chloroform mix to the PGL tube—do NOT vortex.

5. Microcentrifuge at full speed for 2 min.

6. Transfer upper aqueous phase containing the double stranded DNA molecule to a fresh 1.5-mL tube.

3.3. Ethanol Precipitation

1. Add 0.5 vol (~75 µL) of 7.5 M ammonium acetate and 2.5 vol (450 µL) of absolute ice-cold EtOH to each tube and vortex.

2. Immediately centrifuge at ≥12,000g for 20 min. Remove supernatant carefully without disturbing the pellet.

3. Wash pellet with 500 μL of 80% ice-cold EtOH.
4. Centrifuge at 12,000*g* for 5 min at room temperature.
5. Remove the supernatant and repeat.
6. Remove the supernatant and air-dry the pellet.
7. Resuspend pellet in 12 μL DEPC-treated water. Use 1 or 2 μL for agarose gel analysis.

3.4. Synthesis of Biotin-Labeled cRNA (IVT)

1. Use the following table to determine what volume of cDNA to use in the reaction:

Total RNA (μg)	Volume of cDNA to use in the IVT (μL)
5–8	10
8.1–16	5
16.1–24	3.3
24.1–32	2.5
32.1–40	2

2. Add reaction components to RNase-free microfuge tubes in the order indicated in the following table. Keep reactions at room temperature until all ingredients are added.

Reagent	Volume
Template DNA	*See* previous chart
Distilled or deionized water	To give reaction volume of 40 μL
10X HY reaction buffer	4 μL
10X biotin-labeled ribonucleotides	4 μL
10X DTT	4 μL
10X RNase inhibitor mix	4 μL
20X T7 RNA polymerase	2 μL
Total volume	40 μL

3. Carefully mix the reagents and collect the mixture in the bottom of the tube by brief spin.
4. Immediately place tube at 37°C. Incubate for 4–5 h and gently mix the contents of the tube every 30–45 min.
5. Continue to clean up or store at –20°C.

3.5. Cleanup of IVT Product

1. Save an aliquot of the unpurifed IVT product for gel analysis. Proceed to IVT product cleanup using Qiagen total RNA cleanup kit.
2. Use a 1.5-mL, labeled microfuge tube to prepare the following mix:
   a. 80 μL DEPC-treated water.
   b. 350 μL RLT buffer.
   c. 20 μL of IVT product.
3. Mix thoroughly and add 250 μL of 100% ethanol and mix by pipetting.

4. Apply the mixture (~700 µL) to an RNeasy mini spin column setup sitting in a 2.0-mL collection tube.
5. Microfuge for 15 s at 8000*g*.
6. Collect the flow-through and repeat **steps 4** and **5**.
7. Discard the second flow-through and transfer the column to a fresh, labeled collection tube. Add 500 µL of RPE buffer (make sure β-mercaptoethanol has been added to the RPE buffer as per kit instructions).
8. Microcentrifuge for 15 s at 8000*g*.
9. Add 500 µL of RPE buffer to the column and centrifuge again for 2 min at maximum speed to dry out the column (you can discard the previous flow-through).
10. Transfer the column to a new 1.5-mL collection tube.
11. Add 30 µL of DEPC-treated water to the column and let stand for 1 min.
12. Centrifuge for 1 min at 8000*g* and save the eluate containing purified IVT cRNA.
13. Repeat **steps 11** and **12** and add the second eluate to the same collection tube.
14. To the combined eluate (~60 µL) add 0.6 vol (~36 µL) of 7.5 *M* NH$_4$AC and 2.5 vol (~150 µL) of absolute ice-cold EtOH.
15. Add 5–10 µL of glycogen.
16. Let precipitate overnight at –20°C.
17. Centrifuge at 14,000*g* for 30 min at 4°C.
18. Remove the supernatant and wash pellet with 500 µL of ice-cold 80% EtOH.
19. Centrifuge at 12,000–14,000*g* for 5 min and repeat.
20. Remove supernatant and air-dry the pellet.
21. Resuspended the pellet in 22 µL of (use 1 µL for gel electrophoresis and 1 µL for quantification).

3.6. Quantification of cRNA Product

1. Check the optical density at 260 and 280 nm to determine sample concentration and purity.
2. Keep the 260/280 ratio close to 2.0.
3. Proceed to fragmentation or store at –20°C.
4. The cRNA yield for use on the microarray should ideally be 1 µg/µL. Check with the core facility that processes the microarray samples to determine whether an amount less than this can be used.

3.7. Fragmentation of cRNA for Analysis on Microarray

1. This step is usually performed by core facilities at individual institutions (*see* **Note 1**). These laboratories are often created to accommodate the preferred and various microarrays used on site and house the various hybridization ovens necessary for data generation.
2. Fragmentation buffer (purchased from a company of choice) is optimized to break down full-length cRNA samples from 35 to 200 base fragments by metal-induced hydrolysis. This fragmentation step varies based on the array format as well as the specific hybridization oven utilized.

3. Incubate your cRNA with the fragmentation buffer (*see* **step 2**) at 94°C for 35 min and place on ice following the incubation. The cRNA can ultimately be saved and stored at –20°C (or –80°C for longer-term storage).
4. There are many formats that can be utilized for hybridization based on what is available. We have used the 49 Format (Standard)/64 Format Array. The individual components in the mix (for a final volume of 300 µL) are:
   a. Fragmented cRNA (15 µg).
   b. Control oligonucleotide B2 (3 nM).
   c. 20X Eukaryotic hybridization controls (bioB, bioC, bioD, cre).
   d. Herring sperm DNA (10 mg/mL).
   e. Bovine serum albumin (BSA) (50 mg/mL).
   f. 2X hybridization buffer.
   g. Dimethylsulfoxide (DMSO) (30 µL).
   h. H$_2$O.
5. Wet the array by filling it through one of the septa with 1X hybrization buffer using a micropipetor (amount is based on your specific chip) and incubate for 10 min at 45°C with rotation.
6. Heat the hybridization cocktail prepared in **step 3** to 45°C for 5 min. Quick-spin at maximum speed for 5 min to remove any insoluble material from the mixture.
7. Remove the 1X hybridization buffer from the microarray and replace with your targeted cRNA cocktail (at the appropriate volume for your microarray).
8. Set the hybridization oven to 45°C and rotate at 60 rpm for 16 h.
9. Scanning the resultant hybrization of the cRNA probes will depend on the specific oven utilized.

3.8. Hybridization/Staining/Washing

This procedure is performed by a core facility at individual institutions.

1. Quality assessment of the fragmented cRNA preparation by hybridization to Affymetrix Test Chips carrying reference genes (*see* **Note 2**).
2. Overnight hybridization to Affymetrix Gene Chips of interest using a Stovall Hybridization oven.
3. Following overnight hybridization, the Test Chip or the GeneChip is washed and stained with a fluorescent-tagged streptravidin-phyco-erythrin conjugate using the Affymetrix Gene Chip Fluidics Station 400 controlled by a dedicated computer workstation containing Affymetrix software. The initial staining procedure is followed by an antibody amplification step and an additional staining with the fluorescent-tagged conjugate.

3.9. Scanning/Data Processing

This procedure is performed by a core facility at individual institutions. The degree of hybridization is quantified and analyzed using a scanning laser spectrophotometry (Hewlett Packard Gene Array Scanner), which is controlled by the computer workstation. Primary data are transferred to the investigator for analysis.

3.10. Data Analysis

The microarray data can be analyzed using many different software programs, and new programs are also continuously developed. We present here one method that was used to analyze our expression profiling data from nine severely atherosclerotic coronary arteries and six normal coronary arteries (*see* **Note 3**).

1. Once the raw data is obtained from the Gene Array Scanner, it must be entered into a program of choice for further analysis. We used GeneSpring 7.0 for this purpose and will detail how to analyze the data with this specific program.
2. One needs four essential columns of data that are originally generated from the microarrays for the data analysis (*see* **Notes 4–6**). These are: gene assignment number, raw score, Flag ("P" present; "M" marginally present; or "A" absent), and the gene description. These data may need to be saved in a text-delimited Microsoft Excel® worksheet.
3. All of the individual microarray files are to be placed into one folder located on the desktop of a computer with an identifying name. The folder is to be dragged over and dropped over the "navigation window" displaying all 23 sets of chromosomes. The GeneSpring program will automatically load the data into the program and create an experiment with these microarrays.

3.11. Experimental Normalization

1. The microarrays must be normalized or designated into groups comparing one set with the other (i.e., "diseased" vs "controls"). This is accomplished by selecting the command "experimental normalization," which allows one to assign which samples are from the experimental group and which are controls (*see* **Note 7**).
2. Standard comparisons that are made among all the chips and should be selected in the program are as follows. Per chip: normalize to the 50th percentile; per gene: normalize to the median value (*see* **Note 8**).

3.12. Experimental Parameters

1. The microarrays are often run in "replicates" to be able to reproduce the data from the same sample or group. In the navigation window menu "experimental parameters," the microarrays must be assigned a new name (i.e., cell-line, tissue type, time, or weight) according to your data. All of the replicates from the experimental group are designated the same name (i.e., "1") and all the replicates from the control group are designated the same name (i.e., "2").
2. The "parameter order value" will automatically be set to include two groups exclusively: the experimental group and the control group. However, based on the program one is using to analyze the data, this may need to be designated with a separate step.

3.13. Experiment Interpretation

1. The microarrays will be analyzed by comparing two groups. In this step, one can choose how the raw data is to be analyzed (ratio [signal/control], log of ratio, or fold-changes).
2. In the navigation window of GeneSpring, one should select the variable "noncontinuous" to analyze the two groups of replicates as well as select "do not display" the original samples and file name.
3. The "error model" to be utilized is the "cross-gene error model" (*see* **Note 9**).

3.14. Tools

1. The microarray data are now ready to be analyzed to generate gene lists for inspection.
2. In the navigation window under "tools" is the statistical tests and clustering commands to search for statistically significant genes between the two groups of samples.
3. The basic statistical test can be the ANOVA. One must select the Parameter to test (the file name containing the two groups of microarrays), the test type (parametric test—do not assume variances are equal; parametric test—assume variances are equal; parametric test—use all available error estimates; or a nonparametric test). At the same time, the *p* value is selected (for example, 0.05 vs 0.001), as well as any multiple testing corrections (Benjamini and Hochberg False Discovery Rate, Bonferroni, Bonferroni Step-down [Holm], Westfall and Young Permutation [slow], or none at all; *post hoc* tests can also be selected including a Tukey Test or Student-Newman-Keuls test).
4. With the specific statistical tests selected, the command "start" is selected and the gene list will be generated and saved into a Gene List File.
5. With the final gene list is generated, the data can be further manipulated to create: K-mean clusters, gene tree, condition tree, self-organizing map (SOM), or QT clustering. One can also create gene lists with specific fold-changes in gene expression (*see* **Note 10**).

4. Notes

1. Protocols for fragmentation for the microarray, which creates segments of the cRNA molecule to bind to oligonucleotide primers affixed to the array, will vary depending on your array and the specific ovens used for hybridization and the source of your specimens. The process involves the fragmentation of the intact cRNA molecules to represent the 3′, middle, and 5′ component of the molecules. These fragments hybridize to the probes specifically designed on the chips to represent the mRNA. The core facility that does fragmentation will tailor this process to the specific protocol used to synthesize the cRNA molecule.
2. Most institutions require that a "test chip" be analyzed with your cRNA material before proceeding to the microarray. The test chip analyzes the quality of the cRNA including the detection of housekeeping genes and the intactness of the

cRNA molecule. The actual fragmented cRNA molecule used for the official chip is placed on this mini-microarray to assess the binding and gene expression of specific house keeping genes. It also determines the representation of the 3′, middle, and 5′ aspect of the cRNA to ensure equal representation of the original mRNA molecule. This step is important, because if the cRNA is contaminated or degraded, it will save the expense of utilizing the official chip.

3. A major limitation of microarray analysis is that it is usually difficult to distinguish whether the identified differential gene expression patterns are the cause of the disease or the consequence of the disease. Follow-up studies with transgenic overexpression or knockout of an interesting gene in animal systems are needed to solve this issue. Data interpretation should proceed cautiously before any cause-and-effect relationships are hypothesized.

4. Microarray analysis is biased to the genes on the arrays, and cannot be used to evaluate low abundant transcripts. However, this technology is still important, as it offers one at this time more than 25,000 genes to study in the context of one's specific gene of interest. Alternatively, microarrays can be purchased or designed to study specific genes (i.e., cardiochip). If the gene of study is not detected on the array and called "absent," one can still evaluate gene expression patterns and see the raw data score for each gene.

5. Microarray analysis results in many false-positives; thus, it is crucial that results are confirmed using conventional technologies such as quantitative RT-PCR, quantitative RT-PCR, Northern blot, Western blot, or immunostaining analyses. It is a standard practice now to do confirmation studies with the microarray data. However, many studies do consistently show a correlation between the microarray data generated and those seen in an independent study to confirm the gene expression levels and intensity.

6. The expression level of mRNA does not necessarily reflect the expression of the protein, and the pathogenic mechanism of a disease may involve protein modifications such as phosphorylation and glycosylation. Under these circumstances, proteomics will be a powerful, alternative technology *(4)*.

7. There are several ways to normalize the data in GeneSpring. The most common approach is to do per-chip normalization (normalize to the 50th percentile of the measurements taken from that chip) and per-gene normalization (normalize to the median of the measurements for that gene), and data transformation (set measurements less than 0.01–0.01). These three parameters can be considered the standard requirement often used for data analysis. One may need to consult his individual data-mining program for the recommended setting as well as that for the microarray selected.

8. The normalization to the median accounts for the difference in the detection efficiency between each of the genes spotted on the microarray. It selects a value that represents a signal that falls in the middle of all of the signals detected for one gene. This avoids the significant standard deviations that can be generated when using the mean as well as significant biological variability.

9. The cross-gene error model accounts for error by assuming the amount of variability among all the microarrays is a function of the control strength within all of the

measurements for a specific condition. The advantage of making this assumption is that the number of measurements used to estimate the global error is equal to the total number of genes on each of the microarrays.

10. K-means clustering divides genes into groups based on their expression pattern and whether they have a high degree of similarity. It has been assumed that genes that fall into a specific group may share a common mechanism of regulation. A gene tree is based on the concept of phylogenetic trees, in which organisms sharing properties tend to be clustered together. A branch containing two or more genes can be considered a measure of how similar the genes are. A conditional tree is like a gene tree except that is shows the relationships between the genes in terms of their expression level. The SOM is a clustering technique that is similar to the K-means clustering except that it illustrates the relationship between groups by arranging them in a two-dimensional map in addition to dividing genes into groups based on expression patterns.

Acknowledgment

This work was supported by the National Institutes of Health (NIH) grants R01 HL65630, R01 HL66251, and P50 HL77107 and an American Heart Association Established Investigator award (to Q.W.).

References

1. Archacki, S. R. and Wang, Q. (2004). Expression profiling of cardiovascular disease. *Human Genomics* **1,** 355–370.
2. Shen, G. Q., Archacki, S. R., and Wang, Q. (2004) The molecular genetics of coronary artery disease and myocardial infarction. *Acute Coronary Syndrome* **6,** 129–141.
3. Archacki, S. R., Angheloiu, G., Tian, X. L., et al. (2003) Identification of new genes differentially expressed in coronary artery disease by expression profiling. *Physiol. Genomics* **15,** 65–74.
4. You, S. A., Archacki, S. R., Angheloiu, G., et al. (2003) Proteomic approach to coronary atherosclerosis shows ferritin light chain as a significant marker: evidence consistent with iron hypothesis in atherosclerosis. *Physiol. Genomics* **13,** 25–30.

2

Proteomics With Two-Dimensional Gel Electrophoresis and Mass Spectrometry Analysis in Cardiovascular Research

Sun-Ah You and Qing K. Wang

Summary

Proteomics is a large-scale, comprehensive study of the proteins of a cell or organism. It is a unique means of characterizing proteins that are expressed in a cell or tissue at any given time-point and of identifying any modifications that they may undergo. Thus, it is a powerful technology that can detect and identify the changes of the structure and function of proteins in response to intra- and extracellular environmental signals or disease states. As proteomics can establish a link for genes and proteins with a disease, it will play an important role in defining the molecular determinants of a disease and in identifying targets for drug discoveries and diagnostics. We have carried out the first proteomics study for coronary artery disease (CAD) and found that the expression of the ferritin light chain was significantly increased in CAD tissues. In this chapter, we use the CAD study as an example to demonstrate the procedures involved in proteomics analysis. The proteome is visualized by two-dimensional gel electrophoresis, a powerful and widely used method for proteomics, and the proteins of interest are then identified by mass spectrometry. This technique should be useful in characterizing cardiovascular diseases and in defining signaling pathways for cardiovascular development and physiology.

Key Words: Proteomics; two-dimensional (2D) gel electrophoresis; proteome; cardiovascular disease; signaling; mass spectrometry; protein structure and function.

1. Introduction

Proteomics is the large-scale analysis of the structure and function of proteins expressed in cells, tissues, and fluids *(1)*. The proteome, the total protein output encoded by a genome, is far more complex than the genome because there are more proteins than genes as a result of the alternative splicing of genes and posttranslational modification of proteins (~22,000 genes vs

From: *Methods in Molecular Medicine, vol. 129:*
Cardiovascular Disease: Methods and Protocols, Volume 2: Molecular Medicine
Edited by: Q. K. Wang © Humana Press Inc., Totowa, NJ

~400,000 proteins). This discrepancy makes proteomics a necessary tool to characterize the complex network of proteins involved in cellular regulation and signaling.

Proteomics permits the detection of proteins that are associated with specific cellular functions by means of their altered levels of expression. It allows a comparison of two or more different states of a cell or an organism (e.g., diseased vs nondiseased tissues) in order to identify specific qualitative and quantitative protein changes *(2)*. In addition, proteomics can be applied in basic research, for example, the profiling of drug effects, molecular diagnostics, and various other therapeutic areas.

The experimental strategy most often employed in proteomics is to separate the proteins expressed in comparable systems (e.g., diseased vs nondiseased tissues) using two-dimensional (2D) gel electrophoresis and quantify the amounts of each protein in each cell system by the density of staining of each respective protein band (**Fig. 1**). The 2D gel electrophoresis possesses a sufficient resolving power for proteome analysis *(3,4)*. This technique separates proteins in two steps: the first-dimension and the second-dimension gel electrophoresis. In the first dimension, proteins are separated by their isoelectric point (pI), the pH at which a protein carries no net charge and will not migrate in an electrical field. The technique is also called isoelectric focusing (IEF) electrophoresis *(5)*. A sample preparation is the key to successful IEF. In the second dimension, proteins after IEF are further resolved by their molecular weight (MW) using sodium dodecyl sulfate (SDS)-polyacrylamide gel electrophoresis (PAGE). The resulting gel is then stained with Coomassie Blue or silver to visualize the protein spots.

Protein patterns on 2D gels are analyzed using software programs to statistically and scientifically determine meaningful spots. Proteins of interest can then be excised from the gel for further identification and full characterization using mass spectrometry (MS).

2. Materials

2.1. Sample Preparation (see Note 1)

1. Lysis buffer: 8 M urea, 1% Triton X-100, 0.1 M dithiothreitol (DTT), 0.1 M NaCl, 0.045 M Tris-HCl, pH 7.4, 4% "complete" protease inhibitor cocktail (Roche Molecular Biochemicals, Indianapolis, IN). Dissolve with shaking, but do not use any heat (*see* **Note 2**).
2. Tris stock buffer: 0.5 M Tris-HCl, pH 8.0, 50 mM MgCl$_2$.
3. DNAse stock: 10 mg/mL bovine pancreatic DNAse (Sigma, St. Louis, MO) in Tris stock (*see* **Note 3**).
4. RNAse stock: 10 mg/mL bovine pancreatic RNAse (Sigma) in Tris stock.
5. Nuclease reagent: 1 mg/mL DNAse, 1 mg/mL RNAse in Tris stock.
6. Tri-*n*-butylphosphate:acetone:methanol (1:12:1).

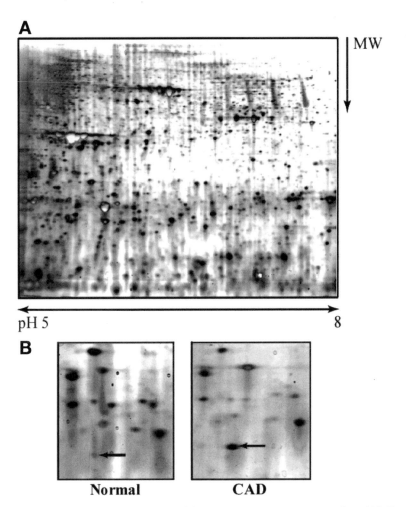

Fig. 1. Two-dimensional (2D) map of human coronary artery proteins. (**A**) Protein extract was prepared from a normal human coronary artery using the delipidation method. Reproducible 2D patterns were obtained from protein samples from other coronary arteries. The resolution of protein spots was optimized using pH 5.0–8.0 immobilized pH gradient strips. (**B**) Enlarged areas from 2D gel images of a normal individual and a coronary artery disease (CAD) patient. The protein spot indicated by the arrow shows a higher level of expression in CAD than in their normal counterparts. This result is reproducible from many other samples. The protein spot has an isoelectric point of 5.5 and molecular mass of about 20 kDa, and has been identified as the ferritin light chain by mass spectrometry.

7. Tri-*n*-butylphosphate (Sigma).
8. Methanol: high-performance liquid chromatography (HPLC)-grade.
9. Acetone: HPLC-grade.

10. Boiling buffer: 0.325 *M* DTT, 4% CHAPS, 0.045 *M* Tris-HCl, pH 7.4 (*see* **Note 4**).
11. Dilution buffer: 8 *M* urea, 4% CHAPS, 0.1 *M* DTT, 0.045 *M* Tris-HCl, pH 7.4.
12. Bio-Rad protein assay kit I: contains 450 mL of dye reagent concentrate and a bovine γ-globulin standard (Bio-Rad, Hercules, CA) (*see* **Note 5**).
13. Whatman no. 1 filter paper or equivalent.
14. Concentrated HCl to make a 0.12 *N* stock.

2.2. First-Dimension IEF

1. Rehydration buffer: 7 *M* urea, 2 *M* thiourea, 1% DTT, 1% CHAPS, 1% ampholytes, 1% Triton X-100. Dissolve with shaking, but do not use any heat (*see* **Note 6**).
2. 1% bromophenol blue (BPB): 1% BPB in water.
3. Immobilized pH gradient (IPG) gel strips (Bio-Rad) (*see* **Note 7**).
4. Mineral oil.
5. Wick (Bio-Rad) (*see* **Note 8**).
6. PROTEAN® IEF cell (Bio-Rad): a first-dimension instrument.

2.3. Second-Dimension Gel Electrophoresis

1. Equilibration buffer: 5.4 g urea, 0.3 g SDS, 3.8 mL 1.5 *M* Tris-HCl, pH 8.8, 3 mL glycerol in a 50-mL centrifuge tube. Adjust the total volume to 15 mL with water. Dissolve with shaking, but do not use any heat (*see* **Note 9**).
2. Reducing reagent: 120 mg DTT in 7.5 mL equilibration buffer.
3. Alkylation reagent: 150 mg iodoacetamide in 7.5 mL equilibration buffer, 100 µL 1% BPB.
4. Agarose sealing solution: 0.5 g agarose, 10 mL of 10X Tris-glycine running buffer (Bio-Rad), 30 mL glycerol. Adjust the total volume to 100 mL with water. Add 1 mL of 1% BPB. This reagent can be stored at room temperature and used repeatedly over several months.
5. Running buffer (1X): 100 mL of 10X Tris-glycine buffer, 900 mL water. Cool on ice before use.
6. Criterion gel (Bio-Rad): the gels are stored at 4°C (*see* **Note 10**).
7. Mini-PROTEAN 3 cell (Bio-Rad): a second-dimension instrument.

2.4. Silver Staining (see Note 11)

1. Fixing solution: 50% methanol, 5% acetic acid in water (v/v).
2. Washing solution: 50% methanol in water (v/v).
3. Sensitizing solution: 0.02% sodium thiosulfate ($Na_2S_2O_3$) in water (make fresh).
4. 0.1% silver solution: 0.1% silver nitrate in water. It takes time to completely dissolve silver nitrate in water.
5. Developing solution: 0.04% formalin, 2% sodium carbonate in water (make fresh).
6. Terminating solution: 5% acetic acid in water (v/v).
7. Storing solution: 1% acetic acid in water (v/v).

2.5. Protein Sequencing and Identification

1. Gel washing solution: 50% acetonitrile, 50 mM ammonium bicarbonate.
2. 50 mM ammonium bicarbonate: 3.96 mg/mL.
3. Protease digestion solution: resuspend lyophilized trypsin (20 µg/vial, Promega, Madison, WI) in 20 µL of the 50 mM acetic acid solution provided with trypsin, yielding a 1 µg/µL stock solution. Dilute that stock to 1 µg/50 µL with 50 mM ammonium bicarbonate (50-fold dilution, 20 ng/µL). Aliquot and store at –70°C. Do not repeat freeze-thaw of trypsin stock solutions more than once.
4. Reducing reagent: 10 mM DTT in 0.1 M ammonium bicarbonate.
5. Alkylation reagent: 50 mM iodoacetamide in 0.1 M ammonium bicarbonate.
6. Extraction solution: 50% acetonitrile, 5% formic acid.

3. Methods

Sample preparation is the key to successful 2D gel electrophoresis *(6–8)*. Sample preparation and solubilization of any protein mixture for subsequent 2D separation is of major importance, as it will affect the overall performance of the technique. It should follow three important rules. First, as many proteins as possible, including hydrophobic proteins, must be solubilized. Second, protein aggregates must be solubilized. Third, sample preparation must be reproducible in order to reduce misleading results.

3.1. Protein Delipidation and Extraction From Tissues

1. 0.1 g of tissue is homogenized in 1 mL of lysis buffer.
2. Incubate for 15 min at 34°C and cool on ice for 10 min.
3. Add nuclease reagent, mix well, and incubate on ice for 10 min.
4. Centrifuge the homogenate at 4°C for 15 min at 10,000g.
5. Collect the aqueous phase between the upper lipid phase and lower cellular debris phase.
6. Mix the collected aqueous phase with 14 mL of ice-cold tri-n-butylphosphate: acetone:methanol (1:12:1) and incubate at 4°C for 90 min.
7. Centrifuge at 2800g for 15 min and remove supernatant.
8. Wash the pellet sequentially with 1 mL of tri-n-butylphosphate, acetone, and methanol, and then air-dry.
9. Boil the precipitate in 0.1 mL of boiling buffer and cool to room temperature.
10. Dilute the cooled sample in 1.5 mL of dilution buffer and incubate at 34°C for 15 min.
11. To quantify total proteins, prepare the bovine γ-globulin standard at 14 mg/mL by reconstituting the lyophilized protein in 1 mL of water. This is 10X of the concentration that is recommended in the kit instructions.
12. Prepare a 1:4 dilution of the dye reagent concentrate by mixing one part dye with three parts water, and filter the dye through Whatman no. 1 filter paper. Each assay point requires 3.5 mL of diluted dye reagent.
13. Prepare 0.12 N HCl (nominal) by diluting concentrated HCl.

14. Prepare standards covering the range of 0.1–14 μg protein/μL by diluting the 14 mg/mL standard in the same buffer as the sample.
15. Mix 20 μL of each standard or sample with 80 μL of 0.12 N HCl in separate assay tubes. It is a good idea to make duplicates for each sample or standard.
16. Add 3.5 mL of diluted dye reagent to each tube. Vortex gently.
17. After 5 min, measure the absorbance of each sample or standard at 595 nm.
18. Plot the absorbance values vs the amount of protein (in micrograms) to generate the standard curve. Expect a nonlinear relationship.
19. Compare the absorbance reading for each sample with the standard curve to determine the concentration of the sample.

3.2. First-Dimension IEF

1. Prepare the samples in 1.5-mL microcentrifuge tubes. For silver-stained gels, add 30 μL of sample (5 mg/mL) to 220 μL of rehydration buffer and 10 μL of 1% BPB (*see* **Note 12**).
2. Transfer the samples to a well in the IEF tray. Place all of samples at one end of the well and coat the entire well by tipping the tray and slowly allow the sample to move to the other end of the tray. Repeat to go back and forth several times. Pop any bubbles with a Kimwipe.
3. Place the IPG gel strip side down in the channel of a focusing tray that contains the sample. Gently move back and forth a bit to ensure good wetting of the gel surface. Force out any bubbles under the gel with a pair of forceps.
4. Cover the strip with oil to prevent evaporation.
5. Rehydrate the strip overnight at room temperature, applying 50 V (program the PROTEAN IEF cell for active rehydration). Typical rehydration time is 12–16 h.
6. Stop the rehydration. Take the tray out of the IEF cell.
7. Take the IPG strips out of the channel of a focusing tray and put them on wet Kimwipe (put the gel side up) (*see* **Note 13**).
8. Wet the electrode wicks with water. Put the wicks on both positive and negative ends of the well.
9. Put the IPG strips back in the wells (face down).
10. Cover the strips and adjacent wells with mineral oil.
11. Set voltage. IEF is conducted at 10°C at 300 V for 3 h, followed by 1500 V for 3 h, and finally 3000 V for 18 h (*see* **Note 14**).

3.3. Second-Dimension Gel Electrophoresis

1. After the first dimension gel electrophoresis, the IPG strip is equilibrated with equilibration buffer (*see* **Note 15**). Place the strip face up in the equilibration tray.
2. Cover each strip with approx 3.5 mL of the reducing reagent.
3. Incubate the strip at room temperature with shaking for 15 min (time is important).
4. Remove the reducing agent.
5. Cover the strip with approx 3.5 mL of the alkylation reagent.
6. Incubate the strip at room temperature with shaking for 15 min (time is important).
7. Proceed directly to the gel assembly. While the strips are equilibrating, prepare the running buffer and cool it on ice.

8. Melt the agarose sealing solution in a microwave oven. Heat to >65°C, but do not boil.
9. This reagent must be used at approx 45°C, but it will begin to solidify at approx 40°C. Therefore, some timing is needed. It is easier to cool the reagent just before use than to heat it just before use.
10. Prepare the gel. Remove the Criterion gel from its package and wash briefly with water. Place the gel in a stand. Remove the green comb and rinse the well (five times) with running buffer. Leave the well covered with running buffer.
11. At the end of equilibration, check the temperature of molten agarose. Carefully cool the agarose sealing solution on ice as needed, until the temperature reaches approx 45°C.
12. Pour buffer out of the gel. Remove the strip from the alkylaton reagent. Blot away any excess reagent and place the strip in the well. Note the orientation (+) end of the strip.
13. Cap the well with agarose. Using a glass pipet, force the agarose over the strip, filling the well. A vigorous action will help minimize the number of bubbles that are trapped in the agarose. These bubbles may disturb protein migration and must be removed. Cool the agarose briefly with ice (*see* **Note 16**).
14. Add approx 5 mL of cold running buffer to the top chamber.
15. To assemble the gel system, pour the buffer out of the top chamber of the gel.
16. Remove the tape covering the bottom of the gel.
17. Place the gel in the criterion cell, and fill each bottom chamber with cold running buffer to the fill lines.
18. Fill each top chamber with cold running buffer to the top of the chambers.
19. Place the ready precast gels in the Mini-PROTEAN 3 cell, taking care to properly orient the electrodes.
20. Following Bio-Rad's instructions, run the gel at 200 V constant voltage. The total running time will be approx 70 min. Stop the run when the tracking dye just leaves the bottom of the gel. If two gels are being run at the same time, it is possible to pause the run, remove one gel, and restart the run if one gel gets ahead of the other.

3.4. Silver Staining

1. Place 300 mL of the fixing solution in the clean Pyrex dish.
2. When the SDS-PAGE run is complete, remove the gel from the cassette.
3. Break the Criterion gel cassette using the green plastic comb taken out of the IPG well.
4. Immerse the broken cassette in the fixing solution and begin removing one plate of the cassette. Being very careful so as not to tear the gel, remove one plate from the cassette.
5. Cut the gel in the top corner at the acidic (+) end of the strip.
6. Carefully cut the gel along the top to remove the IPG strip. Discard the strip.
7. Immerse the second plate, with the gel on it, in the fixing solution. Being very careful so as not to tear the gel, remove the gel from the second plate.
8. Fix the gel for 20 min at room temperature with gentle shaking.
9. Aspirate the fixing solution off of the gel. Be careful so as not to tear the gel.
10. Add 200 mL of washing solution to the gel and wash for 10 min.

11. Aspirate the washing solution off the gel. Be careful so as not to tear the gel.
12. Add 500 mL of water for 2 h. Additional washing overnight will reduce background staining.
13. Aspirate the water off of the gel. Be careful so as not to tear the gel.
14. Add 200 mL of sensitizing solution to the gel and incubate for 1 min.
15. Aspirate the sensitizing solution and wash the gel in 500 mL of water for 1 min.
16. Aspirate the water and wash the gel in 500 mL of water for 1 min.
17. Aspirate the water, add 200 mL of silver solution to the gel, and incubate the gel for 20 min.
18. Aspirate the staining solution and wash the gel with 500 mL of water for 1 min.
19. Transfer the gel to new glass chamber, and wash the gel with 500 mL of water for 1 min.
20. Aspirate the water and add 200 mL of developing solution to the gel. Observe the color and change the solution when the developer turns yellow. Terminate when the staining is sufficient.
21. Aspirate the developing solution and add 200 mL of terminating solution to the gel. Change the solution a couple of times.
22. Leave the gel at 4°C in storing solution.

3.5. Protein Sequencing and Identification (see Note 17)

1. Analyze the 2D gels with an image analysis software. Excise the protein spot of interest from the gel as closely as possible and transfer it into a clean 1.5-mL microcentrifuge tube.
2. Add 500 μL of wash solution and incubate at room temperature for 15 min with gentle agitation. Remove the solution with pipet tips. Repeat this washing step up to three times or until the Coomassie dye has been completely removed.
3. Remove the solution and dehydrate gels in acetonitrile. At this point, the gel pieces should shrink and become an opaque-white color. If they do not, remove the acetonitrile and replace with fresh acetonitrile.
4. Discard the acetonitrile and vacuum centrifuge for 3–5 min (*see* **Note 18**).
5. Add 50 μL of reducing solution at room temperature for 30 min.
6. Remove the reducing solution and add 50 μL of alkylation solution at room temperature for 30 min.
7. Remove the alkylation reagent and dehydrate the gel pieces in 200 μL of acetonitrile.
8. Remove the acetonitrile. The gel pieces should shrink and become an opaque-white color. If they do not, remove the acetonitrile and repeat the washing–dehydration cycle until they do.
9. Remove the acetonitrile and wash the gel pieces by rehydration in 200 μL of 0.1 *M* ammonium bicarbonate.
10. Dehydrate the pieces in 200 μL of acetonitrile and remove the acetonitrile.
11. Dry the gel pieces in a vacuum centrifuge for 3–5 min.
12. Rehydrate the gel pieces in 20 μL of trypsin solution and place them on ice for 10 min.
13. Remove excess trypsin solution and add 5 μL of 50 m*M* ammonium bicarbonate.

14. Incubate overnight at 37°C.
15. Extract the peptides from the gel in 60 μL of 50 mM ammonium bicarbonate.
16. Spin down samples with brief centrifugation at 12,000g for 30 s and transfer supernatant to a clean microcentrifuge tube.
17. Extract the peptides with additional 60 μL of extraction solution.
18. Spin down samples by brief centrifugation at 12,000g for 30 s and transfer the supernatant containing additional tryptic peptides to tube from **step 16**.
19. Repeat **steps 17** and **18**.
20. Combine the extracts and evaporate to <20 μL for liquid chromatography (LC)-MS analysis. The LC-MS analysis is performed by a core facility with necessary expertise.
21. Analyze the data by searching the National Center for Biotechnology Information (NCBI)'s GenPept database using the computer program SEQUEST (*see* **Note 19**).

4. Notes

1. This protocol is used to remove any interfering lipids in coronary artery tissues. Lipids can bind to proteins and increase artifactual migrations and streaking. This problem can be alleviated by a mixture of organic solvents (1 vol of Tri-*n*-butylphosphate:12 vol of acetone:1 vol of methanol) *(9)*. Sample preparation methods may vary from sample to sample, but generally include reducing agents, chaotropes, and detergents.
2. Urea is the most commonly used chaotropic agent in sample preparation for 2D PAGE. It lowers the cohesion of water, making hydrophobic regions of proteins more soluble in aqueous solution *(10)*. Urea should not be heated because carbamylation of the sample, which is a spontaneous nonenzymatic modification of proteins and amino acids by urea-derived isocyanate, may occur. DTT reduces cystine disulfide bonds within or between proteins *(11)*. DTT is oxidized relatively quickly in aqueous solution. For best results in terms of the reproducibility of 2D-PAGE gels, DTT solutions should be prepared fresh.
3. The presence of nucleic acids, especially DNA, interferes with separation of proteins by IEF. DNA binds to proteins in the sample and causes artifactual migration and streaking.
4. CHAPS is a zwitterionic detergent based on a cholesterol ring. It assists urea in the solubilization of hydrophobic proteins *(10)*.
5. Protein assays are generally sensitive to detergent or reducing agents used at the concentrations found in typical sample solutions. Modified Bio-Rad protein assay is used to determine the protein content in typical sample solutions used to load IPG strips.
6. Ampholytes are added to all IPG rehydration buffers and sample solubilization solutions to help keep proteins soluble. An ampholytes is a molecule possessing both positive and negative charge, or that can function as both an acid and a base. A large number of carrier ampholyte mixtures are available with different pH gradients. The choice of ampholytes is dependent on the pH range of the IPG strip.

7. IPG strips are commercially available and must be rehydrated with the appropriated additives prior to IEF because they are provided dry. The pH-gradient ranges of IPG strips vary; the use of broad-range strips (pH 3.0–10.0) allows the display of the most proteins in a single gel. With narrow-range strips (pH 3.0–6.0, pH 5.0–8.0, pH 7.0–10.0), resolution is increased by expanding a small pH range across the entire width of a gel.

8. Wicks collect salts and other contaminants in the sample. Without wicks, salts collect at the anode and cathode, producing high conductivity that can alter the gradient and cause discontinuities in the gel, "hot spots," or burns.

9. Buffer must be freshly prepared.

10. Be aware that the gels have a limited shelf life. Note the expiration date.

11. To prevent carryover of contamination, staining of proteins must be performed with labware that has never been in contact with nonfat milk, BSA, or any other protein-blocking agent.

12. For Coomassie Blue-stained gels, use 150 µL of sample (5 mg/mL) plus 100 µL of rehydration buffer with 10 µL of 1% BPB.

13. Wash the tray with soap and 95% ethanol. It is important to clean the focusing trays properly between runs. Channel-to-channel leakage is common when salts accumulate in the channels.

14. Focused IPG strips can be stored at –20°C indefinitely without affecting the final 2D pattern.

15. Equilibration process reduces disulfide bonds and alkylates the resultant sulfhydryl groups of the cysteine residues. Concurrently, proteins are coated with SDS for separation on the basis of MW.

16. SDS-PAGE standards can be applied to gels that have no reference lane. Pipet 10 µL of the SDS-PAGE standards onto the wick. Slip the wick into the slot in the gel sandwich next to the IPG strip.

17. Protein sequencing and identification is usually performed in an MS center. This protocol is a procedure for the preparation of Coomassie Blue-stained 2D gel spots. In general, the best results are obtained when using Coomassie Blue-stained 2D gels.

18. Care should be taken when handling the tube once the gel is dry, because the gel may "jump" out as a result of static electricity.

19. In the event that no matches in the databases are identified, the spectra are interpreted manually and further searching of the expressed sequence tag database is carried out using the FASTA program.

20. Always use nonlatex gloves when handling samples and gels; keratin and latex proteins are potential sources of contamination.

21. Never reuse any solutions; abundant proteins will partially leach out and contaminate subsequent samples.

22. The quantification of the amounts of each protein in a 2D gel by the density of staining of each respective protein band can be achieved using sophisticated image analysis systems. However, obvious protein bands that show differential differences between two systems (e.g., diseased vs nondiseased tissues) can be identified by direct visualization of the gels. Commercially available software packages can

be used to compare computer images of 2D gels to determine differential protein expression, and the user's guide should be followed from the specific manufacturer. For example, the Bio-Rad PDQuest image analysis software landmarks proteins for gel alignment and identifies subtle changes in the up- or downregulation of proteins based on the intensity of protein staining. Multiple gels can be compared using the image analysis systems when good reproducibility of the gels is maintained and when known landmark proteins can be employed to correct the positions of each protein band.

23. The MS experiments have the sensitivity to take any detectable protein band out of the gel, and determine the amino acid sequence of the peptides from the band. In general, identity of a protein band visible on a Coomassie Blue-stained gel, typically containing greater than 0.2 pmol of protein, can be defined easily and successfully by MS. Silver-stained bands, typically containing between 0.01 and 0.5 pmol of protein, can also be analyzed, but this is done less routinely.

24. The results from proteomics analysis should be validated using reverse-transcription PCR, Northern blot, or Western blot analyses (if antibodies are commercially available).

25. Proteomics holds great promise in cardiovascular research. It can be used to analyze differential protein expression in diseased hearts (e.g., atrial fibrillation, ischemic heart disease, and dilated cardiomyopathy) in comparison with normal hearts in animal models and humans. Furthermore, cells that are important for the pathogenesis of cardiovascular disease such as cardiac cells, endothelial cells, smooth muscle cells, and macrophages, can be challenged with various environmental agents (e.g., oxidized low-density lipoprotein and C-reactive protein, known risk predictors for atherosclerosis), and proteomics studies can be then used to identify proteins or signaling molecules involved in cell responses. These studies will be particularly helpful to better understand the relations between proteome changes and cardiovascular dysfunctions. Thus, proteomics allows us to examine global alterations in protein expression in the diseased hearts or vascular systems, and will provide new insights into the molecular mechanisms involved in cardiovascular dysfunction and disease.

Acknowledgments

The author would like to thank Dr. Michael Kinter in the Lerner Research Institute Mass Spectrometry Laboratory for technical advice, and Dr. Sandro Yong for help. This work was supported by the National Institutes of Health (NIH) grants R01 HL65630, R01 HL66251, P50 HL77107, and an American Heart Association Established Investigator award (to Q.W.).

References

1. Pandey, A. and Mann, M. (2000) Proteomics to study genes and genomes. *Nature* **405**, 837–846.
2. You, S. A., Archacki, S. R., Angheloiu, G., et al. (2003) Proteomic approach to coronary atherosclerosis shows ferritin light chain as a significant marker:

evidence consistent with iron hypothesis in atherosclerosis. *Physiol. Genomics* **13,** 25–30.

3. O'Farrel, P. (1975) High resolution two dimensional electrophoresis of proteins. *J. Biol. Chem.* **250,** 4007–4021.
4. Gorg, A., Obermaier, C., Boguth, G., et al. (2000) The current state of two-dimensional electrophoresis with immobilized pH gradients. *Electrophoresis* **21,** 1037–1053.
5. Garfin, D. E. (2000) Isoelectric focusing, in *Separation Science and Technology* (Ahuja, S. ed.), Academic, San Diego, CA, pp. 263–298.
6. Rabilloud, T. (1999) Solubilization of proteins in 2D electrophoresis. An outline. *Methods Mol. Biol.* **112,** 9–19.
7. Macri, J., McGee, B., Thomas, J. N., et al. (2000) Cardiac sarcoplasmic reticulum and sarcolemmal proteins separated by two-dimensional electrophoresis: surfactant effects on membrane solubilization. *Electrophoresis* **21,** 1685–1693.
8. Molloy, M. P. (2000) Two-dimensional electrophoresis of membrane proteins using immobilized pH gradients. *Anal. Biochem.* **280,** 1–10.
9. Mastro, R. and Hall, M. (1999) Protein delipidation and precipitation by tri-*n*-butylphosphate, acetone, and methanol treatment for isoelectric focusing and two-dimensional gel electrophoresis. *Anal. Biochem.* **273,** 313–315.
10. Rabilloud, T. (1996) Solubilization of proteins for electrophoretic analyses. *Electrophoresis* **17,** 813–829.
11. Zahler, W. L. and Cleland, W. W. (1968) A specific and sensitive assay for disulfides. *J. Biol. Chem.* **243,** 716–719.

3

Developing and Evaluating Genomics- or Proteomics-Based Diagnostic Tests

Statistical Perspectives

Xuejun Peng

Summary

The completion of the Human Genome Project and the ongoing sequencing of mouse, rat, and other genomes have led to an explosion of genetics-related technologies that are finding their way into all areas of biological research in both basic sciences and clinical applications. High-throughput genomics and proteomics technology has been quickly adapted to develop tools for clinical and pharmacological applications. Because molecular alterations usually occur much earlier than histological, physiological, and clinical abnormality, researchers hope to extend the applications of genomics and/or proteomics technology to early diagnosis of diseases and clinical outcome prognosis. Recently, some successful attempts in molecular diagnosis or prognosis have been published. However, for such tests to be translated from the bench to the bed, they must meet some rigorous standards. To develop a clinically meaningful genomics-based diagnostic test, we must have good study design, appropriate statistical analyses, and valid assessment of its clinical efficacy. In this chapter, we discuss statistical considerations on the process of developing reliable and useful genomics- or proteomics-based tests.

Key Words: Genomics-based diagnostic test; proteomics-based diagnostic test; molecular diagnosis; medical genomics; genomic medicine.

1. Introduction

The completion of the Human Genome Project in April 2003 was an important milestone in biological and medical science *(1)*. This remarkable point in biomedical history marks the beginning of an era in which we hope to learn the molecular basis of all human diseases. The identification of all human genes and their regulatory regions provides the framework to expedite our understanding of the molecular basis of disease. This advance has also formed the foundation for a

From: *Methods in Molecular Medicine, vol. 129:*
Cardiovascular Disease: Methods and Protocols, Volume 2: Molecular Medicine
Edited by: Q. K. Wang © Humana Press Inc., Totowa, NJ

broad range of genomic tools that can be applied to medical science. These developments in global gene and gene-product analysis as well as targeted molecular genetic testing are destined to change the practice of modern medicine. The increasing understanding of molecular medicine will shift clinical practice from empirical treatment to therapy based on a molecular taxonomy of disease. Physicians may soon be prescribing rationally designed drugs that have increased efficacy and reduced toxicity. The pharmaceutical industry may soon be able to discover new drugs or find new uses for old drugs that are tailored to patients with certain genetic profiles. Personalized medicine is on the horizon, as more and more advances have been made rapidly in DNA/RNA-based methods of susceptibility screening, disease diagnosis and prognostication, and prediction of treatment outcome in regard to both drug toxicity and response as they apply to various areas of clinical medicine. The practical utility of molecular genetics has been shown in a spectrum of diseases across several medical disciplines, including hematological tumors (acute myelogenous leukemia [AML], acute lymphocytic leukemia [ALL], chronic lymphocytic leukemia [CLL], and lymphoma), breast cancer, colon cancer, melanoma, prostate cancer, cardiovascular disease, Alzheimer's disease, Parkinson's disease, renal allograft rejections, and so on *(2–27)*. Genomic profiling will complement targeted genetic testing in facilitating presymptomatic identification of individuals who are at risk for a specific disease and, therefore, allow early preventive and therapeutic intervention. Genomic studies will also contribute to the molecular characterization of diseases, which in turn will refine current disease diagnosis and classifications as well as the development of targeted therapies. Treatment strategies rely heavily on the specific prognosis of a given disease in an individual, and molecular prognostication may provide more robust information in that regard. Other clinical opportunities may include the potential for prediction of both adverse effects from and response to drug therapy. The hope is that such personalized medicine, derived from an individual's genomic profile, will replace the traditional trial-and-error practice of medical treatment *(28)*.

One major area for application of genomics and proteomics technology is in molecular diagnostics. The potential benefits include early diagnosis and discovery of disease subtypes. Gene expression profiles can generate molecular signatures that may complement current methods of disease diagnosis and classification. Distinct gene expression profiles suggest different pathways of disease pathogenesis and provide clues to understanding the cause of diseases *(2–5,7–13)*. However, in order for such tests to be clinically useful, there are many statistical issues to be resolved. These issues are discussed in this chapter.

2. Evidence-Based Medicine and Medical Diagnostic Test

Evidence-based medicine (EBM) is defined as the explicit, judicious, and conscientious use of current best evidence from clinical care research in the management of individual patients *(29)*. During the past several decades, medical practice has been shifting from intuitive or informal clinical judgment based on the experience of individual clinician to a more formal, defensible process in which evidence from studies of groups of similar patients augments the judgment of practitioners. Medical diagnostics plays important roles in EBM. When a patient sees a doctor with complaints of some symptoms, the doctor will use his/her knowledge gained from professional literature and personal experience to come up with a pretest probability of some candidate disease(s). Then the physician's interaction with the patient, including history inquiry and physical examination, updates his/her estimated posterior probability of a disease. This probability serves as an initial (pretest) probability that directs what diagnostic test(s) and/or procedures are to be ordered, and then the results from the tests and procedures are used to modify this probability until the post-test probability is such that either the suspected diagnosis is confirmed or ruled out. Therefore, the value of a diagnostic test is often assessed in terms of how accurate this updating of information reveals the true disease status of the patient.

Sox et al. *(30)* pointed out that the main purposes of a diagnostic test are: (1) to provide reliable information about the patient's condition and (2) to influence the health care provider's plan for managing the patient. McNeil and Adelstein *(31)* added a third possible purpose: to understand disease mechanisms and natural history through research. Typically, medical tests are used for early screening test for asymptomatic diseases or disease-susceptibility, genetic predispositions, diagnosis of diseases when symptoms exist, and monitoring treatment effects and prognosis. For screening purposes, ideally the disease in question should be common enough to justify the attempts to detect it. It should also be accompanied by significant morbidity or mortality if not treated. Also, detection and treatment in the presymptomatic state should result in benefits beyond those obtained through treatment during the early symptomatic state. When symptoms already exist for a disease, diagnostic tests serve as tools to find the subtypes of the disease and direct to appropriate treatment. They can also be used to predict and monitor clinical outcome with or without treatments.

What characteristics do we want for an ideal medical (screening or diagnostic) test? With details to be discussed later in this chapter, here, we briefly mention some key features of a good medical test. The technology should be reliable so that results can be reproducible. The statistical measurements of diagnostic accuracy should be good. The test results should be meaningful enough to affect a clinician's judgment of patient's disease status and his/her course of action. Consequently, the test results should be meaningful in altering patient's outcome as compared with having not done such a test. Finally, the proposed test should be cost effective for both an individual patient and the society as a whole.

How does a genomics- or proteomics-based test fit into the picture of diagnostic tests? Traditionally, diagnostic tests have been developed using radiological imaging, tissue morphological and pathological changes, and measurement of single or small numbers of biological molecules in the body fluid or tissues. Now, we have some new tools thanks to the recent development of genomics and proteomics technology. The main advantages we gain are in two aspects: one is the ability to measure the expression of many genes simultaneously, making it possible to have large predictor profiles and the other is the ability to catch some diseases at an early stage. The main limitations now include immaturity of the technology leading to questionable reproducibility; increased expense; a large number of features with typically a small number of samples, which makes predictive model building a difficult task (*see* **Subheading 4.** for details). These limitations will eventually be overcome, as have been shown in the history of other technologies such as CT and MRI.

3. Designing Studies to Develop Diagnostic Tests

Designing studies to evaluate the accuracy of a diagnostic test can be challenging. Many issues must be considered, including identifying the relevant patient population, determining the gold standard, and choosing the appropriate measure of accuracy. Zhou et al. *(32)* discussed many potential sources of biases: the selection of patient sample, the accessibility and validity of the gold standard, the setting for the interpretation of the tests, and the analysis of results. All of these biases can potentially affect the design and analysis of genomics-based diagnostic tests and must be carefully considered in the plan phase. The authors listed 10 steps for the process of designing diagnostic accuracy studies. Although not all of the 10 steps are feasible or necessary for genomics-based diagnostic test, we do think the following steps are important: determining the objective of the study, identifying the target patient population, selecting a sampling plan for the patients, selecting the gold standard, choosing a measure of accuracy, planning the data collection, planning data analysis, and determining sample size either statistically or empirically.

The same authors proposed three phases in assessing the accuracy of a diagnostic test. In the *exploratory phase,* we get the first approximation of a new technology's diagnostic ability. This can be done with a retrospective study with small sample sizes. The next phase is the *challenge phase,* when we challenge the test's accuracy to potentially difficult subgroups of patients with or without the diseases. We may consider many covariates such as pathological, clinical, and comorbid conditions. In the third phase, the *clinical phase,* we use carefully designed prospective, randomized, controlled clinical trials for the diagnostic test in order to measure the test's accuracy in a representative sample of patients while tying to avoid most biases. This can be expensive and of long duration, but it is this type of study that will provide strong confidence for clinicians. For this phase, the sample of patients must closely represent the target population(s), and biases that commonly occur in selecting patients and in determining the true diagnosis must be avoided *(33)*.

4. Statistical Methods for Building Predictive Models

Predictive model building plays a pivotal role in developing diagnostic tests using genomic or proteomic data. In statistical terms, we are mainly interested in classification of the samples using genomic or proteomic profiles as predictors. In a typical classification scenario, we have an outcome measure, either categorical, such as heart attack/no heart attack, or quantitative, such as survival time after surgery for colon cancer, that we wish to predict based on a set of potential predictors. We have a *training set* of data, in which we observe the outcome and the measurement of the predictors for a set of patients. This set of known patients is called the training set because it is used by the classification programs to learn how to classify patients. Using these data, we build a prediction model, or learner, which will enable us to predict the outcome for new unseen patients in a *test set*. A good prediction model is one that accurately predicts such an outcome. Any classification method uses a set of predictors, which should be relevant to the task at hand, to characterize each patient. In general, *unsupervised classification* or *class discovery* means that predictors are used to find classes that are unknown a priori, whereas *supervised classification* or *class prediction* means that one has already determined into what classes a patient may be categorized and also has provided a set of sample patients with known classes. In supervised classification, the presence of the outcome variables guides the learning process. In unsupervised classification, we observe only the features and have no measurement of the outcome. Our task is rather to describe how the data are organized or clustered. Both approaches can be used for genomics-based medical diagnostics (**refs.** *2* and *7*; **Fig. 1**). The former is used when we have knowledge about the disease subtypes, whereas the latter can be used when we do not know the subtypes and want to discover them.

There are a number of standard classification methods in use. For unsupervised classification, the main tools are cluster analysis algorithms, with hierarchical cluster analysis being used the most often in genomics studies. For supervised classification, there are classical statistical methods and newer machine learning algorithms. The former category includes methods such as linear discriminant analysis (LDA), quadratic discriminant analysis (QDA), and logistic regression. The advantages of these methods are that they are probability-based and give explicit relationship between predictors and the outcome variable. Thus, the models are readily interpretable. However,

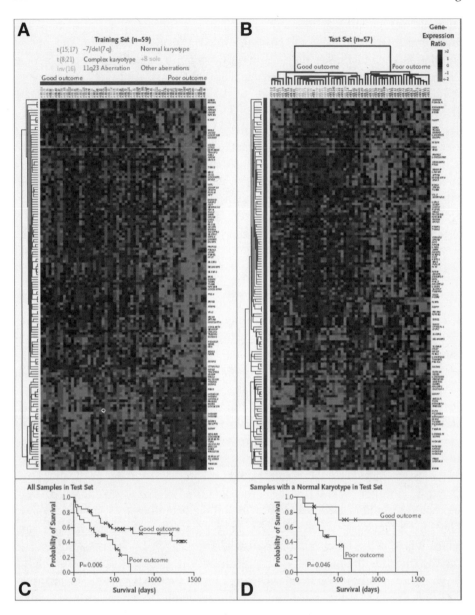

Fig. 1. Gene expression clusters are highly correlated with the survival outcome in patients with acute myeloid leukemia in both training and test set. (Adapted from **ref. 7**. with permission from the Massachusettes Medical Society. Copyright © 2004. All rights reserved.)

there are major limitations for applying these methods to building predictive models with genomics data. The first is that the model assumptions are hardly valid and the second is that they do not handle the "large *p*, small *n* problem" well. Newer machine learning algorithms include *neural networks (NNs)*, the *support vector machine (SVM)*, *classification and regression trees (CART)*, *K nearest neighbors (KNN)*, and so on. The biggest advantage of these methods is that they are general: they can handle problems with very many parameters, and they are able to classify patients well even when the distribution of patients in the high-dimensional parameter space is very complex. Their disadvantage is that they are computational intensive and run slowly, especially in the training phase but also in the application phase. Another significant disadvantage is that it is very difficult to determine how the decision is made in the *"black box."* Consequently, it is hard to determine which of the predictors being used are important and useful for classification and which are worthless. Although the choice of the best predictors is an important part of developing a good classifier, these methods do not give much help in this process. A good in-depth coverage of all these methods can be found in Tastie et al. *(34)*.

If training set and test set are not feasible because of small sample size, leave-one-out or 10-fold cross-validation methods may be used. Resampling-based methods such as boosting, bagging, and random forest can also be used *(34)*.

Because there are many parameters to consider with genomics or proteomics data, the classification problem becomes very difficult. Not only is the resulting high-dimensional space difficult to visualize, but also there are so many different combinations of parameters that techniques based on exhaustive searches of the parameter space rapidly become computationally infeasible. Practical methods for classification always involve a heuristic approach intended to find a "good-enough" solution to the optimization problem. Common strategies to reduce dimensions use either univariate or multivariate techniques. The univariate approach usually ranks genes according to their across-group variances and a certain threshold is used to keep the top *k* genes with the largest variances. The multivariate approach uses some statistical techniques such as *principal component analysis (PCA)* or *multidimensional scaling (MDS)*. Whereas the multivariate approach enjoys more statistical rigor, the univariate approach is more intuitive and easy to implement. Because the final goal is to predict the outcome as accurately as possible, either approach works just as well.

A good example of applying unsupervised classification to find a gene expression profile can be found in Bullinger et al. *(7)*. Using hierarchical cluster analysis, the authors selected a cluster of 133 genes from a total set of 6283 genes to seperate the patients into two groups in both training and test sets. The survival curves were significantly different between the two groups in both sets. The expression profile of this cluster of genes may be used to predict survival outcome in patients with acute mycloid leukemia.

5. Assessment of Efficacy of Genomics-Based Diagnostic Test

Fryback and Thornbury *(35)* proposed a six-level hierarchical model for assessing the efficacy of diagnostic tests in medicine with a focus on the imaging test. Borrowing their tools, we now apply the same principles and discuss levels of assessing efficacy of genomics-based tests.

Level 1 is *technical efficacy*, which is measured by the reliability of genomics or proteomics technology. Given that these technologies are very novel, there are still many concerns over their reliability and reproducibility. Apparently, repeated measurements of the same samples are much more consistent within each platform (e.g., Affymetrix GeneChip®, Amersham Codelink®, and so on), whereas across-platform comparisons are really bothersome *(36–40)*. However, we have reason to expect across-platform comparisons to be greatly improved in the near future, with the fast advance of bioinformatics tools and expansion of our knowledge about more and more genes.

Level 2 is *diagnostics accuracy efficacy*, which has been characterized by such measures as sensitivity, specificity, receive operating characteristic (ROC) curve (*see* **Fig. 2**), area under the ROC curve, likelihood ratio, positive predictive value (PPV), and negative predictive value (NPV). These concepts are briefly discussed here. As shown in **Table 1**, there are four possible outcomes for a diagnostic test, which are true-positive (TP), false-positive (FP), true-negative (TN), and false-negative (FN), respectively. For a diagnostic test T, let $T = 1$ refer to the positive test result and $T = 0$ refer to negative test result. Let $D = 1$ refer to the truth that a disease exists and $D = 0$ refer to the truth that the disease does not exist. Then, *pretest probability* is the probability of a patient having disease before a test is done. Pretest probability often comes from personal experience, published experience, history review, physical examination, and other laboratory or radiological tests.

Sensitivity (Se) is the probability that the test result is positive if the disease exists, i.e., $Se = P(T = 1, given\ D = 1) = \dfrac{TP}{TP + FN} = 1 - False\ negative\ rate.$

Specificity (Sp) is the probability that the test result is negative if the disease does not exist, i.e., $Sp = P(T = 0, given\ D = 0) = \dfrac{TN}{TN + FP} = 1 - False\ positive\ rate.$

PPV is the probability that the disease exists given that the test is positive, i.e.,
$$PPV = P(D = 1,\ given\ T = 1)$$
$$= \frac{Se \times Pretest\ probability}{Se \times Pretest\ probability + (1 - Sp) \times (1 - Pretest\ probability)}.$$

NPV is the probability that the disease does not exist if the test is negative, i.e.,
$$NPV = P(D = 0,\ given\ T = 0)$$
$$= \frac{Sp \times (1 - Pretest\ probability)}{Sp \times (1 - Pretest\ probability) + (1 - Se) \times Pretest\ probability}.$$

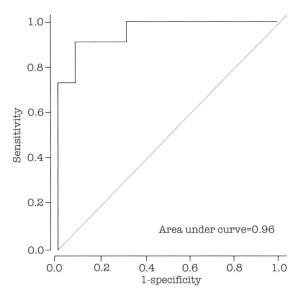

Fig. 2. Receiver operating characteristic (ROC) curve from Chang et al. *(13)*. (Reprinted from **ref.** *13*. Copyright [2003], with permission from Elsevier.)

Table 1
Possible Outcomes From a Diagnostic Test

Test result	Disease present	Disease absent	Total
Positive	*TP*	*FP*	TP + FP
Negative	*FN*	*TN*	TN + FN
Total	*TP + FN*	*FP + TN*	*TP + FP + TN + FN*

TP, true-positive; TN, true-negative; FP, false-positive; FN, false-negative.

A perfect diagnostic test would have all of the sensitivity, specificity, PPV, and NPV equal to 1. However, in reality, we may never have such a utopian test. As we change the cut-off threshold so that the sensitivity increases, usually the specificity will decrease. Thus, we should aim to a threshold with which a good balance between sensitivity and specificity can be achieved. If the goal is to rule-in a disease, i.e., to confirm the presence of a disease, then high specificity (i.e., low false-positive rate) would be desirable. If the goal is to rule out a disease, then a test with high sensitivity (i.e., low false-negative rate) should be desirable. An ROC curve plots the sensitivity as the decision rule of the classification probability is changed. It is thus a good tool to help find the right balance. Both PPV and NPV can be viewed as *post-test* probability. Depending on the consequence of the test result, a clinician may wish to emphasize either PPV or NPV. PPV is important when an action based on a positive test result is serious, such as giving chemotherapy or surgery for cancer. NPV is important when a inaction based on a negative test result has dire consequences, such as when missing diagnosis of a cancer or acute myocardial infarction. A good test or a panel of tests should give us good balance of these probabilities.

Figure 2 shows an example of ROC curve using the gene expression profile to predict resistance to Docetaxel treatment in patients with breast cancer. Docetaxel resistance was considered as the positive outcome. In leave-one out cross-validation analysis with the compound covariate predictor method of Radmacher and colleagues *(42)*, a linear classifier built from the expression profile of 92 genes was able to correctly discriminate 10 of 11 docetaxel-sensitive tumors (90% specificity) and 11 of 13 docetaxel-resistant tumors (85% sensitivity), with an overall accuracy of 88%. All six docetaxel-sensitive tumors in the test set were correctly classified. Despite the limitation of sample size, these results suggest that gene expression profiles may be promising tools to predict drug response in patients with different genetic backgrounds.

Level 3 is *diagnostic thinking efficacy,* which can be measured by, for example, the difference in the clinician's estimated probability of a diagnostic before vs after the test results are known. Although we can compute the normative pretest to post-test change in the probability of a disease if we know the pretest probability, sensitivity, and specificity, whether in the clinical environment the test changes the referring clinician's subjective probability of a disease is an empirical question. A prospective, randomized clinical trial may be helpful to answer such questions, but such trials have rarely been done. Therefore, assessment of the impact of a genomics-based diagnostic test on the diagnostic thinking of the clinician is something that deserves more attention. After all, inducing a change in the clinician's diagnostic thinking is a necessary prerequisite to having an impact on patients.

Level 4 is the *therapeutic efficacy,* which can be measured by the percentage of time that the therapy planned before the diagnostic test is altered by the test results. Note that the alteration does not have to be on the opposite direction, because strengthening confidence for a pretest plan is a special type of "alteration" too. In the context of a genomics-based test, we are asking whether the knowledge that a patient has a certain genomic profile would affect the physician's decision on treatment, which in turn, affects the patient's clinical outcome. The hope is that by giving therapy that is tailored to individual genetic make-up, we can improve treatment efficacy and reduce adverse effects. At this level, the most efficacious diagnostic test would either lead to the institution of new therapies or obviate the need for therapy. These are the most promising aspects of the genomics-based diagnostic test because through them, the disease progress can be caught early and at the fundamental level.

Level 5 is the *patient outcome efficacy,* which can be defined, for example, by the number of deaths prevented or the change in quality of life attributable to the test information. From the patient's point of view, this is really the standard with which the efficacy of a new diagnostic test should be evaluated. What good is a genomics-based test (or, in fact, any test) if it does not benefit the patient? In addition to the absolute efficacy, cost-effectiveness should also be studied because a useful but overly expensive test may be unaffordable to most patients who need it, and thus turn out to be not really useful.

Level 6 is the *societal efficacy,* which is often described by the cost-effectiveness of the test as measured from societal perspective. For the policymaker entrusted with the job of making resource allocations for large groups, the societal question of efficacy goes beyond the question of individual risks and benefits. This has been the focus of health outcomes research.

Two points are worth noting: (1) clearly, lower-level efficacy contributes to higher-level efficacy, but not vice versa; and (2) most diagnostic test literature has been focused on the first two levels, but the higher levels are really important.

6. Conclusion

We have discussed some statistical and clinical perspectives of developing genomics-based diagnostic test in the framework of EBM. Despite all of these complicated issues and challenges, we remain hopeful that the still-evolving genomic and proteomic technology will prove to be powerful in developing reliable diagnostic tests that will be invaluable for personalized medicine. With the publication of more and more exciting results from preliminary studies, the ever-decreasing cost, better understanding of the complexity of the techniques, and the development of better bioinformatics tools, the time when carefully controlled, prospective, large-scale studies will be performed in order to confirm these findings will come. Education of physicians and patients alike is also imperative before routine clinical implementation of genomics- or proteomics-based diagnostic tests becomes a reality.

References

1. Collins, F. S., Green, E. D., Guttmacher, A. E., and Guyer, M. S. (2003) A vision for the future of genomics research. *Nature* **422,** 835–847.
2. Golub, T. R., Slonim, D. K., Tamayo, P., et al. (1999) Molecular classification of cancer: class discovery and class prediction by gene expression monitoring. *Science* **286,** 531–537.
3. Alizadeh, A. A., Eisen, M. B., Davis, R. E., et al. (2000) Distinct types of diffuse large B-cell lymphoma identified by gene expression profiling. *Nature* **403,** 503–511.

 4. Bittner, M., Meltzer, P., Chen, Y., et al. Molecular classification of cutaneous malignant melanoma by gene expression profiling. *Nature* **406,** 536–540.
 5. Perou, C. M., Sorlie, T., Eisen, M. B., et al. (2000) Molecular portraits of human breast tumors. *Nature* **406,** 747–752.
 6. You, S. A., Archacki, S. R., Angheloiu, G., et al. (2003) Proteomic approach to coronary atherosclerosis shows ferritin light chain as a significant marker, evidence consistent with iron hypothesis in atherosclerosis. *Physiol. Genomics* **13,** 25–30.
 7. Bullinger, L., Dohner, K., Bair, E., et al. (2004) Use of gene-expression profiling to identify prognostic subclasses in adult acute myeloid leukemia. *N. Engl. J. Med.* **350,** 1605–1616.
 8. Dave, S. S., Wright, G., Tan, B., et al. (2004) Prediction of survival in follicular lymphoma based on molecular features of tumor-infiltrating immune cells. *N. Engl. J. Med.* **351,** 2159–2169.
 9. Holleman, A., Cheok, M. H., den Boer, M. L., et al. (2004) Gene-expression patterns in drug-resistant acute lymphoblastic leukemia cells and response to treatment. *N. Engl. J. Med.* **351,** 533–542.
10. Lossos, I. S., Czerwinski, D. K., Alizadeh, A. A., et al. (2004) Prediction of survival in diffuse large-B-cell lymphoma based on the expression of six genes. *N. Engl. J. Med.* **350,** 1828–1837.
11. Rassenti, L. Z., Huynh, L., Toy, T. L., et al. (2004) ZAP-70 Compared with immunoglobulin heavy-chain gene mutation status as a predictor of disease progression in chronic lymphocytic leukemia. *N. Engl. J. Med.* **351,** 893–901.
12. Sarwal, M., Chua, M. S., Kambham, N., et al. (2003) Molecular heterogeneity in acute renal allograft rejection identified by DNA microarray profiling. *N. Engl. J. Med.* **349,** 125–138.
13. Chang, J. C., Wooten, E. C., Tsimelzon, A., et al. (2003) Gene expression profiling for the prediction of therapeutic response to docetaxel in patients with breast cancer. *Lancet* **362,** 362–369.
14. Bueno, R., Loughlin, K. R., Powell, M. H., and Gordon, G. J. (2003) A diagnostic test for prostate cancer from gene expression profiling data. *J. Urol.* **171,** 903–906.
15. Guttmacher, A. E. and Collins, F. S. (2002) Genomic medicine—a primer. *N. Engl. J. Med.* **347,** 1512–1520.
16. Burke, W. (2002) Genomic medicine: genetic testing. *N. Engl. J. Med.* **347,** 1867–1875.
17. Khoury, M. J., McCabe, L. L., and McCabe, E. R. B. (2003) Genomic medicine: population screening in the age of genomic medicine. *N. Engl. J. Med.* **348,** 50–58.
18. Goldstein, D. B. (2003) Pharmacogenetics in the laboratory and the clinic. *N. Engl. J. Med.* **348,** 553–556.
19. Evans, W. E. and McLeod, H. L. (2003) Drug therapy: pharmacogenomics—drug disposition, drug targets, and side effects. *N. Engl. J. Med.* **348,** 538–549.
20. Weinshilboum, R. (2003) Genomic medicine: inheritance and drug response. *N. Engl. J. Med* **348,** 529–537.
21. Lynch, H. T. and de la Chapelle, A. (2003) Genomic medicine: hereditary colorectal cancer. *N. Engl. J. Med.* **348,** 919–932.

22. Nussbaum, R. L. and Ellis, C. E. (2003) Genomic medicine: Alzheimer's disease and Parkinson's disease. *N. Engl. J. Med.* **348,** 1356–1364.
23. Staudt, L. M. (2003) Genomic medicine: molecular diagnosis of the hematologic cancers. *N. Engl. J. Med.* **348,** 1777–1785.
24. Wooster. R. and Weber, B. L. (2003) Genomic medicine: breast and ovarian cancer. *N. Engl. J. Med.* **348,** 2339–2347.
25. Nabel, E. G. (2003) Genomic medicine: cardiovascular disease. *N. Engl. J. Med.* **349,** 60–72.
26. Burke, W. (2003) Genomic medicine: genomics as a probe for disease biology. *N. Engl. J. Med.* **349,** 969–974.
27. Guttmacher, A. E., Collins, F. S., and Carmona, R. H. (2004) The family history— more important than ever. *N. Engl. J. Med.* **351,** 2333–2336.
28. Ansell, S. M., Ackerman, M. J., Black, J. L., Roberts, L. R., and Tefferi, A. (2003) A Primer on medical genomics. Part VI, Genomics and molecular genetics in clinical practice. *Mayo Clin. Proc.* **78,** 307–317.
29. Sackett, D. L., Rosenberg, W. M., Gray, J. A., Haynes, R. B., and Richardson, W. S. (1996) Evidence-based medicine, what it is and what it isn't. *Br. Med. J.* **312,** 71, 72.
30. Sox, Jr., H. C., Blatt, M. A., Higgins, M. C., and Marton, K. I. (1989) *Med. Decis. Making.* Butterworths-Heinemann, Boston, MA.
31. McNeil, B. J. and Adelstein, S. J. (1976) Determining the value of diagnostic and screening tests. *J. Nucl. Med.* **17,** 439–448.
32. Zhou, X. H., Obuchowski, N. A., and McClish, D. K. (2002) *Statistical Methods in Diagnostic Medicine.* John Wiley and Sons, New York, NY.
33. Metz, C. E. (1989) Some practical issues of experimental design and data analysis in radiological ROC studies. *Invest. Radiol.* **24,** 234–245.
34. Hastie, T., Tibshirani, R., and Friedman, J. (2001) *The Elements of Statistical Learning, Data Mining, Inference, and Prediction.* Springer-Verlag, New York, NY.
35. Fryback, D. G. and Thornbury, J. R. (1991) The efficacy of diagnostic imaging. *Med. Decis. Making* **11,** 88–94.
36. Tan, P. K., Downey, T. J., Spitznagel, Jr., E. L., et al. (2003) Evaluation of gene expression measurements from commercial microarray platforms. *Nucleic Acids Res.* **31,** 5676–5684.
37. Woo, Y., Affourtit, J., Daigle, S., et al. (2004) A comparison of cDNA, oligonucleotide, and Affymetrix GeneChip gene expression microarray platforms. *J. Biomol. Tech.* **15,** 276–284.
38. Bammler, T., Beyer, R. P., Bhattacharya, S., et al. (2005) Standardizing global gene expression analysis between laboratories and across platforms. *Nat. Methods* **2,** 351–356.
39. Larkin, J. E., Frank, B. C., Gavras, H., Sultana, R., and Quackenbush, J. (2005) Independence and reproducibility across microarray platforms. *Nat. Methods* **2,** 337–344.
40. Irizarry, R. A., Warren, D., Spencer, F., et al. (2005) Multiple-laboratory comparison of microarray platforms. *Nat. Methods* **2,** 345–350.

4

Animal Models for Disease

Knockout, Knock-In, and Conditional Mutant Mice

David F. LePage and Ronald A. Conlon

Summary

Diseases with a genetic basis can be modeled with knockout, knock-in, and conditional mutant gene-targeted mice. In the following, we provide detailed protocols for gene targeting. Gene targeting of embryonic stem cells can be accomplished by laboratories equipped for tissue culture. Alternatively, many gene-targeting services divide the work of targeting with a customer lab. In this collaborative situation, knowledge of the entire process helps ensure a successful outcome. The construction of chimeras for germ-line transmission is not described here, because this procedure is beyond the means of most laboratories, typically is provided by transgenic core facilities, and is best learned through hands-on demonstration.

Key Words: Gene targeting; homologous recombination; embryonic stem cells; ES cells; knockout; knock-in; conditional mutant; animal model of disease; genetically engineered mice.

1. Introduction

The generation of mutant mice by gene targeting takes advantage of the remarkable ability of embryonic stem (ES) cell lines *(1,2)* to participate in the formation of germ cells of mice when the cells are put back into an early embryo *(3)*. Cell lines that have undergone gene targeting are enriched by the incorporation of selectable markers into the targeting vector *(4)*. Out of this enriched set of cell lines, the desired homologous recombination event is identified by molecular analysis of genomic DNA. Targeted ES cell lines that have a normal number of chromosomes are identified and selected to make chimeras.

Targeting can be used to generate knockouts, knock-ins, or conditional alleles. Knockouts, knock-ins, and conditional alleles are generated in a similar

From: *Methods in Molecular Medicine, vol. 129:*
Cardiovascular Disease: Methods and Protocols, Volume 2: Molecular Medicine
Edited by: Q. K. Wang © Humana Press Inc., Totowa, NJ

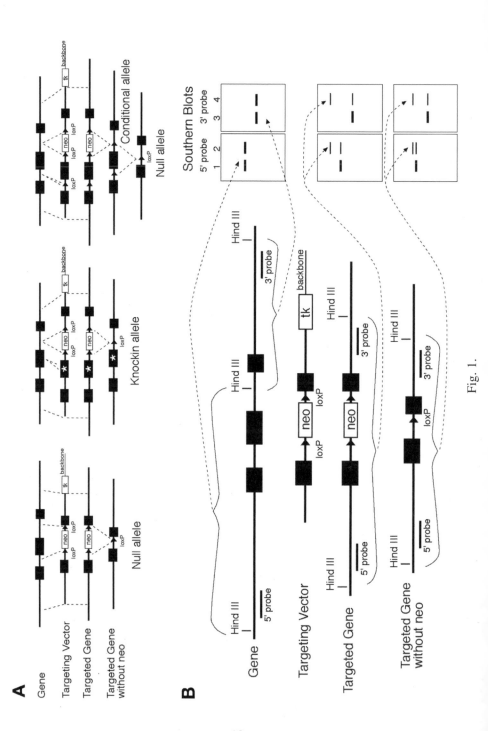

Fig. 1.

fashion using the protocols given here. Knockouts are used to define the overall requirement for a gene and to model loss-of-function mutations. Knock-ins are used to introduce heterologous coding sequences such as reporters or DNA recombinases, to incorporate changes in DNA sequence to "humanize" a mouse gene, or to generate point mutations. Conditional mutations are used to define the organ, tissue, or cellular autonomy of mutant effects, to circumvent embryonic lethality, or to model somatic mutations.

The two major hurdles for the generation of gene-targeted mice are obtaining homologous recombination and obtaining germ-line transmission. Although it has been almost 20 yr since the first gene-targeted mice were constructed *(4,5)*, not all parameters that affect the frequency of homologous recombination and germ-line transmission are known. Nonetheless, we give criteria for the parameters that are known, provide advice on how to ensure success, and provide recovery strategies and trouble-shooting guidance.

The protocols assume a working knowledge of basic tissue culture technique *(6)*.

1.1. Targeting Vector Design

1.1.1. General Principles

Our purpose is to present the most common and widely applicable vector designs (**Fig. 1**). There are a large number of variations possible in the design of targeting vectors and the uses they are put to *(7,8)*. The following concentrates on the most common applications.

For all targeting vectors, the following considerations apply: (1) the vector must be linearized outside of the arms of homology, so provision must be made for a unique recognition sequence for a restriction enzyme at an appropriate place; (2) a strategy to detect gene targeting by Southern blot analysis of

---

Fig. 1. *(Opposite page)* Vector design and detection of targeting. (**A**) Vector designs for gene-targeted null, knock-in, and conditional alleles are shown (left to right). The wild-type allele with three exons is shown at top, the targeting vector on the next line, the correctly targeted allele on the next line, and the targeted allele after excision of the *neo* cassette by transfection of *Cre* recombinase in ES cells. (**B**) Strategy for detection of correctly targeted alleles. DNA probes for Southern blot analysis are selected that are in the gene to be targeted, but external to the targeting vector (5′ and 3′ probes). After targeting, random insertions of the vector that survive the selection do not show alteration of the endogenous gene (lanes 1 and 3), but correctly targeted lines show a wild-type allele and the predicted fragment for a targeted allele. Excision of *neo* is also verified by observing the predicted changes in fragment size (*neo* and *tk* indicate the minigenes consisting of promoters, coding sequences, and polyadenylation signals for the neomycin resistance and herpes simplex virus thymidine kinase genes, respectively.)

genomic DNA must be developed; (3) the greater the amount of sequence match, the more likely the targeting is to succeed.

1.1.2. Targeting Vectors for Null Alleles

We recommend that a targeting vector for construction of a null allele be constructed with genomic DNA from the 129 strain of mice, with at least 7 kb of total homology split in two arms, which are positioned to delete early or critical coding exons of the gene **(Fig. 1)**. Two selectable markers are incorporated into the vector *(4)*. The neomycin-resistance gene (*neo*) should be flanked by *lox*P sites, and located between the two arms. The herpes simplex virus (HSV) *thymidine kinase* (*tk*) gene should be placed outside one of the arms of the vector. The neomycin-resistance gene is removed in ES cells through the activity of *Cre* recombinase acting on the *lox*P sites after gene targeting.

1.1.3. Targeting Vectors for Knock-In Alleles

To create a knock-in allele **(Fig. 1)**, a sequence change or inserted coding sequence is incorporated into one of the arms of the targeting vector *(9)*. The goal is to minimize other disruption of gene function. The neomycin-resistance gene is flanked by *lox*P sites so that it can be excised by expression of *Cre* recombinase, and is typically inserted into an intron. In designing knock-ins, particularly for those generating small or subtle changes, provision must be made to detect whether the knock-in change itself has been integrated as was intended—this is necessary because a homologous recombination exchange could occur internally to the intended change and not incorporate the altered sequence. The *neo* marker is removed in ES cells before constructing chimeras.

1.1.4. Targeting Vectors for Conditional Alleles

A conditional allele has wild-type function, but can be mutated to a null allele in cells in which *Cre* recombinase is expressed *(10)*. To maintain wild-type function, no part of the gene is deleted, and *lox*P sites are inserted into introns away from sequences that might function in splicing and transcription **(Fig. 1)**.

Targeting vectors for conditional alleles should be constructed as for null alleles, except that the neomycin-resistance gene with its flanking *lox*P sites is inserted into an intron, and a *lox*P is inserted into different intron, such that deletion of sequences between the most distal *lox*P sites will remove an essential coding exon.

The neomycin-resistance gene is removed with *Cre* recombinase in ES cells, and alleles with the two *lox*P sites flanking the essential exon are identified. The conditional allele is introduced into mice through chimeras, and the gene is mutated to a null allele through the action of *Cre* recombinase on the two remaining *lox*P sites, deleting the sequences between them.

1.2. Construction of Vectors

1.2.1. Isogenic DNA

The frequency of homologous recombination depends on the degree of sequence match and the length of the matching sequences *(11,12)*. Greater than 7 kb of DNA of perfect sequence match usually is needed to obtain homologous recombination at practical frequencies. The relationship between sequence divergence and targeting rates has not been examined systematically, but about 0.5% sequence divergence was shown to result in a 20-fold decrease in targeting frequency for constructs targeting the Rb locus *(11)*. In a targeting vector, the exact sequence match typically is interrupted by a gap and/or an insertion, with each of the two parts of the match approximately halved. The apparent paradox that the sequence match with the target gene must be near exact whereas the gap or insertion can be as large as 10 kb probably arises because there are two independent homologous recombination events that occur in gene targeting, one for each arm.

The genomic sequences of different inbred strains of mice diverge enough that DNA from the same strain as the ES cells is needed to construct the targeting vector. Most ES cells are made from the 129 strain of mice, thus targeting vectors are made from 129 genomic DNA. There are several different substrains of the 129 strain, but differences between them are unlikely to be great enough to affect gene targeting. Genomic libraries of 129 mice are available in λ phage vectors from commercial vendors (Stratagene, cat. no. 946313), and in bacterial artificial chromosome (BAC) vectors from the BACPAC Resources Center (http://bacpac.chori.org).

Alternatively, long-range PCR can be used to isolate construct arms from ES cell genomic DNA. DNA recovered by PCR should be sequenced to ensure that PCR did not introduce unintended mutations into the targeting vector, particularly for knock-in and conditional gene targeting.

1.2.2. Selectable Markers

Heterologous genes are incorporated into the targeting vector for enrichment of targeting events. Between the arms of the targeting vector, a gene consisting of a promoter, coding sequence for a drug-resistance protein, and a polyadenylation signal is incorporated. The neomycin-resistance coding sequence is typically used, as this confers resistance to the neomycin analog G418. Outside of one arm, a gene to express HSV *tk* is placed. In a successful homologous recombination, the *tk* gene is not integrated into the genome and is lost. Cells in which *tk* has integrated into genomic DNA can be killed by selection with the drug 1-2′-deoxy-2′-fluoro-β-D-arabinofuranosyl-5-iodouracil (FIAU). In most transfections, the majority of cells incorporating the targeting vector do not do so by homologous recombination, so most cells incorporate the *tk* selectable marker, and the FIAU selection kills these cells. Alternative drug selection genes are available as well *(8)*.

The orientation of the selectable marker gene transcription units relative to each other and the targeted gene do not appear to be important.

1.2.3. Avoiding Unintended Consequences

It is important to anticipate the consequences of gene targeting to ensure that the targeted gene lacks all function as intended. Examine the splicing patterns that might be expected to occur in the targeted allele, looking for in-frame splicing, which could result in aberrant protein products with altered activity. Avoid designs that might give rise to proteins with dominant negative or other gain-of-function activities.

The neomycin-resistance coding sequence and its PGK1 promoter can have unintended consequences on the targeted gene and on adjacent genes if they are left in the gene *(13–16)*. The neomycin-resistance gene contains cryptic splice acceptors and donors, which can be utilized by transcripts from the targeted gene. In addition, the function of genes adjacent to the targeted gene can be altered by the neomycin gene inserted at the targeted locus. In one case, this interference has been shown to be due to transcription from the PGK1 promoter and aberrant splicing of *neo* sequences into the adjacent gene, but other mechanisms are possible, including interference through enhancer competition. If the targeting vector is designed with recognition sequences for a site-specific DNA recombinase flanking the *neo* gene as described previously, it can be removed after gene targeting by expression of the DNA recombinase. The *Cre* site-specific DNA recombinase recognizes a 34-bp sequence, the *lox*P site. Sequences between a pair of matched sites in direct repeat orientation are deleted, leaving a single *lox*P sequence.

1.2.4. Planning for Detection of Gene Targeting

A strategy for identifying the targeted locus by Southern blot analysis must be developed in parallel with vector design (**Fig. 1**). Two DNA probes from the gene on each side outside the targeting vector must be able to detect a change in fragment size.

Avoid the use of restriction enzymes, which have recognition sequences that have 5′CG3′ dinucleotides, because this sequence is most often methylated in ES cell genomic DNA and will be resistant to cutting. For example, the recognition sequence for *Xho*I is 5′CTCGAG3′, and thus *Xho*I should be avoided; *Hind*III recognizes the sequence 5′AAGCTT3′ and is suitable. Before transfecting ES cells with the targeting vector, test the probes by Southern blot analysis on a genomic digest of ES cell DNA to verify that they work well.

It is important to verify the homologous recombination event from both sides with probes external to the targeting vector, because recombination can occur on one side only *(17,18)*. In practice, the initial identification of homologous recombination events is done with one external probe, then the candidate targeted cell lines are thawed, larger amounts of genomic DNA are prepared, and targeting is verified by extensive genomic Southern blot analysis using multiple probes and digests.

1.2.5. Vector Linearization

Targeting vectors are linearized before transfection, so provision must be made for a unique recognition sequence to linearize the vector. Ideally, this site is placed such that when the vector is cut, the vector has at one end one arm of homology, and at the other end the vector backbone is external to the *tk* gene.

1.2.6. Assembling the Targeting Vector

We do not provide a protocol describing construction of the targeting vector, but the technology involved is that common to most molecular biology subcloning. Alternatively, companies that provide targeting vector construction services include inGenious, genOway, and Genomatix. For plasmids carrying the *neo* selectable marker flanked by *lox*P sites, pflox *(19)*, and the *tk* selectable marker, pPNT *(20)*, can be obtained from the labs they originated in.

2. Materials

The key material for successful gene targeting is an early passage, germ line-competent ES cell line. Because germ line-competency can be lost during culture, and because the only way to assay germ line-competency is by the construction of chimeras, it is strongly recommended that ES cells be obtained from a lab that is active in gene targeting. Most ES cell lines are from the 129 inbred strain of mice, which historically was most amenable to the establishment of lines *(21)*, and which may be more stable in culture *(22)*. There are a number of different substrains of 129, designated as "129" followed by additional letters. A number of cell lines have been established more recently that derive from the embryos of a cross between 129 and a second strain of inbred mice *(23–25)*. These F1 hybrid cell lines are generally more robust in their growth and contribution to chimeras and may come to be widely used in the future.

Our experience with a number of different ES cell lines for about two decades led us to recommend the R1 ES cell line, a 129-ES cell line established by the Nagy lab *(26)*. This line is robust and has maintained germ line-competency in a large number of different labs, and has adapted to growth without feeder cells multiple times. The methods we describe have been optimized for the growth of R1 cells in the absence of feeder cells.

On obtaining an ES cell line, a stock of frozen vials of early passage cells should be prepared in order to provide cells for future targeting projects.

2.1. General

A lab equipped for tissue culture is necessary, and should contain the following:

1. Laminar air flow hood.
2. 5% carbon dioxide, humidified 37°C incubator.
3. Inverted microscope.
4. Tabletop clinical centrifuge.
5. Water bath.
6. –20 and –80°C freezers.
7. 4°C refrigerator.
8. Liquid nitrogen freezer that can accept freezer boxes.
9. Source of high-quality water suitable for tissue culture.

2.1.1. Thawing ES Cells

1. 10 mM 2-mercaptoethanol. Add 70 µL of 2-mercaptoethanol (14.3 M 2-mercaptoethanol, Sigma-Aldrich, cat. no. M7522) to 100 mL of high-quality water and filter-sterilize through a 0.2-µm filter. Make 10-mL aliquots and store at 4°C.
2. Fetal bovine serum (FBS). Serum of different lots is tested by comparison against serum from a lot known to be satisfactory. ES cells are grown at normal (20%) and high (30%) serum concentrations, and the lot of serum with the highest plating efficiency and growth at 30% FBS is selected. Serum is kept frozen at –80°C for long-term storage, and heat-inactivated as needed. To heat-inactivate, thaw a 500-mL bottle of serum overnight at 4°C in a refrigerator. Put the bottle into a 37°C water bath such that the water comes to the level of the serum inside the bottle. Allow to thaw until only a large ice cube remains (approx 1 h). Heat-inactivate the serum in a water bath set at 56°C for 30 min, mixing occasionally. At the end of heat-inactivation, mix and aliquot the serum into 40-mL aliquots and freeze at –20°C. Do not refreeze. Some white particulate matter floating in the serum after heat-inactivation is normal.
3. ES cell medium: to make 100 mL of ES cell medium, combine in the order listed:
   a. 80 mL Iscove's modified Dulbecco's medium (IMDM; Invitrogen, cat. no. 12440-046).
   b. 20 mL heat-inactivated FBS.
   c. 1 mL 10 mM 2-mercaptoethanol.
   d. 1 mL 10 mM MEM nonessential amino acids solution (Invitrogen, cat. no. 11140-050).
   e. 1 mL 50 U/mL penicillin 50 µg/mL streptomycin (Invitrogen, cat. no. 15070-063).

f. 10 μL of 10^7 U/mL leukemia inhibitory factor (LIF; Chemicon, cat. no. ESG1107) or recombinant protein purified from *Escherichia coli* as described *(27)*.

Store protected from light at 4°C for less than a week. Before use, warm in the tissue culture hood at room temperature for 10–20 min, protected from light.

4. Gelatinized 60-mm tissue culture plates (Falcon, cat. no. 1007). Briefly cover dish with 0.1% gelatin solution (Sigma, cat. no. G9382, autoclaved in water) and then aspirate off. Allow to air-dry in the tissue culture hood for at least 30 min. Use within 24 h.

5. If feeder cells are required to thaw a cell line obtained from another lab, it may be preferable to purchase them (e.g., from Chemicon/Specialty Media, cat. no. PMEF-N) rather than to prepare them yourself *(28)*.

2.2. Passaging ES Cells

1. ES cell medium (*see* **Subheading 2.1.1.**, **item 3**).
2. Gelatinized tissue culture plates (*see* **Subheading 2.1.1.**, **item 4**).
3. PBS: Dulbecco's phosphate-buffered saline, calcium and magnesium-free, made from powder (Invitrogen, cat. no. 21600-010) in high-quality water, stored at 4°C, and brought to room temperature before use.
4. Trypsin: 0.25% trypsin 0.02% EDTA in Hanks' Balanced Salt Solution (JRH Biosciences, cat. no. 59428), stored frozen at −20°C, used freshly thawed at room temperature and not refrozen.

2.3. Freezing ES Cells From 35-mm Plates or Larger

1. ES cell medium (*see* **Subheading 2.1.1.**, **item 3**).
2. PBS (*see* **Subheading 2.2.**, **item 3**).
3. Trypsin (*see* **Subheading 2.2.**, **item 4**).
4. Cryoprotective medium (CPM): IMDM (Invitrogen, cat. no. 12440-046) containing 10% FBS and 10% dimethylsulfoxide (DMSO) (Sigma-Aldrich, cat. no. D2650). Add the serum first, and mix; then, add the DMSO and filter-sterilize through a 0.2-μm filter. Aliquots can be stored frozen at −20°C, protected from light. Before use, thaw and bring to 4°C.
5. Cryovials: 1.8-mL screw-cap round-bottom tubes for liquid nitrogen storage (Nunc, cat. no. 363401).
6. Nalgene slow-freeze container (Nalgene, cat. no. 5100-0001) filled with isopropanol. Replace the isopropanol after five uses.

2.4. Gene Targeting

1. ES cell medium (*see* **Subheading 2.1.1.**, **item 3**).
2. A device suitable for electroporation of eukaryotic tissue culture cells. The models sold by Bio-Rad are widely used in gene targeting labs. The current model is the Gene Pulser Xcell electroporation device, and requires the capacitance extender (CE) module for electroporation of ES cells.

3. G418: 50 mg/mL Geneticin (G418) solution (Invitrogen, cat. no. 10131-019) frozen at $-20°C$ in 1-mL aliquots. Because activity varies with lot and ES cells vary in their sensitivity, batches are purchased in bulk from the same lot number and the activity of the lot is determined empirically. Mock-electroporated (electroporation without DNA) cells are plated and subjected to G418 selection at different concentrations for 7–10 d. The minimum concentration that yields 100% killing in 7–10 d is chosen. For R1 ES cells grown in IMDM without feeders, a final concentration of 100 µg/mL has proven the optimal concentration for most lots of G418.

4. FIAU (Moravek Biochemicals, cat. no. M-251). To make a 100 mM stock, add 388 mg of FIAU to 9 mL of PBS and add NaOH until the FIAU has dissolved. Make total volume to 10 mL. Dilute in PBS to give a 200 µM (1000X) stock. Aliquot and store at $-20°C$. The working concentration in ES cell medium is 0.2 µM FIAU.

5. 500 µg purified, linearized targeting vector: purify the targeting vector using a maxi-prep protocol, for example a Qiagen kit protocol. Cut the vector to completion with the appropriate restriction enzyme, and purify by phenol/chloroform and chloroform extraction and ethanol precipitation. Dissolve the purified, linearized plasmid in low EDTA TE (10 mM Tris, pH 8.5, 0.1 mM EDTA) at a concentration of 2 µg/µL.

6. 0.1% (w/v) erythrosin B (Sigma-Aldrich, cat. no. E-7379) in PBS.

7. Hemacytometer/counting chamber (Fisher, cat. no. 02-671-10).

8. Gelatinized 100-mm tissue culture plates (Falcon, cat. no. 3003).

9. Methylene blue/basic fuchsin: 0.33% (w/v) methylene blue (Fisher, cat. no. M291), 0.11% (w/v) basic fuchsin (Fisher, cat. no. F98) in methanol.

2.5. Picking Colonies Into 96-Well Plates

1. ES cell medium (*see* **Subheading 2.1.1.**, **item 3**).
2. G418 (*see* **Subheading 2.4.**, **item 3**).
3. Gelatinized, 96-well flat-bottom tissue culture plates (Falcon, cat. no. 3072).

2.6. Tryplating 96-Well Plates

1. ES cell medium (*see* **Subheading 2.1.1.**, **item 3**).
2. G418 (*see* **Subheading 2.4.**, **item 3**).
3. PBS (*see* **Subheading 2.2.**, **item 3**).
4. Trypsin (*see* **Subheading 2.2.**, **item 4**).
5. Eight-well multichannel pipetor, adjustable, 10 µL maximum volume.
6. Eight-well multichannel pipetor, adjustable, 50 µL maximum volume.
7. Eight-well multichannel pipetor, adjustable, 300 µL maximum volume.
8. Eight-well multichannel aspirator (Inotech, cat. no. IV-596).

2.7. Splitting ES Cells for DNA and Freezing in 96-Well Plates

1. U-bottom polypropylene 96-well plates (ABgene, cat. no. AB-0796) and sealing mat lids (ABgene, cat. no. AB-0674).

2. 2X freezing medium: IMDM containing 20% FBS and 20% DMSO (Sigma-Aldrich, cat. no. D2650), made fresh and placed on ice.
3. Mineral oil, mouse embryo tested (Sigma-Aldrich, cat. no. M8410).

2.8. Preparing Genomic DNA From ES Cells Grown in 96-Well Plates

1. 96-well plate lysis buffer: 10 mM Tris-HCl, pH 7.5, 10 mM EDTA, 10 mM NaCl, 0.5% Sarkosyl, 1 mg/mL proteinase K.
2. Plastic wrap.
3. Humidified container: a plastic container large enough to hold the 96-well plates, with wet paper towels on the bottom.
4. 55°C incubator.
5. Ethanol + salt, made fresh: combine 10 mL of 95% ethanol and 0.15 mL of 5 M NaCl stock; put on ice.
6. Paper towels.
7. 70% EtOH.
8. Low EDTA TE: 10 mM Tris-HCl, pH 8.4, 0.1 mM EDTA.

2.9. Digestion of Genomic DNA in 96-Well Plates for Southern Blot Analysis

1. Restriction enzyme cocktail:

Genomic DNA in low-TE in well	20 µL
10X restriction enzyme buffer	4 µL
Water	To bring total volume to 40 µL
100 mg/mL bovine serum albumin (BSA)	0.4 µL
50 mM Spermidine	0.8 µL
10 mg/mL DNase-free RNase A	0.2 µL
Restriction enzyme	20–40 U

2. Humidified container.
3. 37°C oven.

2.10. Recovering Candidate Targeted Clones and Verifying Homologous Recombination

1. 37°C water bath.
2. Gelatinized 24-well plates (Falcon, cat. no. 3047).

2.11. Extracting Genomic DNA From ES Cells in Quantity

1. Large-scale lysis buffer: 200 mM NaCl, 100 mM Tris-HCl, pH 8.5, 5 mM EDTA, 0.2% sodium dodecyl sulfate (SDS), 100 µg/mL proteinase K.
2. Nutator (Becton Dickinson, cat. no. 421105).
3. Orbital shaker.

2.12. Digestion of High-Molecular-Weight DNA

1. Restriction enzyme cocktail:

Genomic DNA in low EDTA TE	10 μL
10X restriction enzyme buffer	20 μL
Water	To bring volume to 200 μL total
10 mg/mL BSA	2.0 μL
50 mM Spermidine	4 μL
High concentration restriction enzyme	20–100 U

2. 5 M NaCl.
3. Microcentrifuge.
4. 70 and 95% EtOH.

2.13. Counting ES Cell Chromosomes

1. ES cell medium (*see* **Subheading 2.1.1.**, **item 3**).
2. Colcemid: 3.125 μL of 10 μg/mL colcemid (Invitrogen, cat. no. 15212-012) per milliliter of medium.
3. 37°C water bath.
4. 0.075 M KCl warmed to 37°C.
5. Methanol/acetic acid fix: 2 mL glacial acetic acid and 5 mL methanol, prepared fresh.
6. Microscope slides: plain, precleaned slides (Fisher, cat. no. 12-549) labeled with etching tool.
7. Coplin jar (Fisher, cat. no. 08-813).
8. Giemsa: 2.5 mL of Giemsa solution (Invitrogen, cat. no. 10092-013) in 47.5 mL of Gurr's pH 6.8 buffer (Invitrogen, cat. no. 10582-013).
9. Glass cover slips.
10. Permount® mounting medium (Fisher, cat. no. SP15-100).
11. Compound microscope with ×40 and ×100 objectives.

2.14. Transient Transfection of ES Cells With Cre Recombinase to Excise the neo Cassette

1. Supercoiled pOG231 plasmid *(29)* for the expression of *Cre* Recombinase, 25 μg per cell line.
2. ES cell medium (*see* **Subheading 2.1.1.**, **item 3**).
3. Gelatinized 100-mm plates.

3. Methods

ES cells lose their ability to colonize the germ line with increased time in culture. Because the only reliable means of testing germ line competency is by constructing and breeding chimeras, and because gene-targeted cell lines

Table 1
Culture Plate Size, Area, and Volumes

Plate size	Surface area (cm^2)	Medium volume (mL)	Trypsin volume (mL)
96 wells	0.2/well	0.2–0.3/well	
24 wells	2/well	0.5/well	
35 mm	9.5	1.5–2.0	0.7–1
60 mm	21	3.5	1.5–2
100 mm	56	10	3–4

represent a large investment of time and money, great care must be taken in the culture of the ES cells to avoid subjecting the cells to less than optimal culture conditions. Avoid overgrowth by passaging ES cells before they become confluent; change media frequently; and keep the total passage number as low as possible.

ES cells grow as a colony of cells tightly apposed to each other through extensive cell–cell contacts. When ES cells differentiate, they attach and spread on the surface of the tissue culture plate. Differentiated cells have lost the stem cell character, cannot be propagated, and will not colonize the germ line of chimeric mice.

3.1. Thawing ES Cells

1. Loosen the cap of the vial and quickly warm in a 37°C water bath (*see* **Note 1**). Before all of the ice has disappeared, transfer the cells to a tube containing 8 mL of ES cell media and gently invert the tube a few times to mix.
2. Recover the cells by centrifugation at 300*g* for 5 min.
3. Promptly resuspend the cells in 3.5 mL of ES cell medium and plate on a 60-mm gelatinized tissue culture plate.

3.2. Passaging ES Cells

1. Replace the medium daily, and passage the cells every second day. ES cells are split typically into six equivalent plates (*see* **Table 1** for plate sizes, medium, and trypsin volumes). Aspirate the medium from the plate.
2. Add an equal or greater volume of PBS to the plate.
3. Aspirate the PBS from the plate.
4. Add trypsin and place the plates in the incubator for 5 min.
5. Using a plugged Pasteur pipet with a bulb, vigorously pipet each plate in order to break up the colonies into single cells. With a circular stream, pipet all around the dish, avoiding bubbles as much as possible. The goal is an even suspension of single cells. Examine the plates on the microscope to see that the colonies are well broken up and consist mostly of single cells (*see* **Note 2**).
6. Transfer the suspension of cells to a tube with an equal volume of medium. Draw the suspension up and down in the pipet three times to mix.

7. Centrifuge at 300*g* for 5 min.
8. Promptly aspirate the medium and thoroughly disperse the cells in the appropriate amount of ES cell medium.
9. Gently add the cells to gelatinized plates, splitting the original plate onto six equivalent plates (*see* **Note 3**).

3.3. Freezing ES Cells From 35-mm Plates or Larger

1. Four hours before freezing, replace the medium on the cells with fresh medium and place them back in the incubator (*see* **Note 4**).
2. Bring a sufficient volume of CPM and the slow-cool freezing container to 0–4°C on ice (*see* **Note 5**).
3. Trypsinize the cells exactly as for passaging cells under **Subheading 3.2.**, and add the cells in trypsin solution to a tube with an equal volume of ES cell culture medium.
4. Pellet the cells by centrifugation at 300*g* for 5 min.
5. Promptly remove the supernatant and resuspend the cells in ice cold CPM, using 1.5 mL CPM for each 35-mm confluent plate equivalent. Add the cells to labeled vials on ice.
6. When all vials are ready to freeze, place them in the prechilled Nalgene slow-cool freezing container.
7. Promptly place the slow-cool freezing container in a –70°C freezer, and leave in the freezer for at least 24 h.
8. Transfer the vials to liquid nitrogen storage.

3.4. Gene Targeting

1. Thaw a vial of early pass ES cells onto a 60-mm plate as described in **Subheading 3.1.** (*see also* **Note 6**).
2. On the second day, replace the medium.
3. On the third day, passage the plate onto two 100-mm plates (a 1:6 split) as described under **Subheading 3.2.**
4. On the fourth day, replace the medium.
5. On the fifth day, passage the cells (*see* **Subheading 3.2.**), splitting them 1:2.
6. Early on the sixth day, replace the medium.
7. Four hours later, remove the medium, wash the cells with PBS, and trypsinize each plate with 3–4 mL of fresh trypsin as described previously to obtain a single-cell suspension, and mix with an equal volume of medium. Recover the cells by centrifugation at 300*g* for 5 min, and promptly and gently resuspend the cells in 1 mL of cold PBS for each plate of cells. Pool the cells, storing on ice.
8. Remove 0.1 mL of cells and add to 0.9 mL of 0.1% erythrosin B in PBS. Mix, and apply a small volume to the assembled hemacytometer and count the number of cells. Adjust the concentration of the pooled cells to 7×10^6 cells/mL by adding cold PBS.
9. There should be enough cells for 6–12 electroporation cuvets containing 0.8 mL of cell suspension each. Place the cuvets on ice, and add 0.8 mL of cells and 40 µg of linearized vector to each.

10. Electroporate at 240 V, 500 µF, and place the cuvets on ice for 20 min.
11. Using a plugged Pasteur pipet, gently resuspend the cells of each cuvet and pool with 1.5 mL of prewarmed medium per cuvet. Wash each cuvet with 1 mL of medium, add to the pool, and mix.
12. Mark a single 100-mm gelatinized plate to monitor transfection efficiency, then add 0.3 mL of the cell suspension to 9.7 mL of medium in the dish: this plate will be used for monitoring transfection efficiency as the one-tenth quantitation plate. For the remainder of the plates, add 3 mL of cells to 7 mL medium in each 100-mm plate.
13. Approximately 24 h after the cells were plated out, start the drug selection by replacing the medium with medium with G418 and FIAU together, or G418 alone for the plate used to monitor transfection efficiency.
14. Feed the cells daily with media supplemented with the appropriate fresh drugs. Most colonies will grow and die; a small number of colonies will survive. For a brief period of time, it may appear that nothing has survived under double selection, but after 7–10 d of selection, colonies should be clearly visible.
15. After 7–10 d of selection, when colonies are visible to the naked eye as specks on the plate and debris has been cleared from the plates, feed the cells every other day with medium containing only G418 (no FIAU).
16. Pick cells (*see* **Subheading 3.5.**) at 10–14 d, depending on the rate of growth. When the plate for monitoring transfection efficiency has grown clear colonies, remove the medium from the plate, wash with PBS, fix/stain with methylene blue/basic fuchsin for 5 min, wash with water, and air-dry (*see* **Note 7**).

3.5. Picking Colonies Into 96-Well Plates

1. For each 100-mm plate, prepare a 96-well gelatinized plate with 180 µL per well of medium with G418. Warm the 96-well plates for 10–15 min in the incubator (*see* **Note 8**).
2. Remove one 100-mm plate and one 96-well plate from the incubator. Using an inverted or stereo microscope, pick up and place each colony into one well of the 96-well plate, and mark the well with an air bubble. To pick up a colony, use a small-volume (20 or 10 µL maximum volume) pipetor with a yellow tip set at 10 µL and dislodge and pick up an intact colony. Place the pipet tip in the corner of the well of the 96-well plate, and draw the colony up and down in the pipet tip to break the colony into three to five pieces.
3. Use a fresh tip for each colony. Repeat for 10–20 colonies from the same plate, then place the paired 100-mm dish and 96-well plate into the incubator and pick another plate for 10–20 colonies.
4. Place the picked cell lines in the incubator, and discard any 100-mm plates from which colonies have been completely picked.
5. Leave the plates undisturbed in the incubator for about 48 h.

3.6. Tryplating 96-Well Plates

1. Aspirate the medium from a 96-well plate using a multichannel aspirator (usually, the clumps of cells will collect on one side of all of the wells; the aspirator tips can

be inserted on the opposite side, and there will be no need to change tips between columns) (*see* **Note 9**).

2. Add 180 μL of PBS to each well with a multichannel pipet, and aspirate.
3. Add 50 μL of fresh trypsin to each well, and place the plate in the incubator for 5 min.
4. Stop the trypsin digestion by adding 180 μL of medium to each well. The chunks of colonies should be floating.
5. With a multichannel pipet set at 150 μL, disperse the cells to a single cell suspension by vigorously drawing the cells of a column up and down five or six times. Change the tips for each column.
6. Examine the plate carefully to ensure that a single cell suspension has been achieved. If cells are not completely dispersed, continue to triturate the cells until dispersed. If a single cell suspension cannot be obtained by trituration, let the cells attach and repeat the tryplating procedure the following day. Place the plates in the incubator.
7. Early the next day, replace the medium on the cells. Grow the cells for 3–5 d with daily changes of medium containing G418 until the cells are confluent.

3.7. Splitting ES Cells for DNA and Freezing in 96-Well Plates

1. Replace the medium on the cells with fresh medium without G418 2–4 h before trypsinizing the cells (*see* **Note 10**). Prepare the plates as described in **step 2** while the cells are feeding.
2. Prepare two gelatinized 96-well plates, and one freezing plate for each of the original plates. In the gelatinized plates, place 100 μL of medium without G418 in each well and place these plates in the incubator. To each well of the U-bottom polypropylene freezing plates, add 30 μL of 2X freezing medium. Overlay each well with 100 μL of mineral oil. Put the labeled mat cap on loosely and place the plate on ice protected from light.
3. Remove the fed cells from the incubator and aspirate the medium from the wells.
4. Wash each well of the plate once with 100 μL of PBS.
5. Add 25 μL of fresh trypsin to each well. Place the plates in the incubator for 5–10 min. Gently agitate the plates. The colonies should have detached from the plate.
6. Apply 25 μL of medium per well to stop the trypsinization. From this point on, work with two plates at a time.
7. Put the appropriate pair of labeled freezing plates on a shallow tray with flat compacted ice. Set the multichannel pipetor to 30 μL and vigorously break up a column of colonies. Transfer 30 μL to the appropriate column of the freezing plate, stabbing under the oil and mixing gently by drawing up and down three times. Repeat using fresh tips for each column. Fully place the matt cap on the freezing plate and return it to ice. Process the second plate. When both freezing plates are finished, transfer both sealed freezing plates to a Styrofoam box and place the box inside the –80°C freezer. Place the original 96-well plates (which have 20 μL per well remaining) back in the incubator.
8. Repeat the processing steps until all the plates are in the –80°C freezer.

9. Now return to the original plates and add 80 μL of medium to each well. Return them to the incubator temporarily.
10. Remove an original plate and two gelatinized 96-well plates to split it into (do not attempt to do more than one original plate at a time).
11. Gently mix the original plate and transfer 50 μL of suspension to each replicate, mixing gently each time. The replicates should now have all the cells. Return the replicates to the incubator. Discard the original. Repeat for each original plate. The replicate plates for DNA can usually be ignored the next day, fed the second day, and fed every day thereafter (without drug selection).
12. After the freezing plates have been in the –80°C freezer for 2 d, they can be transferred to liquid nitrogen. Wrap each plate in aluminum foil (so that the lid will not float off in the liquid nitrogen) and place on dry ice for transport to the liquid nitrogen freezer. Two capped plates can fit into a large freezer box.

3.8. Preparing Genomic DNA From ES Cells Grown in 96-Well Plates

1. Grow the cells to very high density, changing medium (without G418) daily. When the cells are at sufficiently high density, the media will have turned yellow daily for four to five consecutive days (*see* **Note 11**).
2. Aspirate the medium from each well, and wash each well with 180 μL PBS.
3. Aspirate the PBS from each well, and wash again with 180 μL PBS per well.
4. Add 50 μL of 96-well lysis buffer to each well, and cover the plate with plastic wrap followed by the lid. Stack plates and wrap the stack with plastic wrap. Place the stack in a humidified container in an oven at 55°C overnight.
5. Add 100 μL of ethanol + salt to each well *without mixing*. Put the lid back on.
6. Leave the plates undisturbed at room temperature for 30–60 min, preferably on a dark background to visualize the DNA. The DNA should become visible as a white filamentous network or a white sheet.
7. Drain the plates by gently inverting the plates onto a stack of paper towels.
8. Wash gently three times with 150 μL of 70% EtOH per well, inverting gently each time onto fresh paper towels.
9. After the last wash, make certain that all the ethanol has drained, then air-dry the plates tilted upside down for 20 min at room temperature. Do not overdry the plates, as this makes the DNA hard to dissolve.
10. Add 20 μL of low-EDTA TE to each well and cover the plate with plastic wrap. Put the lid back on and stack the dishes, then wrap the stack in plastic wrap. Store overnight at 4°C. The DNA is stable for several months at 4°C.

3.9. Digestion of Genomic DNA in 96-Well Plates
for Southern Blot Analysis

1. Add 20 μL of the digestion cocktail to each well. Stir the column of wells with the tips of the multichannel pipetor, and slowly and gently draw the mixture up and down once or twice. Take note of the degree of viscosity of the DNA, because the viscosity will be lost when the DNA is cut, so it can be a helpful sign that digestion has occurred (*see* **Note 12**).

2. Seal each plate with plastic wrap and put the lids on. Stack several plates and wrap the stack with plastic wrap. Place in a humidified container and place in a 37°C oven overnight.

3. The next day, check the state of digestion of a few wells by drawing them up in a yellow pipet tip and seeing that they drip down, and that the viscosity is lost. If they seem too viscous, add more enzyme up to but not exceeding a volume of 4 μL of enzyme per well when all enzyme additions are considered. Alternatively, run a few microliters from a row on a mini-gel to see if the DNA forms the continuous smear indicative of a complete digest (*see* **Note 13**).

3.10. Recovering Candidate Targeted Clones and Verifying Homologous Recombination

1. Set up a 37°C water bath for thawing 96-well plates by stacking empty yellow tip racks such that there are only a few millimeters of warm water above the rack (the water level should not be so high that it seeps into the lid—practice with an old plate). Prepare sufficient gelatinized 24-well plates to accept all the candidate lines and a few extra lines as negative controls. Add 0.5 mL of medium (without G418) to each well of the 24-well plate (*see* **Note 14**).

2. Work with one plate at a time. Put the plate on the rack in the 37°C water bath. To keep it in close contact with the water, put a weight on it. It will take 8–10 min for the plate to thaw.

3. Once you can see that the majority of clones have thawed (the wells will be translucent), remove the dish from the water bath. Place the plate on top of 70% EtOH-soaked tissues and wipe dry all around the top and edges.

4. Clearly mark all positive clones. Also mark one or two nontargeted lines to serve as negative controls.

5. Using a 200-μL pipetor set at 105 μL, stab under the oil and gently stir to mix. Draw up the entire volume of medium plus a little oil. Place the cells in a well of the 24-well plate. Draw medium up and down in the tip to disperse cells evenly and remove 105 μL of the 24-well plate and put it back under the oil of the well of the 96-well plate that the cells came from. Draw up repeatedly to mix and get most of the cells. Return this to the 24-well plate. Repeat with each cell line you wish to recover.

6. Culture at 37°C.

7. Replace the medium on the cells daily. The growth of the individual cell lines will vary. Those lines that are growing well can be passaged to a 35-mm dish (a 1:5 split). Those lines that are growing more slowly can be passaged to one or two wells of a 24-well plate. Passage all lines by the fourth day.

8. After each line is established in a 35-mm plate, the next split is into two 60-mm plates and two 35-mm plates. The 60-mm plates will be used to freeze the line into four vials **(Subheading 2.3.)**, one 35-mm plate will be used to prepare DNA **(Subheading 3.11.)**, and one 35-mm plate will be used to obtain a chromosome count **(Subheading 2.13.**; pause at **step 7** until targeting has been confirmed).

Table 2
Volumes for DNA Digestion by Plate Size

Dish size	Lysis buffer volume (mL)	Low-EDTA TE volume (mL)
1 well of a 24-well plate	0.5	0.05
35 mm	2.0	0.2
60 mm	4.0	0.4
100 mm	10.0	1.0

3.11. Extracting Genomic DNA From ES Cells in Quantity

1. Grow the cells until they are confluent (*see* **Note 16**).
2. Aspirate medium and wash twice with PBS.
3. Add large-scale lysis buffer using the volumes listed in **Table 2**.
4. Wrap the dishes in plastic wrap and enclose inside a humidified container. Incubate overnight at 55°C.
5. For 24-well plates, the precipitation can be done in the dish. For larger plates, transfer the lysate to either a 15-mL (35 or 60 mm) or a 50-mL (100 mm) conical capped plastic tube, using a cut blue tip or large-bore pipet.
6. Add an equal volume of isopropanol to the dish or tube without making an effort to mix.
7. Cover the 24-well plates with plastic wrap and put the lids on. Tape the dish to an orbital shaker, and start the shaker at low speed, gradually turning up until it is going as fast as possible without spilling. The tubes are mixed on a rocking or rotating mixer such as a nutator.
8. Mix for at least 20 min at room temperature. A large white "jellyfish" of precipitated DNA will begin to appear at the interface of the alcohol with the lysate. The longer it is rotated the tighter and easier to manage the "jellyfish" will become.
9. Using a Pasteur pipet, carefully remove the fluid leaving the DNA precipitate behind. Add an equal volume of 70% EtOH and rotate for another 20 min at room temperature.
10. Lift the precipitate out with a clean pipet tip. Put the DNA into a tube with the appropriate amount of low-EDTA TE (*see* **Table 2**). Sometimes the precipitate sticks to the tip. Carefully scrape the DNA off on the side of tube.
11. Incubate the tubes at 50–60°C for 30 min with the lids off to evaporate trace ethanol.
12. Place the tubes in a refrigerator at 4°C overnight or longer before use. The DNA can be stored for months at 4°C.

3.12. Digestion of High-Molecular-Weight DNA

1. Assemble a 200-μL digestion reaction for each sample and incubate overnight at the temperature appropriate for the restriction enzyme.
2. Check to see if the DNA is still viscous by drawing it up with a pipetor and dripping it back down into the tube drop-wise. If the DNA is still viscous, add

more enzyme, keeping the total enzyme added to less than 10% of the total volume and continue incubating. Once you are satisfied that the DNA is cut, proceed to the next step.

3. To each reaction, add 8.3 μL of 5 *M* NaCl and mix.
4. Add 530 μL 95% EtOH and precipitate 20 min at −20°C.
5. Spin down for 10 min at top speed in a microcentrifuge and remove the supernatant.
6. Wash the pellet with 530 μL of 70% EtOH and spin down for 5 min.
7. Remove the supernatant.
8. Dry the pellet by placing the open tube in a dry bath at 37°C for 5 min.
9. Dissolve the DNA pellet in 36 μL of TE, and add 4 μL of 10X gel loading dye.
10. Load the entire reaction in a well of a 0.7%/0.5X TBE gel and perform Southern blot analysis.

3.13. Counting ES Cell Chromosomes

1. Culture cells for 24 h after they have been passaged onto a 35-mm gelatinized plate.
2. Culture for 4 h in medium containing colcemid (*see* **Note 17**).
3. Remove the medium from the plate and transfer it to a 15-mL conical capped tube. Wash the plate with 2 mL PBS, and add the wash to the tube. Trypsinize the plate with 1.5 mL trypsin, and add the cell suspension to the tube and mix.
4. Pellet the cells by centrifugation at 300*g* for 5 min. Aspirate the supernatant and flick the tube to disperse the cells in the residual supernatant.
5. Add 37°C 0.075 *M* KCl drop by drop, flicking the tube to mix the cells with each drop for the first 10–15 drops. Bring the total volume up to 7 mL with 0.075 *M* KCl, invert several times, and incubate in the 37°C water bath for 10 min.
6. Centrifuge at 300*g* for 5 min.
7. Aspirate the supernatant and flick the tube to loosen the pellet. In the next step, be careful to disperse the cells thoroughly in the fix. Add fresh methanol/acetic acid fix drop by drop, flicking the pellet with every drop for the first 10–15 drops, bringing the total volume to 7 mL. Cap and incubate at 4°C overnight. The fixed cells can be stored at 4°C indefinitely.
8. Centrifuge at 300*g* for 5 min and aspirate the old fix. Resuspend the cells in 0.5–0.75 mL of fresh methanol/acetic acid fix.
9. Dip labeled glass slides in water, leaving a puddle of water on the slide. Gently draw the cell suspension up in a Pasteur pipet. Each tube will have enough cells to make four to five slides.
10. From a height of about 1 foot above the slide, drop three drops of cell suspension per slide.
11. Leave the slides to air-dry.
12. Stain the slides for 10 min with 50 mL of Giemsa in a Coplin jar.
13. Rinse with water three to four times until the excess stain is removed.
14. Thoroughly air-dry the slides.
15. Mount glass cover slips with Permount.

16. After the Permount has dried, count the chromosomes in the metaphase spreads of widely separated fields. Scan slides with a ×40 objective and count the chromosomes with a ×100 objective. Five metaphase spreads on each of four different slides gives a good sample. A cell line with a majority of metaphases with 40 chromosomes is a good candidate for germ-line transmission (*see* **Note 18**).

3.14. Transient Transfection of ES Cells With Cre Recombinase to Excise the neo Cassette

1. Thaw (**Subheading 3.1.**) and grow (**Subheading 3.2.**) a targeted line that has been thoroughly characterized by Southern blot analysis and has been shown to have 40 chromosomes (**Subheading 3.13.**) (*see* **Note 19**).
2. Electroporate one cuvet of cells (**Subheading 3.4.**, **steps 1–10**) with 25 µg supercoiled pOG231 *Cre* expression plasmid, resuspending the cells in 10 mL of ES cell medium (*see* **Note 20**).
3. From the 10 mL of electroporated cells, plate out 0.1, 0.250, and 0.5 mL into 10 mL of medium each on gelatinized 100-mm plates.
4. Allow the cells to grow in ES cell medium, changing the medium every second day, for 10–14 d in the tissue culture incubator.
5. Select a plate with well separated colonies, and pick (**Subheading 3.5.**) about 96 colonies into a 96-well plate.
6. Tryplate (**Subheading 3.6.**) and propagate the lines in the 96-well plate and split (**Subheading 3.7.**) to freeze and prepare DNA.
7. Prepare DNA from the 96-well plates (**Subheading 3.8.**), analyze by Southern blot or PCR, and retrieve the desired cell lines from the frozen plate (**Subheading 3.10.**) (*see* **Notes 21** and **22**).

4. Notes

1. Frozen cells must be thawed rapidly and removed quickly from the freezing medium. Thawed cells should be returned to the culture conditions that they experienced before freezing, so if a frozen cell line is obtained from a commercial source or another lab, use the culture conditions (media, supplements, and feeder cells) that the cells are accustomed to before attempting to passage them into new conditions, for example, growth without feeder cells.
2. ES cells grow as clonal colonies. In passaging ES cells, it is important to disperse the colonies down to single cells so that growth of the culture is even and rapid, and so that differentiation is prevented.
3. For routine splitting into 60- or 100-mm dishes, add a bolus of concentrated cells to one side of a dish that is covered with medium. Resuspend the cells in a convenient volume of medium—say 0.5 or 1.0 mL for each plate. Because the cells are coming out of a stressful spin, be gentle. Mix cells by running them along the side of the tube. When thoroughly resuspended, apply the cells to one side of the receiving dish and gently rock the plate back and forth so that a wave front goes from side to side. When first starting out, do only one plate at a time and keep the dish down on the table—eventually, you can do three or four plates by rocking

them gently in the air. Do not swirl the dishes, as this concentrates the cells in the middle. Thirty-five-millimeter dishes (and smaller) are too small to rock back and forth—gently resuspend cells with their full volume of medium and apply to the dish. Incubate plates overnight and evaluate your technique the next morning. If there are large numbers of clumps, or cells are not evenly distributed, then repeat the passaging onto fresh plates. ES cells have a plating efficiency of only about 20%; therefore, expect a lot of floating debris the day after plating.

4. ES cells are slowly frozen in a CPM in cryovials and stored indefinitely in liquid nitrogen, or stored for less than 6 mo at –70°C. Each vial contains the equivalent of one confluent 35-mm dish (or two vials per 60-mm dish and six vials per 100-mm dish).

5. A cold Styrofoam box with a lid can be used in place of the Nalgene slow-cool freezing container.

6. A total of about 400 μg of linearized targeting vector is electroporated into 6×10^7 ES cells (about five dense 100-mm plates of ES cells) in several electroporations. A day after plating the cells, drug selection is started. Several hundred colonies should survive the double selection.

7. The expected outcome is that each plate under double selection will have about 40 colonies, and the one-tenth quantitation plate under G418 selection alone will have about 50 colonies, representing a 12.5-fold enrichment ($50 \times 10 / 40 = 12.5$). A low transfection efficiency indicated by a substantially lower number of colonies on the one-tenth quantitation plate indicates either that the *neo* gene is defective or that the context of the targeting arms does not allow for efficient expression of the *neo* gene. A low transfection efficiency may need to be corrected by construction of a new targeting vector. Enrichments that are too low (2-fold) or too high (100-fold) can indicate that something is awry with the selection. Although extremes in the enrichment ratio can still result in gene targeting, most often a fresh round of electroporations will result in a more typical enrichment ratio and bona fide gene targeting events. Targeting frequencies in the enriched cells surviving double selection typically range from one-tenth to one-hundredth. Therefore, to ensure that several targeted cell lines are recovered, several hundred colonies are picked, and cell lines are grown and screened for gene targeting. If thorough analysis of several hundred cell lines fails to identify targeted cell lines, and the transfection and enrichment are close to the expected values, consider building a new targeting vector with a greater length of sequence match or with *neo* in a different position. The targeting frequency of a targeting vector is reproducible. Low frequencies may be owing to a failure of homologous recombination to occur, or poor expression of *neo* from the targeted locus.

8. Colonies that survived the double selection are propagated as individual cell lines. Several hundred lines of cells should be analyzed to ensure that several gene targeted cell lines can be identified. Each colony is used to establish a cell line propagated in a well of a 96-well plate. It takes about an hour for an experienced individual to pick a full 96-well plate.

9. The key to propagating cells in 96-well plates is ensuring comparable growth rates in all wells by dispersing colonies to individual cells by the technique of tryplating about 48 h after picking colonies. Tryplating disperses the roughly broken colonies from picking into a single cell suspension. The cells are allowed to attach to the same plate.

10. The cell lines in 96-well plates are split three ways into one freezing plate and two DNA plates. Analysis of the DNA is used to retrieve targeted cell lines from the frozen copy, so be sure to clearly mark the plates so that the correct cell lines can be retrieved. G418 selection is removed just before splitting.

11. In order to obtain enough DNA from each cell line, and because the cells in these replicates will not be used to make chimeras, the DNA replicate plates are grown to very high density. If the plates and their lids are not all clearly marked in order that sibling cell lines in the freezer can be easily identified, do this now. The DNA preparation protocol involves lysis, digestion, DNA precipitation, and washing *in situ* in the plate the cells grew in.

12. The genomic DNA of the ES cell lines is digested in the wells of the plate. Each plate should have enough DNA for two Southern blots. Typically, only one external probe is used to identify candidate cell lines from this round of Southern blot analysis. The strategy is to narrow down the cell lines to a smaller number that can be thoroughly analyzed and to freeze the lines in a format in which there is near certainty that they can be reestablished after thawing. We do not provide a detailed protocol for performing Southern blots, as there are many good descriptions to be found elsewhere, and there are no exceptional requirements for the analysis of ES cell genomic DNA other than that a large number of samples (several hundred) will be analyzed. Thus, it is useful to have large gel boxes that can accommodate multiple combs with many wells, for example 12×8 inch gels with three combs with 36-well combs (thus, an entire plate can be loaded onto a gel with 4×8 columns = 32 samples with room for markers on each third of the gel).

13. Once the Southern blot analysis is complete, and the films have been exposed long enough to identify all possible candidate targeted clones, thaw and recover the candidate cell lines from the frozen 96-well plates as soon as possible.

14. The cells are grown without selection from the recovery from freezing in the 96-well plate to freezing again in vials. The cells grow faster in the absence of selection, and this improves the chances of recovering all lines. Cells are also grown without selection after thawing from the vials up to injection into blastocysts, because there are data that indicate that growth in G418 is detrimental to the chimeras. However, long-term growth without selection can lead to loss of the targeted allele in some or all of the cells of a line. If cells are propagated in culture beyond the number of passes indicated here, it would be best to grow them under G418 selection, at least for one passage, to kill any cells that have lost the targeted allele, or that survived the original selection.

15. The yield of DNA prepared by this protocol is about 0.5 µg/µL. For analysis by PCR, make a 1:5 dilution with water and store frozen at –20°C. Use 1 µL of the

diluted DNA for each PCR reaction. For analysis by Southern blot, cut 10 µL of undiluted DNA in a 200-µL reaction as described under **Subheading 3.12.**

16. Because the cells on these DNA plates will not be propagated further, it is permissible to let them grow to a density beyond which would be desirable for cells that would be used to make chimeras. Thus, if multiple cell lines are progressing at different rates, the fast growers can be allowed to grow very dense until the slow growers are at sufficient density such that all dishes can be processed at one time.

17. Cells are grown in the presence of colcemid to arrest them at metaphase. The colcemid treatment causes cells to detach from the plate, so the medium from the cells is collected from the plates after the colcemid treatment, in addition to the cells released by trypsin treatment.

18. A normal number (40) of chromosomes is not a guarantee that a cell line is euploid, but identifying cell lines with a normal number of chromosomes should greatly enrich for euploid cell lines. Two or three targeted cell lines with 40 chromosomes should be used to generated chimeras, in order that the probability of germ line transmission is high.

19. For the construction of conditional mutants and knock-ins, the *neo* cassette can be removed in ES cells by transiently transfecting a targeted line that has a normal number of chromosomes with an expression plasmid for *Cre* recombinase. Although the *neo* cassette could be removed in mice by crossing to mice transgenic for *Cre* recombinase expressed in the germ line or early embryo, there are advantages to removing the *neo* cassette early. There is no need to maintain an additional line of mice, and because the *neo* cassette has cryptic splice acceptors and donors, the possibility that the targeted allele has an unintended gain-of-function activity, which might prevent colonization of the embryo or germ line, is avoided.

20. ES cells are transiently transfected by electroporation with supercoiled expression plasmid for *Cre* recombinase. Because transient transfection and recombination driven by *Cre* are efficient, no selection is necessary to find the desired recombinant. In those instances where there are three *lox*P sites at the targeted locus, recombinants between each pair of *lox*P sites (in addition to nonrecombinants) are recovered.

21. The typical result is that 30–50% of the cell lines have undergone a *Cre*-mediated recombination. In the case of conditional alleles among those lines that have undergone recombination, some proportion will have undergone recombination only between the two *lox*P sites flanking *neo*, leaving *lox*P sites flanking the sequence to be conditionally deleted in mice.

22. Chimeras made by injection of ES cells into host embryos are mosaics of the heterozygous mutant cells and the host embryo cells. The contribution of the ES cells to the chimera is reflected by the coat color of the chimera in most cases, with the ES cells contributing brown (agouti) hairs, and the host black (recessive nonagouti, the mutated version of agouti) hairs. Most ES cells used for targeting are male, and the male ES cells will coopt most female host embryos into participating in male development through the nonautonomous action of the

hormone testosterone. Male chimeras of the brown/black coat color combination are mated to black mice such as C57BL6. Both brown and black offspring are possible, and the brown offspring indicate that a sperm derived from an ES cell fertilized the C57BL6 egg (agouti over recessive nonagouti, so a brown mouse). Because sperm are haploid and the ES cells are heterozygous, a brown pup could be either heterozygous mutant or wild type for the targeted gene. Thus, the brown offspring must be analyzed for their genotype at the targeted locus, preferably by one of the Southern blot assays developed by targeting. Once a few heterozygous founder mice are obtained, a PCR assay for the allele can be developed with confidence. The best PCR assays identify a unique DNA junction specific to the mutant. Heterozygous mutant offspring of the chimeras can be bred to each other to obtain homozygotes for analysis. Quite often, the heterozygous mutants are bred for nine or more generations to C57BL6 mice to place them fully on the standard inbred genetic background to minimize the effect of segregation of other gene variants.

References

1. Martin, G. R. (1981) Isolation of a pluripotent cell line from early mouse embryos cultured in medium conditioned by teratocarcinoma stem cells. *Proc. Natl. Acad. Sci. USA* **78,** 7634–7638.
2. Evans, M. J. and Kaufman, M. H. (1981) Establishment in culture of pluripotential cells from mouse embryos. *Nature* **292,** 154–156.
3. Bradley, A., Evans, M., Kaufman, M. H., and Robertson, E. (1984) Formation of germ-line chimaeras from embryo-derived teratocarcinoma cell lines. *Nature* **309,** 255–256.
4. Thomas, K. R. and Capecchi, M. R. (1987) Site-directed mutagenesis by gene targeting in mouse embryo-derived stem cells. *Cell* **51,** 503–512.
5. Doetschman, T., Gregg, R. G., Maeda, N., et al. (1987) Targeted correction of a mutant HPRT gene in mouse embryonic stem cells. *Nature* **330,** 576–578.
6. Davis, J. (Ed.) (2002) *Basic Cell Culture: A Practical Approach.* Oxford University Press, Oxford, UK.
7. Nagy, A., Gertsenstein, M., Vintersten, K., and Behringer, R. (2003) *Manipulating the Mouse Embryo.* Cold Spring Harbor Laboratory Press, Cold Spring Harbor, NY.
8. Hasty, P., Abuin, A., and Bradley, A. (2000) Gene targeting, principles, and practice in mammalian cells, in *Gene Targeting. A Practical Approach,* Vol. 212 (Joyner, A. L., ed.). Oxford University Press, Oxford, UK, pp. 1–35.
9. Hanks, M., Wurst, W., Anson-Cartwright, L., Auerbach, A. B., and Joyner, A. L. (1995) Rescue of the En-1 mutant phenotype by replacement of En-1 with En-2. *Science* **269,** 679–682.
10. Gu, H., Marth, J. D., Orban, P. C., Mossmann, H., and Rajewsky, K. (1994) Deletion of a DNA polymerase beta gene segment in T cells using cell type-specific gene targeting. *Science* **265,** 103–106.
11. te Riele, H., Maandag, E. R., and Berns, A. (1992) Highly efficient gene targeting in embryonic stem cells through homologous recombination with isogenic DNA constructs. *Proc. Natl. Acad. Sci. USA* **89,** 5128–5132.

12. Hasty, P., Rivera-Perez, J., and Bradley, A. (1991) The length of homology required for gene targeting in embryonic stem cells. *Mol. Cell. Biol.* **11,** 5586–5591.
13. Meyers, E. N., Lewandoski, M., and Martin, G. R. (1998) An Fgf8 mutant allelic series generated by Cre- and Flp-mediated recombination. *Nat. Genet.* **18,** 136–141.
14. Nagy, A., Moens, C., Ivanyi, E., et al. (1998) Dissecting the role of N-myc in development using a single targeting vector to generate a series of alleles. *Curr. Biol.* **8,** 661–664.
15. Olson, E. N., Arnold, H. H., Rigby, P. W., and Wold, B. J. (1996) Know your neighbors: three phenotypes in null mutants of the myogenic bHLH gene MRF4. *Cell* **85,** 1–4.
16. Ren, S. Y., Angrand, P. O., and Rijli, F. M. (2002) Targeted insertion results in a rhombomere 2-specific Hoxa2 knockdown and ectopic activation of Hoxa1 expression. *Dev. Dyn.* **225,** 305–315.
17. Hasty, P., Rivera-Perez, J., Chang, C., and Bradley, A. (1991) Target frequency and integration pattern for insertion and replacement vectors in embryonic stem cells. *Mol. Cell. Biol.* **11,** 4509–4517.
18. Moens, C. B., Auerbach, A. B., Conlon, R. A., Joyner, A. L., and Rossant, J. (1992) A targeted mutation reveals a role for N-myc in branching morphogenesis in the embryonic mouse lung. *Genes Dev.* **6,** 691–704.
19. Chui, D., Oh-Eda, M., Liao, Y. F., et al. (1997) Alpha-mannosidase-II deficiency results in dyserythropoiesis and unveils an alternate pathway in oligosaccharide biosynthesis. *Cell* **90,** 157–167.
20. Tybulewicz, V. L., Crawford, C. E., Jackson, P. K., Bronson, R. T., and Mulligan, R. C. (1991) Neonatal lethality and lymphopenia in mice with a homozygous disruption of the c-abl proto-oncogene. *Cell* **65,** 1153–1163.
21. Robertson, E. J. (1987) Embryo-derived stem cell lines, in *Teratocarcinomas and Embryonic Stem Cells: A Practical Approach*, Vol. 212, (Robertson, E. J., ed.), Oxford University Press, Oxford, UK, pp. 71–112.
22. Auerbach, W., Dunmore, J. H., Fairchild-Huntress, V., et al. (2000) Establishment and chimera analysis of 129/SvEv- and C57BL/6-derived mouse embryonic stem cell lines. *Biotechniques* **29,** 1024–1032.
23. You, Y., Bersgtram, R., Klemm, M., Nelson, H., Jaenisch, R., and Schimenti, J. (1998) Utility of C57BL/6J x 129/SvJae embryonic stem cells for generating chromosomal deletions: tolerance to gamma radiation and microsatellite polymorphism. *Mamm. Genome* **9,** 232–234.
24. Thomas, J. W., LaMantia, C., and Magnuson, T. (1998) X-ray-induced mutations in mouse embryonic stem cells. *Proc. Natl. Acad. Sci. USA* **95,** 1114–1119.
25. Brook, F. A., Evans, E. P., Lord, C. J., et al. (2003) The derivation of highly germline-competent embryonic stem cells containing NOD-derived genome. *Diabetes* **52,** 205–208.
26. Nagy, A., Rossant, J., Nagy, R., Abramow-Newerly, W., and Roder, J. C. (1993) Derivation of completely cell culture-derived mice from early-passage embryonic stem cells. *Proc. Natl. Acad. Sci. USA* **90,** 8424–8428.

27. Mereau, A., Grey, L., Piquet-Pellorce, C., and Heath, J. K. (1993) Characterization of a binding protein for leukemia inhibitory factor localized in extracellular matrix. *J. Cell. Biol.* **122,** 713–719.

28. Matise, M. P., Auerbach, W., and Joyner, A. L. (2000) Production of targeted embryonic stem cell clones, in *Gene Targeting. A Practical Approach*, Vol. 212, (Joyner, A. L., ed.), Oxford University Press, Oxford, UK, pp. 101–132.

29. O'Gorman, S., Dagenais, N. A., Qian, M., and Marchuk, Y. (1997) Protamine-Cre recombinase transgenes efficiently recombine target sequences in the male germ line of mice, but not in embryonic stem cells. *Proc. Natl. Acad. Sci. USA* **94,** 14,602–14,607.

5

Generation of Transgenic Mice for Cardiovascular Research

Xiao-Li Tian and Qing K. Wang

Summary

The transgenic mouse technology is a powerful tool that can be used for creating animal models for cardiovascular disease to identify molecular pathogenic mechanisms and for identifying the physiological functions of a novel gene. A transgenic animal can be generated by several methods, which include microinjection of a DNA fragment into the pronucleus, embryonic stem cell manipulation and injection, sperm-mediated transgenesis, and viral infection of preimplanted embryos. The microinjection method is one of the most widely used approaches. This method involves four steps: (1) collection of fertilized eggs from the superovulated female, (2) injection of DNA into the pronucleus of fertilized eggs, (3) transfer of the injected eggs back into the oviduct of a pseudo-pregnant foster recipient, allowing the eggs to develop into pups, and (4) identification of the transgenic founder and establishment of transgenic lines through further breeding.

Key Words: Transgene; cardiovascular disease; animal model; fertilized egg; foster; super-ovulation; pronucleus; breeding; pseudopregnant.

1. Introduction

A transgenic animal is generated by introducing a specific gene or DNA fragment into animal's genome at the developmental stages from the fertilized egg to blastocyst. This technique allows for the functional characterization of a gene from cellular to the whole animal level, and more importantly, it permits elucidation of the target gene functions more faithfully under physiological or pathophysiological conditions than other in vitro methods. Transgenic animal models for a number of human diseases have proven to be useful tools in illustrating the role of gene(s) in the pathogenesis and in screening new drugs for treatments of the diseases.

In 1980, the first transgenic mouse was generated by microinjection of DNA into the pronucleus of fertilized mouse oocytes (*1*) and the injected DNA was

From: *Methods in Molecular Medicine, vol. 129:*
Cardiovascular Disease: Methods and Protocols, Volume 2: Molecular Medicine
Edited by: Q. K. Wang © Humana Press Inc., Totowa, NJ

transmitted into the descendants. The transgene is usually integrated as a cluster (head to head, head to tail, or tail to tail) at a single site, but rarely at multiple sites on the chromosome(s) *(2)*. The transgene functions as an endogenous gene *(3)*. In addition to transgenic mice, transgenic rats, rabbits, sheep, pigs, goats, and cows have been successfully generated, too *(4–9)*.

Transgenic animals can be generated using various methods. The conventional procedure is to inject DNA into the pronuclei of fertilized eggs at the one-cell stage *(4,10)*. In addition, the other methods include the infection of blastocysts with retrovirus *(11)*, sperm-mediated DNA transfer *(12,13)*, and embryonic stem (ES) cell-mediated DNA transfer *(14–16)*. This chapter focuses in creation of a transgenic mouse using the microinjection of transgene DNA into fertilized eggs.

A transgene consists of three parts: a promoter region, a structural gene (target gene), and a polyadenylation signal sequence. Depending on the experiment, the transgene can be designed for overexpression, inducible expression, or suppression in specific tissues or at the whole-animal level. It can also be used as a reporter to trace the expression pattern of a given gene.

1.1. Overexpression

The transgene can be overexpressed in the specific tissues/organs or in the whole body. Tissue-specific overexpression of a given gene can be achieved by using either a tissue- or organ-specific promoter to direct the expression of the transgene. There are several tissue-specific promoters available, such as the cardiac *myosin heavy chain (MHC)*-α promoter specific for cardiac tissues (both ventricles and atria) *(17)*, the *cardiac MHC-2* promoter specific for ventricles *(5)*, and *tie* (*tie*1 and *tie*2) promoters selective for endothelial cells *(18,19)*. Some promoters, such as the cytomegalovirus *(CMV)* and rous sarcoma virus *(RSV)* promoters, are strong but of less selectivity in tissue expression, and give high expression levels in most parts of the body. The high expression of a gene in the various tissues or organs can allow one to investigate a spectrum of functions of the gene. The enhanced expression of a gene in its natively expressed tissues can be accomplished by using its genomic DNA, including bacterial artificial chromosomes (BACs), phage P1 artificial chromosomes (PACs), and yeast artificial chromosomes (YACs) *(20)* or its natural promoter-directed cDNA as the transgene.

1.2. Inducible Expression

The tetracycline (Tc)-resistance operon was modified and used in the regulation of a transgene's expression, a system referred to as *tet-off/tet-on*. The expression of the transgene can be initiated when the animal is treated with Tc or doxycycline (Dc) *(21)*.

1.3. Reporter Gene

The spatial and temporal expression pattern of a given gene during embryogenesis as well as adulthood can be analyzed by using its promoter to drive the expression of a reporter gene, such as *Lac Z* or *GFP* in transgenic animals. The expression pattern of the gene of interest can be mapped by determining the expression of the reporter gene *(22)*.

1.4. Dominant Negative, Antisense, and Small Interfering RNA

The functions of a gene of interest can be arrested if a dominant negative mutant is used as the transgene. Typically, the dominant negative mutant is a truncated fragment or a mutant form of a given gene that antagonizes the normal function of the endogenous gene *(23)*. The function of a gene can also be suppressed by employing an antisense construct as the transgene *(24)*. More recently, small interfering RNA (siRNA) was used to knock down the gene's expression in transgenic animal, providing a potent tool to study a gene's function *(25,26)*.

2. Materials

2.1. Equipment

1. Microscope, type 307-148.004, with objective ×10, ×20, and ×40, and ocular ×16 (Leitz Microsystems, Inc.).
2. Stereo microscope, Wild M18, MDG17, with objective from ×6–50 and ocular ×10 (Leica Microsystems, Inc.).
3. Needle puller, needle/pipet puller (Kopf Instruments, cat. no. 750).
4. Holder maker (Kopf Instruments, cat. no. 750).
5. Injectors: Eppendorf Microinjector 5242 (Leitz).
6. Falcon 3001 CO_2 incubator (Falcon).
7. Minipump, osmotic pump, Alzet Model 2001 (Alza Corporation).
8. Freezer (–20°C, –80°C).
9. Silicon tubes for connections.
10. Rubber mad for holding microinjection needles and holders.
11. Diamond pencils.
12. Alcohol burner.
13. 35-mm Petri dishes.
14. Depression slides.
15. Surgical instruments.
16. Holding pipet and injection pipet.

2.2. Reagents

1. Media: M2 and M16 (*see* **Table 1** and **Note 1**). Adjust the pH to 7.4 for both M2 and M16 and check that the osmolarity is about 300 mOsmol. The media can be stored at 4°C for up to 1 wk.

Table 1
M2 and M16 Media

Component	M2 g/L	M16 g/L
$CaCl_2 \cdot 2H_2O$	0.251	0.251
$MgSO_4$	0.165	0.165
KCl	0.356	0.356
KH_2PO_4	0.162	0.162
$NaHCO_3$	0.35	2.101
NaCl	5.532	5.532
Lactic acid (Na)	4.35	4.35
Phenol red (Na)	0.01	0.01
Pyruvic acid (Na)	0.036	0.036
HEPES	5.43	–
D-Glucose	1	1
Albumin, bovine fraction v	4	4

2. Hormones (both pregnant mare's serum gonadotropin [PMSG] and human chorionic gonadotropin [hCG] are 50 U/mL in saline; aliquot and store at $-20°C$).
3. Hyaluronidase (100 µg/mL in saline; aliquot and keep at $-20°C$).
4. Microinjection buffer: 10 mM Tris-HCl, 0.5 mM EDTA, pH 7.4, filtered through a 0.22-µm filter, then stored at $-20°C$.
5. Anesthesia: Avertin, or Rampu/Kataven.
6. 70% ethanol.
7. Suprarenin.
8. Antibiotic powder (neomycin).

2.3. Animals

Mice from either NMRI, CB6F1, or C57BL6 are hosted with a constant light-cycle of 6:00 AM to 6:00 PM and temperature of 20–25°C. Several types of mice should be prepared: donor female (23–32 d old, providing fertilized eggs), stud male (2- to 6-mo-old healthy male, for mating with donor female), sterile male (2- to 6-mo-old vasectomized male, for mating with foster female), and foster female (2- to 6-mo-old pseudopregnant healthy female; after mating with the sterile male, it serves as a recipient for injected eggs).

3. Methods

In order to illustrate the process of producing a transgenic animal model by microinjection method in detail, here we use the generation of a transgenic mouse model, TGM(NS31), with cardiac selective expression of the human mutant cardiac sodium channel gene (*hSCN5A*) as an example *(27)*.

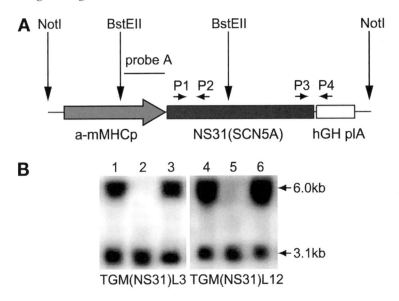

Fig. 1. Generation and genotyping of TGM(NS31) transgenic mice. (**A**) Transgenic construct for the engineering of transgene, *NS31(SCN5A)* (human SCN5A with long QT syndrome-associated mutation, N1325S), into the mouse genome. The *Not*I fragment consists of the mouse *myosin heavy chain-α* promoter (*a-mMHCp*), transgene NS31(SCN5A), and the *human growth hormone* poly(A) signal (*hGH* plA). Probe A (1.7 kb), a portion of α-*mMHCp*, was used as a marker for Southern blot analysis. Probe B, a junction fragment between NS31 and *hGH* plA, was used for Northern blot analysis to determine the expression profile of the transgene. PCR primer pairs P1–P2 and P3–P4 were used to identify transgenic mice during breeding. (**B**) Southern blot analysis to determine the copy of the transgene. Mouse genomic DNA was digested with *BstE II* and hybridized with probe A (*see* **A**). The 6.0- and 3.1-kb fragments represent, respectively, the transgene, *NS31(SCN5A)* and the endogenous *MHC-α* gene. Two transgenic lines, TGM(NS31)L3 and TGM(NS31)L12, were generated. The following genotypes are listed: Lanes 1 and 3, TGM(NS31)L3; Lanes 4 and 6, TGM(NS31)L12; and Lanes 2 and 5, nontransgenic mice.

3.1. DNA Purification for Microinjection

To obtain cardiac-specific expression, we placed the full-length *hSCN5A* cDNA with a mutation (N1325S causing long QT syndrome) into vector Clone 26 *(28)*, forming an expression vector for *hSCN5A* (pMHC-hSCN5A). In this construct, the *hSCN5A* is under the control of mouse *MHC*-α promoter and followed by the human growth factor polyadenylation signal sequence (**Fig. 1A**). The entire transgenic fragment including the *MHC*-α promoter (5.5 kb), *hSCN5A* cDNA (6.2 kb),

Table 2
Restriction Reaction

NEB buffer 3	10 μL
H$_2$O	X μL (make up to 100 μL)
Bovine serum albumin (100X)	1 μL
pMHC-hSCN5A	10 μg
*Not*I	100 U

Table 3
Dilution of Injection Samples

Transgenic fragment (kb)	Working concentration
<5	2 μg/mL
5–10	3–4 μg/mL
>10	5 μg/mL

and the polyadenylation signal sequence (0.6 kb) was excised by restriction digestion with *Not*I and purified for microinjection as follows:

1. Set up restriction reaction (*see* **Table 2**).
2. Incubate the reaction mixture at 37°C overnight.
3. Separate the transgenic fragment (12 kb) from the vector backbone (3 kb) by a 0.8% agarose gel (in 1X TAE buffer).
4. Excise the agarose gel containing 12-kb band (the transgenic fragment) and purify the DNA by either β-agarose digest or gel extraction kits (*see* **Note 2**).
5. The purified transgenic fragment is then dialyzed against microinjection buffer overnight at 4°C.
6. Transfer the dialysate into a fresh tube, and centrifuge at 12,000*g* for 10 min at 4°C.
7. Gently transfer two-thirds volume of DNA solution into a fresh tube. This will be the DNA stock solution for microinjection.
8. Estimate the concentration of the DNA stock solution by comparing band densities of 10 μL DNA stock with a quantified DNA standard, for example, λ DNA/ *Hind*III.
9. Dilute the DNA stock by microinjection buffer to a working concentration (*see* **Table 3**). The transgenic fragment at working solution is aliquoted at 20 μL per tube, and kept at –20°C prior to use.

3.2. Superovulation

Day 1: At 11:00 AM, the donor females are intraperitoneally administered with PMSG at the dose of 5 U (100 μL) per mouse (*see* **Note 3**).

Day 3: At 11:00 AM, hCG is given to PMSG-treated females at the dose of 5 U (100 μL) per female. At 3:00–5:00 PM, set up mating by placing each hormonized female

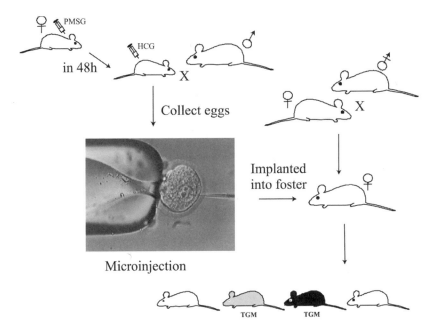

Fig. 2. General scheme for generating transgenic mice.

with one stud male in one cage; set mating such that the 10 pairs of females and sterile males get fosters (usually one to three plugged females).

Day 4: At 9:00 AM, check the female vaginal plugs to determine whether copulation occurred. The plugged hormonized females are ready for the collection of fertilized eggs while the plugged females by sterile males will be the fosters for egg transplantation after microinjection. Usually, at 10:30 AM egg collection can be started, and at 2:00–5:00 PM, microinjection is performed. After a brief culture around 7:00 PM, start to transfer the microinjected eggs into oviduct of fosters.

A general scheme for generation of a transgenic animal is shown in **Fig. 2**.

3.3. Collection of Fertilized Eggs

1. Prewarm 10 mL of M2 and M16 at 37°C/CO_2 incubator for 0.5–1 h.
2. Transfer 3 mL of M2 into a Petri dish and mix with 100 µL of hyaluronidase (hy-M2). Place the several large separated drops of hy-M2 in the second dish, several large separated drops of M2 in the third dish, and several large separated drops of M16 in the fourth dish. The fourth dish is covered with mineral oil.
3. The plugged female is sacrificed. Open the abdominal cavity, cut the oviducts out by scissors, and transfer into hy-M2 drops (one oviduct per drop).
4. The superovulated oviduct presents swollen and clear ampulla under the stereomicroscope. Use watchmaker forceps to break the ampulla, after which a cloudy mass containing fertilized eggs will be released. Discard the oviduct.
5. Gently shake the dish and watch the eggs that are releasing (*see* **Note 4**). Transfer the eggs into a fresh drop of M2 to wash out hyaluronidase when most of the eggs

are separated. After an additional wash, transfer the eggs into a drop of M16 and put this back into a CO_2 incubator until use.

6. Repeat **steps 3–6** to collect the eggs from all plugged females.

3.4. Microinjection and Implantation of Injected Fertilized Eggs

1. Set up the injection chamber: put one drop of M2 at the center of a depression slide, and cover the M2 drop with mineral oil.
2. The holder and syringe (10 mL) are connected by hard silicon tube and filled with mineral oil. Mount the holding pipet and fill it with oil. Add 1–2 µL of DNA sample into the injection needle from the open end, and mount the injection needle into the second holder that is connected with a 10-mL syringe and filled with oil; or, the second holder can be connected with a injector.
3. Transfer 20–40 eggs (*see* **Note 5**) into the injection chamber at the upper position, and place the holding and injection pipets at the center of the chamber. Adjust the position of the pipets to focus the eggs and pipets.
4. By adjusting the syringe, the egg can be held by the holding pipet. Change the position of the egg by catching and releasing until the pronucleus is well focused. Punch the injection pipet into the pronucleus and inject DNA by injector or by adjusting the syringe. Once the pronucleus becomes slightly swollen, stop the injection and withdraw the needle carefully. Move the injected egg down to separate it from the noninjected eggs.
5. After the eggs in the chamber are injected, transfer them into M16 and put them back into the incubator.
6. Repeat **steps 3–4** to inject all of the eggs.
7. At the completion of the injection, the surviving eggs are transferred into the double oviducts of the fosters (10–15 eggs for each side; *see* **Note 6**). If there is no the same-step foster, the eggs can be cultured overnight, and then transferred into fosters from the next day.

3.5. Detection of Transgene From Biopsies

After gestation of 21–23 d, fosters produce pups that are developed from the injected fertilized eggs. Some of them will carry the transgene and, therefore, become the transgenic founders. Each founder represents one transgenic line, which differs from the other lines by different integration sites and copy numbers of the transgene in the mouse genome.

The pups can be numbered by ear-punch or toe-cut. Tissue biopsies from the ear or the toe can be used for the detection of the transgene. Because the founders are usually chimera, we recommend using PCR to detect the founders. In the detection of our transgenic mice, two pairs of PCR primers were used. They were located at the 5′ end (P1/P2) and 3′ end (P3/P4) of the *SCN5A* transgene, respectively, to make sure that the transgene was intact in each transgenic line (**Fig. 1**).

To extract toe or ear biopsy DNA:

1. Toe–ear buffer (*see* **Table 4**). Before use, add proteinase K to a final concentration of 0.5 mg/mL.

Table 4
Toe–Ear Buffer

Tris-HCl	10 mM
NaCl	100 mM
EDTA	10 mM
SDS	0.25%

2. One to two pieces of toe or ear are digested in 50 µL toe–ear buffer (overnight in 55°C oven with shaking).
3. Heat at 95°C for 5 min, then mix with 950 µL H$_2$O.
4. Centrifuge at 12,000g for 10 min. Take 1–3 µL for PCR (*see* **Note 7**).

3.6. Establishment of Transgenic Lines

Three founders for *hSCN5A* transgene were obtained and bred with wild-type mice. Pups were genotyped by PCR. Eventually, two founders demonstrated the germline transmission, and resulted in the creation of two transgenic lines (L3 and L12). Different transgenic lines from the same transgene should not bred together to avoid confusion. The transgenic lines are maintained as heterozygousity to get littermate controls for the future experiments.

3.7. Estimation of Transgenic Copy Number

Once transgenic lines are established, the copy numbers of the integrated transgene can be estimated by quantitative Southern blot analysis. Two types of quantitative Southern blot analysis can be used for this purpose.

One type of Southern blot requires a series of dilution of transgenic DNA fragments (standard). Based on the estimation that one nucleus contains 7 pg of genomic DNA, 10 µg of genomic DNA should carry 5×10^{-6} pmol of a single copy of a gene. For a 5-kb long standard, for example, 15 pg will be similar to a single copy, 30 pg will be similar to two copies, and so on, at radioactive density. When performing Southern blot, load 10 µg of genomic DNA in one lane, and the diluted standards in the other lanes separately. Following Southern blot, the copy number of the transgene can be estimated by measuring which standard produces a signal strength similar to that of 10 µg of genomic DNA.

The other type of Southern blot analysis is to choose a common region shared by mouse endogenous gene and transgene as a probe. On Southern blot, this probe identifies two bands from the endogenous gene and transgene, respectively. If the endogenous gene is a single-copy gene, then the copy number of the transgene can be estimated by comparing the radioactive density of two bands. It should be noted that the first type of Southern blot is recommended if the copy number is more than 10.

For instance, we used a 1.7-kb *MHC*-α promoter fragment as a probe, which recognized two bands at 3.1 and 6.0 kb, representing endogenous *MHC*-α promoter

Table 5
Tail Buffer

Tris-HCl	10 mM
NaCl	100 mM
EDTA	20 mM
SDS	0.5%

Table 6
Genomic DNA Digestion

10X buffer	3 µL
H$_2$O	Make up to 30 µL
BstEII	50–100 U
Tail DNA	5–10 µg

and transgene, respectively (*see* **Fig. 2B**). After Southern blot, we compared the radioactive densities of the 6.0 and 3.1-kb bands, and estimated that the copy number was about 1 in L3 and 10 in L12.

3.7.1. Extraction of Tail Genomic DNA

1. Tail buffer (*see* **Table 5**). Before use, add proteinase K to a final concentration of 0.5 mg/mL.
2. Each tail biopsy (0.5–1 cm long) is digested in 600 µL tail buffer (overnight in 55°C with shaking).
3. Put the digest tube on ice for 10 min, add 300 µL saturated NaCl (6 M), and mix well by inversion. Leave the tube on ice for additional 10 min.
4. Centrifuge at 12,000g for 10 min, transfer the supernatant (700 µL) into a fresh tube, and add 350 µL isopropanol. Mix by inversion until DNA fiber is well formed.
5. Carefully pick up the DNA fiber with pipet tips and dissolve it into 150 µL TE buffer; or, DNA fiber can be centrifuged down and dissolved in 150 µL TE buffer following an additional wash by 70% ethanol.

3.7.2. Southern Blot

1. Digestion of genomic DNA (for each tail DNA sample; **Table 6**). Mix well, and perform digestion overnight at 37°C.
2. After adding 6 µL of loading buffer, all samples are subjected to agarose gel electrophoresis (0.8%) until the molecular weight markers are properly separated.
3. Put the gel into 0.2 N HCl for 15 min; afterward, transfer the gel into 0.4 M NaOH.
4. The alkaline blot method is used to transfer the DNA onto prewetted Hybond-N+ membrane. The blotting buffer is 0.4 M NaOH.
5. After the blot, mark and crosslink the membrane by ultraviolet crosslinker twice with 1200 (Stratalinker® 2400; Stratagene).

Table 7
Membrane Wash Buffer and Procedure

Wash buffer	Temperature/time
1X SSC,	Rinse five times
0.5X SSC, 0.5% SDS	60°C/three times for 15 min
0.1X SSC	Rinse once

6. Place the blotted membrane into a hybridization tube and add 20 mL of 6X SSC. Mount the hybridization tube in the oven, set temperature to 60°C, and run about 30 min.
7. Make prehybridization buffer (3 mL of 20X SSC, 1 mL of 100X Denhardt's solution, 0.5 mL of denatured sperm DNA [10 mg/mL], 1 mL of 10% sodium dodecyl sulfate [SDS], and 5 mL of H_2O).
8. Replace 6X SSC with prehybridization buffer, and let prehybridization run for 0.5–1 h. Meanwhile, radioactively label 1.7 kb MHC probe A using the random-priming kit (Stratagene). After labeling, the probe is purified though the column (Micro Bio-Spin 30, Bio-Rad).
9. Heat the labeled probe at 95°C for 5 min, then place it on ice for 5 min and add to prehybridization tube. Hybridization is usually performed at 60°C overnight.
10. Membrane wash and exposure (*see* **Table 7**). Expose the membrane to a film, and use intensive screen to enhance the signal (–80°C). Exposure time is about one to several days, depending on the strength of the signal.
11. Develop the film, scan the image, and calculate signal intensity (**Fig. 2B**).

3.8. Detection of Expression of Transgene

Expression of the transgene can be detected by the typical methods, which include quantitative reverse-transcription (RT)-PCR, Northern blot and RNase protection assays at the mRNA level, and Western blot analysis at the protein level *(29)*.

4. Notes

1. Media can be purchased from Specialty Media, Sigma-Aldrich, or others.
2. Either way is good for purification of DNA. For large DNA fragments, we suggest the use of the agarose method.
3. The number of the females is determined by the size of the transgenic facility and the number of injectors. Usually, four to six females are suitable for one injector.
4. The amount of hyaluronidase should be optimized for separation of eggs. If the eggs are released in 3–5 min, this indicates that the dose of hyaluronidase is sufficient.
5. To keep the eggs fresh, do not transfer too many eggs into the chamber. The injection media should be changed at a regular time interval of 30–45 min.
6. The number of the implanted eggs depends on the skill with which the injections are performed and the quality of the eggs. The survival rate of the injected eggs should be tested by overnight culture after injection.

7. A 50-µL PCR reaction system should be used, and PCR buffer should contain Triton X-100 to protect the Taq polymerase from SDS and other impurities that can inhibit Taq polymerase activity.

Acknowledgments

This work was supported by the National Institutes of Health (NIH) grants R01 HL65630 and R01 HL66251, and an American Heart Association Established Investigator award (to Q.W.).

References

1. Gordon, J. W., Scangos, G. A., Plotkin, D. J., Barbosa, J. A., and Ruddle, F. H. (1980) Genetic transformation of mouse embryos by microinjection of purified DNA. *Proc. Natl. Acad. Sci. USA* **77,** 7380–7384.
2. Wagner, E. F., Stewart, T. A., and Mintz, B. (1981) The human beta-globin gene and a functional viral thymidine kinase gene in developing mice. *Proc. Natl. Acad. Sci. USA* **78,** 5016–5020.
3. Palmiter, R. D., Brinster, R. L., Hammer, R. E., et al. (1982) Dramatic growth of mice that develop from eggs microinjected with metallothionein-growth hormone fusion genes. *Nature* **300,** 611–615.
4. Tian, X. L., Chen, L. Y., and Hu, R. L. (1995) *Transgenic Animals: Principles, Techniques and Application.* Changchun Science and Technology, Changchun.
5. Tian, X. L., Pinto, Y. M., Costerousse, O., et al. (2004) Over-expression of angiotensin converting enzyme-1 augments cardiac hypertrophy in transgenic rats. *Hum. Mol. Genet.* **13,** 1441–1450.
6. Wall, R. J., Kerr, D. E., and Bondioli, K. R. (1997) Transgenic dairy cattle: genetic engineering on a large scale. *J. Dairy. Sci.* **80,** 2213–2224.
7. Denman, J., Hayes, M., O'Day, C., et al. (1991) Transgenic expression of a variant of human tissue-type plasminogen activator in goat milk: purification and characterization of the recombinant enzyme. *Biotechnology (N.Y.)* **9,** 839–843.
8. Hammer, R. E., Pursel, V. G., Rexroad, C. E. J., et al. (1985) Production of transgenic rabbits, sheep and pigs by microinjection. *Nature* **315,** 680–683.
9. Mullins, J. J. and Ganten, D. (1990) Transgenic animals: new approaches to hypertension research. *J. Hypertens. Suppl.* **8,** S35–S37.
10. Hogan, B., Beddington, R., Costantini, F., and Lacy, E. (1994) *Manipulating the Mouse Embryo: A Laboratory Manual.* Cold Spring Harbor Laboratory, Cold Spring Harbor, NY.
11. Jaenisch, R. and Mintz, B. (1974) Simian virus 40 DNA sequences in DNA of healthy adult mice derived from preimplantation blastocysts injected with viral DNA. *Proc. Natl. Acad. Sci. USA* **71,** 1250–1254.
12. Maione, B., Lavitrano, M., Spadafora, C., and Kiessling, A. A. (1998) Sperm-mediated gene transfer in mice. *Mol. Reprod. Dev.* **50,** 406–409.
13. Lavitrano, M., Forni, M., Varzi, V., et al. (1997) Sperm-mediated gene transfer: production of pigs transgenic for a human regulator of complement activation. *Transplant. Proc.* **29,** 3508–3509.

14. Zhao, S., Maxwell, S., Jimenez-Beristain, A., et al. (2004) Generation of embryonic stem cells and transgenic mice expressing green fluorescence protein in midbrain dopaminergic neurons. *Eur. J. Neurosci.* **19,** 1133–1140.

15. Psarras, S., Karagianni, N., Kellendonk, C., et al. (2004) Gene transfer and genetic modification of embryonic stem cells by Cre- and Cre-PR-expressing MESV-based retroviral vectors. *J. Gene Med.* **6,** 32–42.

16. Guglielmi, L., Battu, S., Le Bert, M., Faucher, J. L., Cardot, P. J., and Denizot, Y. (2004) Mouse embryonic stem cell sorting for the generation of transgenic mice by sedimentation field-flow fractionation. *Anal. Chem.* **76,** 1580–1585.

17. Rindt, H., Subramaniam, A., and Robbins, J. (1995) An in vivo analysis of transcriptional elements in the mouse alpha-myosin heavy chain gene promoter. *Transgenic. Res.* **4,** 397–405.

18. Loughna, S., Yuan, H. T., and Woolf, A. S. (1998) Effects of oxygen on vascular patterning in Tie1/LacZ metanephric kidneys in vitro. *Biochem. Biophys. Res. Commun.* **247,** 361–366.

19. Schlaeger, T. M., Bartunkova, S., Lawitts, J. A., et al. (1997) Uniform vascular-endothelial-cell-specific gene expression in both embryonic and adult transgenic mice. *Proc. Natl. Acad. Sci. USA* **94,** 3058–3063.

20. Schedl, A., Beermann, F., Thies, E., Montoliu, L., Kelsey, G., and Schutz, G. (1992) Transgenic mice generated by pronuclear injection of a yeast artificial chromosome. *Nucleic. Acids. Res.* **20,** 3073–3077.

21. Imhof, M. O., Chatellard, P., and Mermod, N. (2000) A regulatory network for the efficient control of transgene expression. *J. Gene Med.* **2,** 107–116.

22. Franz, W. M., Breves, D., Klingel, K., Brem, G., Hofschneider, P. H., and Kandolf, R. (1993) Heart-specific targeting of firefly luciferase by the myosin light chain-2 promoter and developmental regulation in transgenic mice. *Circ. Res.* **73,** 629–638.

23. London, B., Jeron, A., Zhou, J., et al. (1998) Long QT and ventricular arrhythmias in transgenic mice expressing the N terminus and first transmembrane segment of a voltage-gated potassium channel. *Proc. Natl. Acad. Sci. USA* **95,** 2926–2931.

24. Schinke, M., Baltatu, O., Bohm, M., et al. (1999) Blood pressure reduction and diabetes insipidus in transgenic rats deficient in brain angiotensinogen. *Proc. Natl. Acad. Sci. USA* **96,** 3975–3980.

25. Hasuwa, H., Kaseda, K., Einarsdottir, T., and Okabe, M. (2002) Small interfering RNA and gene silencing in transgenic mice and rats. *FEBS Lett.* **532,** 227–230.

26. Lu, W., Yamamoto, V., Ortega, B., and Baltimore, D. (2004) Mammalian Ryk is a Wnt coreceptor required for stimulation of neurite outgrowth. *Cell* **119,** 97–108.

27. Tian, X. L., Yong, S. L., Wan, X., et al. (2004) Mechanisms by which SCN5A mutation N1325S causes cardiac arrhythmias and sudden death in vivo. *Cardiovasc. Res.* **61,** 256–267.

28. Gulick, J., Subramaniam, A., Neumann, J., and Robbins, J. (1991) Isolation and characterization of the mouse cardiac myosin heavy chain genes. *J. Biol. Chem.* **266,** 9180–9185.

29. Tian, X. L. and Paul, M. (2003) Species-specific splicing and expression of angiotensin converting enzyme. *Biochem. Pharmacol.* **66,** 1037–1044.

6

Quantitative Assay for Mouse Atherosclerosis in the Aortic Root

Julie Baglione and Jonathan D. Smith

Summary

The mouse has become the preferred species for genetic manipulation aimed at creating and studying models for human disease. Although mice are highly resistant to atherosclerosis, dietary induction and, more frequently, gene knockout and transgenic mice have been widely used to study factors that alter the susceptibility to atherosclerosis. Although there are several ways to assess atherosclerosis in mice, measurement of the aortic root lesion area is a commonly used, medium-throughput method that allows for histological examination of the lesions. Here, we provide the detailed methods for the quantitative analysis of mouse aortic root lesion area.

Key Words: Atherosclerosis; mouse; histology; image analysis; lesion area measurement.

1. Introduction

1.1. Development and Use of Diet-Induced and Genetically Modified Mouse Models of Atherosclerosis

Most of the plasma cholesterol in mice is found on high-density lipoprotein (HDL), which is protective against atherosclerosis, whereas in humans, most of the plasma cholesterol is found on low-density lipoprotein (LDL), which plays a direct role in atherogenesis. Thus, wild-type mice fed a chow diet do not develop atherosclerotic lesions. Although mouse atherosclerosis was first studied in the 1960s (for review, *see* **ref.** *1*), the modern era of mouse atherosclerosis study was initiated in 1985 by Beverly Paigen, who used a high-fat (15%), high-cholesterol (1.25%), cholic acid (0.5%)-containing diet to induce hypercholesterolemia and atherosclerosis in susceptible mouse strains *(2,3)*.

From: *Methods in Molecular Medicine, vol. 129:*
Cardiovascular Disease: Methods and Protocols, Volume 2: Molecular Medicine
Edited by: Q. K. Wang © Humana Press Inc., Totowa, NJ

The assay for quantitative assessment of atherosclerosis in the aortic root was also initially described by Paigen in 1987 *(4)*, and with modification, this is the assay that is described next. The discovery of susceptible and resistant strains allowed the application of classical mouse genetic techniques to map the position of genes that influence atherosclerosis susceptibility. In 1987, Paigen's laboratory defined the first atherosclerosis susceptibility locus, *Ath1,* on mouse chromosome 1 *(5)*. It then took 18 yr before Paigen and colleagues identified the *Tnfsf4* gene, encoding the Ox40 ligand, as the gene responsible for atherosclerosis susceptibility in the *Ath1* locus *(6)*.

In 1992, Breslow's and Maeda's laboratories independently reported the generation of apoE-deficient mice via homologous recombination using embryonic stem cells, and both groups reported that these mice develop hypercholesterolemia and atherosclerosis, even on chow diets *(7,8)*. Now, there are a variety of gene knockout and transgenic mice that are susceptible to atherosclerosis; a catalog of these mice, their phenotypes, and the choice of diets for these models is beyond the scope of this chapter. However, the other most frequently used model along with the apoE-deficient mouse is the LDL receptor-deficient mouse created by Herz et al. *(9)*. These genetically modified models have been used extensively to identify atherosclerosis susceptibility modifying genes by two methods: (1) the testing of candidate genes by breeding atherosclerosis-prone mice with mice that over- or under-express a specific candidate gene; and (2) by unbiased mouse genetic methods that allow positional identification of these genes. For the latter method, the availability of the mouse genome sequence and other shortcuts via the use of microarray expression analysis should greatly shorten the time needed to identify additional atherosclerosis genes. Other uses for these models include tests of therapeutic reagents, the study of arterial remodeling, the development of models of plaque rupture, and the study of pathogenic mechanisms.

1.2. Protocol Considerations

Atherosclerotic lesions in all species develop focally at specific sites where there is nonlaminar flow. Thus, quantitative atherosclerosis assays must be performed using anatomical landmarks to keep the area under study constant. There are several different assays to quantitatively assess mouse atherosclerosis at various locations; however, the aortic root assay is still considered the standard assay in many laboratories, one reason being that this site is highly susceptible to atherosclerosis in mice and thus lesions develop here at earlier ages than in other areas. The second most commonly used assay is analysis of *en face* lesion surface area in the entire aorta, from the arch to the iliac bifurcation or limited just to the arch area. This method, described by Palinski's laboratory, yields results that are generally well correlated with measurement of lesions at the aortic root *(10)*.

It is often not sufficient to only assess atherosclerosis in the aortic root, as there are examples of an aortic root lesion area not being altered while the *en face* lesion area is affected, and these effects may occur selectively in the thoracic or abdominal regions of the aorta *(11,12)*. Limitations of the *en face* assay are that it does not take into account lesion thickness or allow analysis of cellular composition, and thus two lesions of very different volumes may take up equal surface area. It is also possible to measure atherosclerosis biochemically, by determining cholesterol ester content of the aorta *(13)*. Limitations of this assay are the lack of volume or area measurements and the inability to gather histological information.

Other sites besides the aorta can also be quantitatively assessed for lesions. ApoE-deficient mice also develop lesions in the carotid, pulmonary, femoral, and innominate (first branch off of the aortic arch) arteries, the latter being a good site for quantification as it is a site of early lesion predilection in young mice and plaque hemorrhage in older mice *(14–16)*. Getz et al. have recently reviewed the site-specific modulation of atherosclerosis in mouse models and the importance of examining more than one location *(17)*.

We provide here a detailed protocol for the assessment of mouse atherosclerosis in the aortic root, and many of the methods described here can be applied to cross-sectional lesion area measurements at other locations as well. Diagrams of the anatomy of aortic root have been published previously *(4,17)*. This method, although difficult to master, requires very little surgical time compared with the other methods that require the surgical isolation of the aorta or innominate artery, enabling the processing at a medium throughput level of approx 30 or more mice per day. It is possible to make many modifications of this protocol: for example, it may be necessary to eliminate fixation for immunohistochemical staining with certain antibodies. For a description of alternate methods of atherosclerosis assays, we refer the reader to the excellent article by Daugherty and Whitman *(18)*.

2. Materials

2.1. Mouse Sacrifice, Heart Removal, and Fixation

1. Ketamaine/xylazine anesthesia is prepared by adding 10 mL of ketamine stock (100 mg/mL; Fort Dodge Animal Health, Fort Dodge, IA) and 1.5 mL xylazine stock (20 mg/mL; Vedco, St. Joseph, MO) to 35.5 mL sterile phosphate-buffered saline (PBS), yielding a solution of 21.25 mg/mL ketamine and 0.625 mg/mL xylazine.
2. Small animal surgical tools: fine scissors, fine forceps, and coarse forceps with serrated tips.
3. PBS or normal saline in a 10-mL syringe with a 24-G needle for perfusion.
4. 10% phosphate buffered formalin (Fisher, Pittsburgh, PA). Care should be taken to minimize exposure to formalin vapors.

2.2. Gelatin Embedding and Sectioning

1. Embedding capsules (HistoPrep Tissue Capsules; Fisher, cat. no. 15-182-218).
2. Gelatin type A (ICN Biomedicals, Aurora, OH; cat. no. 901771) used to make 5, 10, and 25% solutions in water.
3. Optimal cutting temperature (OCT) embedding medium (Sakura Finetechnical Co, Torrence, CA).
4. Fisher Plus coated microscope slides (Fisher, cat. no. 12-550-15).
5. Cryostat. We use and recommend the Leica model CM 1850.

2.3. Staining and Quantification

1. Glass Staining racks with removable trays and wire handles (Fisher, cat. no. 08-812).
2. Oil red-O stain (0.24%): 1 g oil red-O powder (Sigma Aldrich, St. Louis MO) and 250 mL 2-propanol are combined and mixed for 10 min. 150 mL of double-distilled (dd)H_2O is added and mixed for an additional minute, allowed to stand for 6 min, and then filtered through a 0.45-µm Stericup (Millipore, Billerica, MA). Oil red-O stain should be made freshly and used within 2 h of preparation.
3. Harris hematoxylin (2.4%): 100 mL Harris hematoxylin stock solution (Sigma Aldrich) is combined with 98 mL of ddH_2O and 2 mL of glacial acetic acid and filtered.
4. Bluing solution: five drops of ammonium hydroxide reagent in 1 L of ddH_2O.
5. Light Green solution (0.25%): 50 mL of a 1% stock solution (2 g Light Green SF powder [Fisher], 198 mL ddH_2O, and 2 mL acetic acid) is added to 150 mL ddH_2O. 0.25% solution is good for 2–3 wk and 1% solution 2–4 wk when kept in a brown bottle.
6. Glycerol gelatin (Sigma Aldrich).
7. 22 × 60 mm no. 1 cover slips (Fisher).
8. Image Pro Plus software, packaged as Olympus MicroSuite software, Soft Imaging System (Lakewood, CO).
9. Microscope equipped with video imaging camera, video capture card, and personal computer (PC): we use an Olympus CX41 microscope (Melville, NY), a Panasonic Industrial Color charge-coupled device (CCD) camera, model no. GP-KR222 (Secaucus, NJ), Pincacle Systems video capture card, and software in a Dell PC.

3. Methods

3.1. Mouse Sacrifice, Heart Removal, and Fixation

1. Each mouse is weighed and a 25-g mouse is anesthetized by intraperitoneal injection with 200 µL of the ketamine/xylazine stock (delivered from a 1-cc tuberculin syringe with a 30-G needle). Adjust the volume according to the weight of the mouse using approx 8 µL of anesthesia stock per gram body weight. The depth of anesthesia is tested by lack of response to a firm squeeze of the hind foot. Additional anesthesia should be administered in 50-µL increments until this depth is achieved. The age of the mice under study should be kept constant ±0.5 wk, as lesion area is extremely age-dependent (*see* **Note 1**).

2. The legs of the supine mouse are taped down onto several folded paper towels, and the ventral surface is wet with water or 70% ethanol (to keep the hair matted down). A lateral skin incision is made at the base of the abdomen extending to the width of the rib cage. Wrap some skin from the top side of the incision around a blunt forceps with serrated tips, hold down the mouse's rear legs, and forcefully tear the skin and pull it up over the mouse's head exposing the peritoneum and chest. Using fine scissors, cut open the peritoneal membrane from the base of the abdomen to the ribcage. Lift the sternum with fine forceps, and penetrate the diaphragm with the tip of fine scissors. Quickly cut through the sternum up the ribcage, make two lateral cuts at the top of the ribcage, and remove the ventral ribs exposing the beating heart. At this point, blood may be removed by intracardiac puncture (*see* **Note 2**).
3. The circulatory system is perfused with 10 mL of PBS or normal saline by placing the needle of the saline-loaded syringe into the left ventricle, using fine scissors to nick the right atrium (allowing drainage of the circulatory system into the chest cavity), and slowly pumping the saline into the heart. The mouse is euthanized at this point by exsanguination.
4. The heart is gently lifted out by the apex, without squeezing the top, which can damage the aortic root, which is completely embedded within the heart. Any fibrous connective tissue attached to the heart is cut, and finally, the aorta is cut just above the level of the heart and the heart is put into a vial (we use glass scintillation vials) containing 5–10 mL of 10% phosphate-buffered formalin (*see* **Note 3**). The vial is placed at 4°C indefinitely, until ready for embedding but for a minimum of 24 h.

3.2. Embedding Hearts in Gelatin

1. The next step for routine quantitative assay is gelatin embedding, which helps maintain the integrity of the friable lesions during sectioning, although this step may also be omitted, particularly for immunostaining. For gelatin embedding, each heart is placed in a labeled histological capsule and washed under cold running tap water for 1 h. Hearts are then placed in a shallow plastic container and floated in a 42°C water bath and covered with 5% gelatin and 10% gelatin sequentially for 2 h each. Twenty-five percent gelatin is incubated with the hearts at 42°C overnight. The hearts in 25% gelatin are refrigerated until the gelatin solidifies.
2. Hearts are removed from the capsules **(Fig. 1A)** and the gelatin is trimmed with a razor blade into a solid block **(Fig. 1B)**. The gelatin embedded hearts are placed back into formalin and stored at 4°C until ready for sectioning.

3.3. Mounting the Hearts on a Pedestal in OCT and Sectioning Hearts With a Cryostat

1. The lower half of the heart is removed by cutting with a razor blade. The alignment of this cut is crucial to getting sections perpendicular to the axis of the aortic root. The cut is made approx 1 mm beneath the base of and parallel to the right and left atria **(Fig. 1C)**.

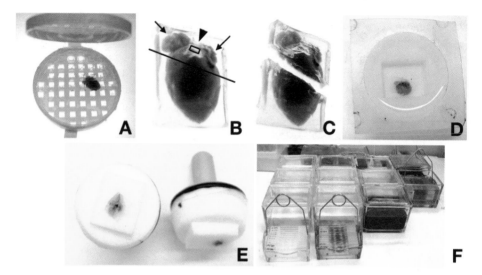

Fig. 1. Setup for embedding, sectioning, and staining of aortic roots. (**A**) Gelatin-embedded heart in tissue capsule. (**B**) Heart in gelatin block. Arrows point to atria, and line shows position of cut critical for proper orientation. (**C**) Heart in gelatin block after cut is made. (**D**). Top half of heart in tissue mold, cut face down, covered with liquid optimal cutting temperature (OCT) medium. (**E**) Two views of heart top mounted on cryostat pedestal in frozen OCT. (**F**) Staining racks with slides in front of staining trays.

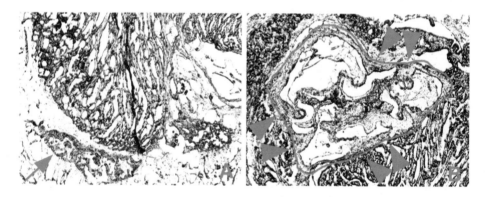

Fig. 2. Appearance of unstained sections used to determine the start of the aortic root. (**A**) Section showing the appearance of an atrium (red arrow) indicating proximity to the aortic root. (**B**) Section at the beginning of the aortic root showing the three bipartite valve bases (red arrowheads) and the complete aortic medial wall (red outline).

2. The top half of the heart is then placed into a plastic tissue mold (lower chamber is 1.5 × 1 × 0.5 cm, L × W × D) with the cut surface at the bottom of the mold, and then covered in OCT compound in both the lower and upper chambers (**Fig. 1D**). If the heart is not gelatin-embedded, the heart is moved around carefully

to fill the aorta with OCT. The mold is placed in the cryostat set at –22°C to freeze the OCT.

3. The heart is removed from the base mold and mounted with the cut side facing up on the sample pedestal, which is mounted on the cryostat freezing stage, on a bed of not-yet solidified OCT (**Fig. 1E**).

4. The pedestal is placed into the chuck of the cryostat and a 30-μm thick section is cut and transferred to a microscope slide (*see* **Note 4**) for observation to check whether this section is parallel to the cut surface of the heart, or oblique, yielding a partial section. If orientation is incorrect, the pedestal angle is readjusted within the chuck. More sections are cut with observation every 10 sections to detect the atria, appearing as appendages, which signal the approach of the aortic sinus (**Fig. 2A**). The aortic sinus should appear as three bipartite valve bases with attached leaflets (these may break in sectioning) along with an intact intima (**Fig. 2B**). Novices may find this is difficult to see, but with practice, this becomes readily apparent.

5. Once the aortic sinus is visible, the section thickness is decreased to 10 μm and every other section is saved, four sections per slide covering a total distance of 80 μm. Six slides are prepared in this manner, covering a total distance of 400 μm, at which point the valve bases are shrunken, but still visible, and the valve leaflets may not all be visible (**Fig. 3A–F**). It is possible to quantify distal to this point, either by taking more slides, or by increasing the section thickness. In this case, one can capture sections going about 600 μm distal to the sinus origin, until the valve bases have disappeared. Slides are labeled, using a solvent resistant marker or a pencil, with the mouse identification number and the slide number and stored at room temperature until ready to stain, or at –20°C for immunostaining.

3.4. Staining Sections for Aortic Root Analysis

1. Twenty slides are placed back to back in the 10 slots of each staining rack. A series of staining trays are set up with the solutions listed next and the slides are immersed for the specified times. **Figure 1F** shows the staining setup.
2. ddH$_2$O for 2 min.
3. 60% 2-propanol for 30 s.
4. Filtered oil red-O staining solution for 18 min, in order to stain neutral lipids.
5. 60% 2-propanol for 30 s.
6. ddH$_2$O for 1 min.
7. ddH$_2$O for 1 min.
8. Harris hematoxylin stain for 2 min.
9. Bluing solution, 10 dips.
10. ddH$_2$O rinse for 1 min.
11. Light Green counterstain for 30 s.
12. ddH$_2$O for 1–15 min to partially destain Light Green.
13. Air-dry slides until ready for cover slipping.
14. For cover slipping, glycerol gelatin is heated to 55°C in a water bath. One drop is placed over each of the four sections on the slide. The cover slip is placed on the slide

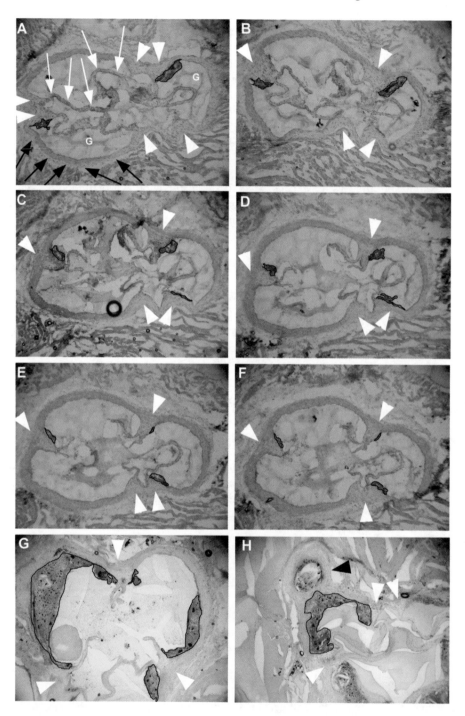

Fig. 3.

and pressed down firmly to remove any air bubbles. After the glycerol gelatin sets for an hour, excess is removed by washing the slides in soapy water (*see* **Note 5**).

3.5. Quantification of Aortic Root Lesion Area

1. The slide is observed microscopically under brightfield illumination using a ×4 or ×10 objective lens. Video images are captured with a video capture card and frame grabber software (in our system, this adds additional magnification).
2. One section on each of the six slides is quantified. Lesions consist of oil red-O staining lipid-filled regions as well as any fibrous regions lumenal to the internal elastic lamina. Lesions can crack and even lift away from the media, these are quantified without the empty space. Using Image Pro or other similar software, and after calibration with a stage micrometer (for each objective lens), the lesions can be circled and the area of each lesion for the quantified section on the slide is exported to a spreadsheet in square micrometers. This is repeated for each of the five remaining slides from the heart, using 80-μm intervals between the sections, if possible.
3. The sum of the lesion areas are calculated for each of the six quantified sections. Then, the mean lesion area is calculated for all of the six quantified sections (*see* **Note 6**).
4. Lesion cellular composition, necrotic area, and fibrotic area should be qualitatively assessed from these slides, but a quantitative analysis requires cell-type specific or collagen specific staining.

3.6. Statistical Analysis

1. For each mouse, the mean aortic root lesion area in square micrometers is used as the primary measurement.
2. Lesion areas vary among individual mice of the same age, gender, and genetic background. High-cholesterol diets also have a pronounced effect on lesion area. For larger lesions (>200,000 μm^2), the coefficient of variation may be approx 25–30%, but for smaller lesions (<50,000 μm^2) the coefficient of variation can be much greater.
3. Gender has an effect on lesion area, and females of most strains have larger aortic lesions than males.

Fig. 3. (*Opposite page*) Stained aortic root sections. (**A–F**) Series of six sections taken at 80-μm intervals through the aortic root of an apoE-deficient mouse with very small lesions to display the anatomy of this region. Large white arrowheads point to the three bipartite valve bases each of which fuse together distal to the origin. White arrows (**A**) point to one valve leaflet in the lumen. Lesions (staining red) were circled in thin black lines. (**G**) Common appearance of aortic root lesions in an16-wk-old apoE-deficient mouse fed a chow diet. Note coun terstain fading in this photograph taken several months after section staining. (**H**) Portion of the aortic root showing moderate sized lesions and the appearance of the proximal coronary artery (black arrowhead), which branches from the aortic root and that also contains lesions. All photographs were taken using a ×4 objective lens. Larger lesions yield outward aortic remodeling to preserve lumen area.

4. For routine analysis, we plot individual lesion areas of each mouse using a log scale graph.
5. Lesion areas may not be normally distributed within a group. If this is the case, it is better to use nonparametric statistical analyses to compare lesion areas between groups. This results in a comparison of the median value rather than the mean value, and also decreases the weighting of values from outliers. If lesion areas are normally distributed, parametric analyses may be used, comparing the mean lesion values. For complex statistical analysis, such as quantitative trait locus analysis, we normalize the distribution by using the log10 of the lesion area.
6. Power calculations can be performed to estimate the number of mice needed for each group (genders cannot be pooled) using StatMate software from GraphPad (San Diego, CA), or other similar software. Assuming a coefficient of variation of 25%, using 10 mice per group yields 90% power to detect a 38% difference between the groups, with a two-tailed α of 0.05. In practice, we find that a group size of 10 is sufficient to detect any reasonably strong (40%) effect on lesion area. In order to detect subtler effects on lesion areas, larger group sizes must be employed.

4. Notes

1. Care must be taken to sacrifice mice on schedule. **Figure 4** shows the dramatic effect of age on lesion area in apoE-deficient mice fed a Western-type diet.
2. Blood can be obtained prior to perfusion by cardiac puncture. For plasma isolation, prepare a 1-cc syringe with a 19-G needle by drawing up a 0.5 M EDTA solution and then expelling it. Puncture the left ventricle with the prepared syringe and very gently pull up on the plunger; if blood does not draw, gently reposition or rotate the syringe until blood comes into the syringe. Do not create a large back pressure, as this will only cause tissue to block the needle. Deliver the blood into a microfuge tube containing 10 µL of 0.5 M EDTA, mix by inversion several times, and place on ice. After all samples are obtained, the plasma can be isolated by centrifugation for 2 min in a microfuge.
3. The OCT-embedded aortic root can be sectioned on a cryostat without fixation or gelatin embedding; this is often required for immunostaining with certain antibodies.
4. Sections are flattened by the anti-roll plate of the cryostat and positioned onto a room temperature slide. If sections start to roll, the plate may be repositioned or the sections may be manually unrolled with a fine paintbrush. As a final option, rolled sections may be floated in room temperature water and positioned on slides.
5. Harris hematoxylin and Light Green staining solutions will diffuse and fade over time in the aqueous glycerol gelatin mounting medium and reduce contrast (*see* **Fig. 3G,H**). It is best to capture the images or make photomicrographs within 2 wk of staining.
6. Lesions areas are not constant over the 400 µm of the aortic root. The lesion area is often greatest on the second or third slide and then decreases in the distal slides. One can estimate the lesion volume from these cross sectional areas by use of the Cavalieri sterologic method.

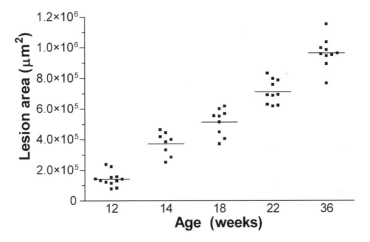

Fig. 4. Effect of age on aortic root lesion are in apoE-deficient mice fed a Western-type diet *(7)*. Mice were started on the western type diet at 6 wk of age and sacrificed for aortic root lesion area at the indicated times. The lesion areas were normally distributed at all of the ages, so a parametric analysis of variance was performed with a Newman-Keuls post-test. The mean lesion area at each age was significantly different from that at every other age, $p < 0.001$. Note that going from 12 wk of age to 14 wk of age increased the mean lesion area by 2.6-fold, demonstrating the need to schedule animal sacrifices as accurately as possible.

Acknowledgments

The authors would like to acknowledge Eddy Rubin, whose lab protocol formed the basis for our current method, and Suey Lee and Helen Yu of Jan Breslow's lab, who taught us how to section and stain mouse aortic roots. This work was supported by grant PO1 HL029582 from the National Heart, Lung, and Blood Institute of the National Institutes of Health.

References

1. Smith, J. D. and Breslow, J. L. (1997) The emergence of mouse models of atherosclerosis and their relevance to clinical research. *J. Intern. Med.* **242,** 99–109.
2. Paigen, B., Havens, M. B., and Morrow, A. (1985) Effect of 3-methylcholanthrene on the development of aortic lesions in mice. *Cancer Res.* **45,** 3850–3855.
3. Paigen, B., Morrow, A., Brandon, C., Mitchell, D., and Holmes, P. (1985) Variation in susceptibility to atherosclerosis among inbred strains of mice. *Atherosclerosis* **57,** 65–73.
4. Paigen, B., Morrow, A., Holmes, P. A., Mitchell, D., and Williams, R. A. (1987) Quantitative assessment of atherosclerotic lesions in mice. *Atherosclerosis* **68,** 231–240.

5. Paigen, B., Mitchell, D., Reue, K., Morrow, A., Lusis, A. J., and LeBoeuf, R. C. (1987) Ath-1, a gene determining atherosclerosis susceptibility and high density lipoprotein levels in mice. *Proc. Natl. Acad. Sci. USA* **84,** 3763–3767.

6. Wang, X., Ria, M., Kelmenson, P. M., et al. (2005) Positional identification of TNFSF4, encoding OX40 ligand, as a gene that influences atherosclerosis susceptibility. *Nat. Genet.* **37,** 365–372.

7. Plump, A. S., Smith, J. D., Hayek, T., et al. (1992) Severe hypercholesterolemia and atherosclerosis in apolipoprotein E-deficient mice created by homologous recombination in ES cells. *Cell* **71,** 343–353.

8. Zhang, S. H., Reddick, R. L., Piedrahita, J. A., and Maeda, N. (1992) Spontaneous hypercholesterolemia and arterial lesions in mice lacking apolipoprotein E. *Science* **258,** 468–471.

9. Ishibashi, S., Brown, M. S., Goldstein, J. L., Gerard, R. D., Hammer, R. E., and Herz, J. (1993) Hypercholesterolemia in low density lipoprotein receptor knockout mice and its reversal by adenovirus-mediated gene delivery. *J. Clin. Invest.* **92,** 883–893.

10. Tangirala, R. K., Rubin, E. M., and Palinski, W. (1995) Quantitation of atherosclerosis in murine models: correlation between lesions in the aortic origin and in the entire aorta, and differences in the extent of lesions between sexes in LDL receptor-deficient and apolipoprotein E-deficient mice. *J. Lipid. Res.* **36,** 2320–2328.

11. Febbraio, M., Podrez, E. A., Smith, J. D., et al. (2000) Targeted disruption of the class B scavenger receptor CD36 protects against atherosclerotic lesion development in mice. *J Clin. Invest* **105,** 1049–1056.

12. Lichtman, A. H., Clinton, S. K., Iiyama, K., Connelly, P. W., Libby, P., and Cybulsky, M. I. (1999) Hyperlipidemia and atherosclerotic lesion development in LDL receptor-deficient mice fed defined semipurified diets with and without cholate. *Arterioscler. Thromb. Vasc. Biol.* **19,** 1938–1944.

13. Rudel, L. L., Kelley, K., Sawyer, J. K., Shah, R., and Wilson, M. D. (1998) Dietary monounsaturated fatty acids promote aortic atherosclerosis in LDL receptor-null, human ApoB100-overexpressing transgenic mice. *Arterioscler. Thromb. Vasc. Biol.* **18,** 1818–1827.

14. Nakashima, Y., Plump, A. S., Raines, E. W., Breslow, J. L., and Ross, R. (1994) ApoE-deficient mice develop lesions of all phases of atherosclerosis throughout the arterial tree. *Arterioscler. Thromb.* **14,** 133–140.

15. Seo, H. S., Lombardi, D. M., Polinsky, P., et al. (1997) Peripheral vascular stenosis in apolipoprotein E-deficient mice. Potential roles of lipid deposition, medial atrophy, and adventitial inflammation. *Arterioscler. Thromb. Vasc. Biol.* **17,** 3593–3601.

16. Rosenfeld, M. E., Kauser, K., Martin-McNulty, B., Polinsky, P., Schwartz, S. M., and Rubanyi, G. M. (2002) Estrogen inhibits the initiation of fatty streaks throughout the vasculature but does not inhibit intra-plaque hemorrhage and the progression of established lesions in apolipoprotein E deficient mice. *Atherosclerosis* **164,** 251–259.

17. VanderLaan, P. A., Reardon, C. A., and Getz, G. S. (2004) Site specificity of atherosclerosis: site-selective responses to atherosclerotic modulators. *Arterioscler. Thromb. Vasc. Biol.* **24,** 12–22.

18. Daugherty, A. and Whitman, S. C. (2003) Quantification of atherosclerosis in mice, *Methods Mol. Biol.* **209,** 293–309.

7

Animal Models for Heart Failure

Sudhiranjan Gupta and Subha Sen

Summary

Heart failure (HF) is a major cause of morbidity and mortality worldwide. Although many therapeutic means are available to prolong the life of HF patients, why HF develops is still poorly understood. Investigators still seek a truly appropriate animal model that will reliably mimic human HF, so that the cause of the disease can be targeted and proper therapeutic modalities implemented. HF is a complex condition in which multiple molecular mechanisms interact, resulting in compromised cardiac function and often death. Once this elusive animal model is found, investigators will be able to translate findings from the model to human disease, thereby allowing analysis of the molecular changes and dissecting out multiple complicated changes in HF cascade. In this chapter, we describe the methodology that is used to analyze both transcriptional and translational molecular changes and correlate them with cardiac function to assess the cause-and-effect relationship to HF. We used one particular animal model of HF as an example (induced by causing overexpression of myotrophin specifically in the heart) that allowed us to analyze the changes during initiation, progression, and transition of hypertrophy to HF. We have also summarized some other animal models of HF currently available to study mechanisms of HF.

Key Words: Genetic alteration; compromised cardiac function; molecular changes myotrophin; gene expression.

1. Introduction

Heart failure (HF) is a major cause of morbidity and mortality the world over. More than 10 million patients are diagnosed with HF in North America and western Europe *(1)*. Although many therapeutic means are available to prolong the life of such patients, the underlying cause of the development of HF is still poorly understood. One reason is the lack of availability of an appropriate animal model to understand the mechanism so that the root causes can be targeted and proper therapeutic modalities implemented. More importantly,

From: *Methods in Molecular Medicine, vol. 129:*
Cardiovascular Disease: Methods and Protocols, Volume 2: Molecular Medicine
Edited by: Q. K. Wang © Humana Press Inc., Totowa, NJ

the prognosis of the patient with HF remains very clear cut because it involves multiple molecular mechanisms and is characterized by a complex of symptoms, which reduce the pumping efficiency of the heart and thereby impede blood supply to target organs. To overcome this deficiency, the heart initially responds by remodeling, usually by becoming enlarged (hypertrophy). Ironically, this initial hypertrophy, resulting from remodeling, helps for some time; over longer periods, however, the heart decompensates by showing compromised function and advancing to HF. Reduced hemodynamic function and pathological remodeling are markers for congestive HF (CHF), but the condition is still poorly understood as a result of multiple molecular mechanisms in the disease process, most of which remain undefined.

Many animal models have been used to study aspects of HF, but most models do not mimic human HF. Commonly used HF models are the mouse or rat models, either of which closely follows a course similar to that of human HF. Therefore, in this article, we will concentrate on animal models available to date to study HF from the initiation of hypertrophy (compensatory phase) to decompensation and transition to full HF.

The advancing state of techniques in molecular biology and genetics has provided a solid foundation for research in cardiovascular diseases. Today, molecular and genetic approaches are routinely used in most scientific laboratories, and physicians have access to various molecular and genetics tools to guide the diagnosis and treatment of patients. In fact, many medications are now produced by commonly used molecular techniques. In recent years, various animal models of cardiac hypertrophy and HF have been created by overexpression or knockout techniques, and applications of such models are increasing. Many models mimic important aspects of human HF, allowing investigators to determine the role of various proteins, cytokines, and growth factors in this process. Data are continually being gathered regarding the upstream and downstream pathways in the signal transduction pathway and thereby refining our understanding of the complex pathways involved during hypertrophy that transition to HF.

The molecular mechanisms underlying cardiac hypertrophy that worsens to HF are poorly understood. The general pathophysiology and therapeutic options of CHF have been revealed recently by Mann and Bristow *(2)* and Hoshijima and Chien *(3)*, as well as McMurray and Pfeffer *(4,5)*. In this chapter, we will discuss how different parameters of HF can be studied using a transgenic (Tg) mouse model.

2. General Methodology

To understand the difference in gene expression or protein expression profile, we used a HF Tg mouse model, in which overexpression of myotrophin resulted in HF over 9 mo; the following methods are used to understand the alteration in the following:

1. Heart weight to body weight ratio.
2. Gene expression.
3. Protein.
4. Hormonal changes.
5. Cytokines.

To understand changes in gene expression, Northern blot analysis is the most commonly used technique to isolate RNA from normal and diseased hearts. To understand changes in proteins corresponding to genes, Western analysis is performed using an antibody to the protein of interest. To understand changes in hormonal (growth factors and cytokines) pattern, the best way to identify the global changes is to perform a ribonuclease (RNase) protection assay (RPA) using a specific probe available commercially. Once the global picture is known, a specific analysis is usually performed by Northern analysis. In the following, we will describe the methodologies generally used.

2.1. Southern Blotting

Southern blotting is designed to locate a particular sequence of DNA within a complex mixture and is used to locate a particular gene within an entire genome. DNA is isolated from mice tail clips using a kit from Qiagen (Valencia, CA). The DNA is then subjected to restriction enzyme digestion and then transferred to Nytran membrane (Genescreen, Perkin Elmer, Inc., Boston, MA) by the downward neutral (20X SSC) capillary transfer method. The membrane is then ultraviolet (UV)-crosslinked using a UV crosslinker (Stratagene, Inc.).

The membrane is then put into prehybridization solution (2 m*M* Tris-Cl, pH 7.4, 10% dextran sulfate, 0.1% sodium dodecyl sulfate [SDS], 4X SSC, 1X Denhardt's solution, 2 µg/mL sheared salmon sperm DNA, and 40% formamide) at 42°C for 3–5 h. The random-primer labeling method is performed using a kit from Roche.

Denatured DNA	50 ng
Random primers (hexanucleotide)	2 µL
dNTPs (except the radiolabeled one)	3 µL
32p dCTP	5 µL
Klenow	1 µL

The components are mixed and incubated at 37°C for 2–3 h. After incubation, unincorporated radionucleotide is removed by using nucleotide removal kit (Qiagen). The probe is then eluted in 100 µL of water and denatured in boiling water for 5 min, chilled on ice for 1 min, and poured into a prehybridization bottle and kept overnight at 42°C. The membrane is then washed two times in 2X SSC and 0.5% SDS for 15 min and finally washed in 0.1X SSC, 1% SDS at 50°C for 15 min. The dried membrane is subjected to autoradiography at –70°C with an intensifying screen for 1–3 d.

2.2. Northern Blot Analysis

Northern blotting allows detection of specific RNA sequences. RNA is fractionated by agarose gel electrophoresis, followed by transfer (blotting) to a membrane support, followed by hybridization with DNA or RNA probes. Total RNA is isolated from wild-type (WT) and Tg mouse hearts following the phenol chloroform extraction method. Total RNA is fractionated on 1% agarose formaldehyde gels, and then transferred to a Nytran membrane as described in Southern blotting. The membrane is then UV-crosslinked using a UV crosslinker (Stratagene, Inc.).

Prehybridization and hybridization procedures are the same as those described in the Southern blotting section.

2.3. Western Blot Analysis

Western blot analysis allows detection of specific size, and quantity of a particular protein from a tissue extract or protein mixture.

2.3.1. Total Protein Extracts

Tg and WT mouse hearts are washed in cold phosphate-buffered saline (PBS), minced with a sterile blade and lysed on ice in a buffer containing 10 mM Tris-HCl (pH 7.5), 150 mM NaCl, 5 mM MgCl$_2$, 1 mM EDTA, 10 mM sodium pyrophosphate, 10% glycerol, 50 mM sodium fluoride, 100 μM Na$_3$VO$_4$, 10 nM okadaic acid, 0.5 mM dithiothreitol (DTT), 1 mM phenylmethylsulfonylfluoride (PMSF), 1% Triton X-100, 1 μg/mL leupeptin, 10 μg/mL aprotinin, and 1 μg/mL pepstatin. The lysates are centrifuged at 14,000g for 20 min at 4°C. The total protein concentration is measured by the Bradford method. Samples containing 50 μg of protein are separated on 10% SDS-polyacrylamide gels and electrophoretically transferred onto polyvinyldifluoride (PVDF) membranes using a wet transfer apparatus (Bio-Rad). Membranes are incubated in a blocking buffer containing 5% nonfat dry milk (Bio-Rad) in TBS with 0.1% Tween-20. Membranes are probed with appropriate antibodies overnight at 4°C, washed three times in TBS-Tween-20 and then detected using a horseradish peroxidase conjugated secondary antibody and ECL (NEN). Actin and histone antibodies (Santa Cruz Biotechnology) are used as an internal protein loading control for cytoplasmic and nuclear protein, respectively.

2.3.2. Preparation of Cytoplasmic and Nuclear Protein Extracts

WT and Tg mice hearts are washed with cold PBS and minced with a sterile blade. Nuclear and cytoplasmic extracts are made according to the method described in **ref. 6**. All buffers are kept on ice. PMSF, DTT, and a protease inhibitor cocktail are added just before use. The cytoplasmic and nuclear extracts are quantified for protein amounts determined by Bradford assay using bovine serum albumin (BSA) as a standard (Bio-Rad Protein Assay Kit). Protein fractions are aliquoted and stored at –70°C.

2.4. Ribonuclease Protection Assay

RPA is a highly sensitive and specific method for the detection and quantitation of mRNA species. The amount of protected probe is directly proportional to the amount of target mRNA in the sample. Total RNA from WT and Tg mouse hearts is extracted and 15 μg is used in an RNase protection assay using templates specific for growth factors and cytokines according to the manufacturer's protocol (RiboQuant, BD PharMingen, San Diego, CA; MCK-3B template set). After RNase digestion, protected fragments are resolved on 6% denaturing polyacrylamide gels and quantified using a PhosphorImager. We normalized the value of each hybridized signals to that of an internal control, GAPDH.

2.5. Determination of Cardiac Function

2.5.1. Data Collection

Mice are assessed in a conscious state, with a familiar handler holding them in a supine position. Echocardiography is performed using Vivid 7 echocardiography machine (GE Medical, Milwaukee, WI). M-mode echocardiography, two-dimensional (2D) echocardiography (frame rate >160 fps), and 2D color tissue Doppler echocardiography (TDE) data (frame rate >220 fps) using 14 MHz pericardial linear transducer. Data are digitized and stored in a proprietary format for further analysis.

2.5.2. Data Analysis

Data are analyzed using Echopac PC (GE Medical, Milwaukee, WI). Left atrial area is measured from the basal short-axis view of the heart that maximizes left atrial appendage size. Left-ventricular (LV) end-diastolic (EDDs) and end-systolic diameters (ESDs) are measured from M-mode data in a standard manner. Fractional shortenings (FSh) are calculated as FSh = 1 – LV ESD/ LV EDD, where LV EDD and LV ESD are measured from M-mode data. LV end-diastolic and end-systolic volumes are measured from the parasternal short- and long-axis view by bullet equation. LV mass is calculated from 2D echocardiography data by bullet equation also.

2.6. Microarray Analysis

Microarray analysis permits detection of genes in a small sample and analysis of the expression of these genes. They are simply ordered sets of DNA molecules of known sequence. Total cellular RNA (10 μg) is reverse-transcribed, and double-stranded cDNA (1 μg) is transcribed into cRNA (Enzo Bioarray RNA transcript labeling kit, Affymetrix, Inc., Santa Clara, CA). Biotin-11-CTP and biotin-16-UTP are incorporated into cRNA during synthesis. Approximately 20 μg of biotinylated cRNA is fragmented in buffer at 94°C for 35 min and added to murine genome U74Av2 arrays, containing approx 12,683 gene probe sets (Affymetrix) and hybridized at 40°C for 16 h. Arrays are washed, stained with streptavidin-phycoerythrin, and read using a confocal microscope scanner with a 560-nm filter. Pair-wise comparisons between the experimental animals of interest and all other animal samples are used to identify genes with consistent up- or downregulation at a particular developmental time. In addition, self-organinzing map (SOM) clustering is used to identify gene clusters with similar expression patterns that might reflect similar modes of regulation within the pertinent samples.

2.6.1. Data Analysis

Data are analyzed using the Microarray Suite and Data Mining Tools software packages (Affymetrix). Genes identified as upregulated are consistently increased in each pair wise comparison between the animals of interest (such as 9-mo-old Tg mice) and all other animals of both age groups (p-values varying from 0 to 0.0025). Upregulated genes are screened to eliminate those with "marginal" or "absent" absolute calls in the induced samples. Fold change is calculated by converting average signal log ratio values (change in the expression level of a transcript between the control and experimental samples) for each probe set to a whole number. This is accomplished by raising 2 to the power of the signal log ratio value ($2^{[\text{signal log ratio}]}$).

Gene clusters with similar expression patterns are identified using the SOM-clustering algorithm *(7)* of the Data Mining Tool software package (v3.0; Affymetrix). Signal values for all genes were imported from the Microarray Suite (v5.0) into the Data Mining Tool after publication using MicroDB software (Affymetrix) *(8)*. SOM clustering is performed using default-filtering values and parameters set to identify up to 81 possible clusters. After clustering, results again are screened to eliminate genes that failed to attain a "present" call in any of the pertinent samples.

In the following pages, we will describe our Tg animal model with cardiac-specific overexpression of myotrophin that showed initiation of hypertrophy at early age and progressed to HF by 9 mo of age. This Tg mouse model can serve as an example of how to systematically study the possible mechanisms that cause the progression of the disease and its transition to HF.

3. Generation of Myotrophin Transgenic Mice

3.1. Myotrophin and its Significance in Cardiac Hypertrophy and HF

Myotrophin, a 12-kDa soluble protein, has been isolated, purified, and sequenced from the hearts of spontaneously hypertensive rats (SHRs) and dilated cardiomyopathic human heart tissue and has been shown to stimulate myocyte growth *(9,10)*. Its effects on in vitro-cultured myocytes include an increase in protein synthesis, cellular hypertrophy, gap-junction formation, increased sarcomere number, induction of early-response genes (e.g., c-*myc*, c-*fos*, and c-*jun*), and, subsequently, the transcription upregulation of skeletal α-actin, β-myosin heavy chain (MHC), and atrial natriuretic factor (ANF) *(11)*. Evidence also suggests that enhanced protein kinase C (PKC) activity occurs with myotrophin-induced myocyte growth *(12)*. A cDNA clone encoding myotrophin has been isolated, and this recombinant form of myotrophin was found to be as biologically active in cultured myocytes as native myotrophin *(13)*. Moreover, a human homolog of myotrophin has been cloned, sequenced, and characterized *(14)*. Our laboratory has demonstrated that elevated levels of myotrophin are expressed in human dilated cardiomyopathic hearts and that recombinant human myotrophin produced cardiomyocyte hypertrophy in cultured neonatal rat myocytes *(9,10,15)*.

Myotrophin has a close structural homology with inhibitory κB (IκB, a regulatory molecule of the transcription factor called nuclear factor [NF]-κB) *(13)*. Moreover, because of the presence of tandem ankyrin repeats in the myotrophin molecule and their resemblance to those found in the IκB/rel protein, a role has also been postulated for myotrophin binding to NF-κB and modulatory activity of the transcription factor NF-κB *(16)*.

3.2. Construction of Myotrophin Transgene Expression Vector

We chose an expression vector known as pcDNA3 to overexpress myotrophin in the hearts of Tg mice. We first designed a 72-base oligomer that carried the 5′ untranslated region (UTR) of skeletal α-actin promoter and generated a chimeric myo-cDNA in pcDNA3 vector. The reason for introducing 72 bp of skeletal α-actin promoter is to achieve good expression, as the Kozak sequence of myotrophin was poor, but the first four amino acid sequence from the ATG shared a homology with skeletal α-actin *(17)*. Therefore, we introduced 72 bp of α-actin promoter before the myotrophin open reading frame (ORF). A high level of myotrophin expression in the heart

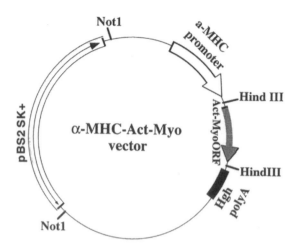

Fig. 1. Construction of an α-myosin heavy-chain myotrophin vector.

was observed by using α-MHC promoter *(18)*. To construct the α-MHC-myotrophin transgene, we used a vector called pBS2SK+, which contains α-MHC promoter and the human growth hormone (HGH) poly (A) tail (kindly provided by Dr. Jeffrey Robbins, University of Cincinnati, Cincinnati, OH). The chimeric myo-cDNA was released from the pcDNA3 vector and was inserted into pBS2SK+ at the *Hind*III site **(Fig. 1)**. The DNA fragment containing the α-MHC promoter with recombinant myotrophin was isolated, purified, and linearized with the *Not*1 enzyme using a Qiagen gel extraction kit.

3.3. Generation of Myotrophin Transgenic Mouse Line

The pronuclear injection was performed at the University of Cincinnati's Tg animal facility. The founder mice were screened for the presence of the myotrophin transgene by Southern blot analysis of genomic DNA extracted from tail clips. We crossed each of the founder mice with WT to maintain a heterozygotic population for further studies. We tested up to 11 generations of transgene expression by Northern and Western blot analysis and found them to have a similar expression level of the myotrophin gene. In addition, we tested myotrophin transgene expression in other tissues (e.g., liver, lung, brain), and we did not observe any overexpression or transgene expression in those organs; overexpression occurred only in the heart.

These Tg mice develop hypertrophy at as early as 4 wk of age and progress toward HF by 36 wk of age *(19)*. They exhibit LV hypertrophy, atrial dilation, myocyte necrosis, multiple focal fibrosis, pleural effusion, and compromised cardiac function associated with significant reduction in ejection fraction

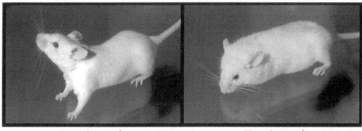

WT - 9 month   Tg - 9 month

Fig. 2. Typical appearance of wild-type and myotrophin transgenic mice.

(EF) and FSh (*see* **Fig. 2**). This model will also help to study the molecular events that occur during the onset and progression of hypertrophy and its transition to HF.

It is evident from the literature that HF does not result only from a single gene; it is associated with the alteration of many factors, including hormones, cytokines, PKC signaling, transcription factor activation, structural protein alteration, calcium protein changes, and mitochondrial dysfunction.

4. Biochemical and Molecular Characterization

4.1. Hypertrophy and HF Marker Gene Expression

Cardiac hypertrophy marker genes (e.g., atrial natriuretic factor [ANF] and β-MHC [and proto-oncogenes]) are the set of genes that are activated during hypertrophic process and also during HF. To study the result of overexpression of myotrophin at early and late stages, RNA was isolated from both WT and Tg mouse hearts at the initiation of the hypertrophic phase (4 wk of age) and at the transition of hypertrophy to the HF phase (36 wk of age), and Northern blot analysis was performed. As a consequence of myotrophin gene overexpression, expression of both ANF and β-MHC and proto-oncogenes (c-*fos*, c-*jun*, and c-*myc*) are also upregulated in Tg mice at the initiation (4 wk of age), during the progression of the disease (12–16 wk of age), and also during the transition to HF (36 wk) *(19)*. We also observed similar changes (tumor necrosis factor [TNF]-α overexpression) in other Tg mouse models that we have developed *(20,21)*.

4.2. Expression Profile for Growth Factors and Cytokines by RNase Protection Assay

To analyze a set of gene expression in a single experiment to get an overview regarding the expression profile, RNase protection assay was performed. In our Tg mouse model, we observed an increase in cytokines and growth factors such as lymphotoxin (LT)-β, TNF-α, interferon (IFN)-γ, interleukin (IL)-6, transforming growth factor (TGF)-β_1, TGF-β_2, TGF-β_3, and migration inhibitory factor (MIF) in 9-mo-old Tg mice, when chronic hypertrophy advanced to HF *(19)*. At 4 wk of age, three genes (*LT*-β, *TGF*-β_2, and *TGF*-β_3) were upregulated in Tg mice, compared with the age- and sex-matched WT mice. These data suggest that the cytokine/growth factor-mediated hypertrophic process is different in young and old Tg mice, especially during the transition to HF.

4.3. Gene Array Studies and Data Analysis

To identify candidate genes that mediate physiological responses to myotrophin overexpression, oligonucleotide gene array analyses were performed on heart samples from Tg and age- and gender-matched WT controls. This analysis gives a global view of alteration of gene expression profiling during the onset of hypertrophy and transition of hypertrophy to HF. Gene array analyses utilized RNA from heart tissue isolated from WT and Tg mice.

In our study, we observed that 80 genes are consistently upregulated in all pair-wise combinations when the 4-wk-old Tg mice are compared with all other mice (9-mo-old Tg and WT and 4-wk-old WT). When just one of the pair-wise combinations is varied with the others, 179 genes are induced. Of those 179 genes, 39 genes are clustered in three major functional categories: extracellular matrix and cytoskeleton, cell signaling, and growth factors/transcriptional regulators. Eleven of 30 upregulated expressed sequence tags (ESTs) have some assigned function. Among these, sarcolemmal-associated proteins, actin crosslinking protein 7, talin, glycogenin 1, and Cdc 5-like protein are elevated during the initiation of cardiac hypertrophy.

Pair-wise comparisons were also used to identify genes that decreased in expression when comparing 9-mo-old Tg hearts with all other samples. One hundred thirty-three genes are consistently elevated in failing hearts compared with nonfailing WT or young Tg hearts. Fifty-one of these genes are functionally clustered into six different categories: cell signaling, growth and transcriptional factors, extracellular matrix and cytoskeleton, cell defense, apoptosis, protein expression regulators, and metabolic enzymes. Out of 82 ESTs, only 11 had unknown functions.

5. Signal Transduction

In recent years, investigation has centered mainly on defining the intracellular signaling pathways that are associated with hypertrophy and HF. The recent advancement in molecular genetics allows the study of various signal transduction pathways involved in cardiac hypertrophy and its transition to HF. Therefore, delineating intracellular signaling pathways in the context of cardiac hypertrophy and HF will have potential implications in drug development for various cardiac diseases. Here, we will discuss a few of the most important signaling cascades using a Tg mouse model.

5.1. Protein Kinase C Signaling

PKC, a lipid-binding serine threonine kinase, acts as a downstream target for the membrane-associated signaling cascade *(22)*. Multiple studies implicate various PKC isoforms in the pathology of cardiac disease, including HF. Elevated expression of PKC has been observed in failing human heart *(23)*. Some studies have shown that Tg overexpression of PKCβ and PKCβ II in the heart engendered myocardial fibrosis, dilation, hypertrophy, poor cardiac function, and sudden death *(24,25)*. However, some controversy exists about the role of PKCβ overexpression in Tg mice in other studies *(26)*. Therefore, the role of PKC in HF can be studied using a Tg mouse model in which HF occurred. In the Myo-Tg model that we have been discussing, total PKC activity is increased during the progression of hypertrophy and also during its transition to HF. In addition, translocation of various isoforms of PKC have also been analyzed, and it has been observed that the translocation of PKCα, β, ε, and λ in Myo-Tg mice occurred during progression of hypertrophy, compared with WT mice. The translocation of various isoforms of PKC into the subcellular membrane pool during the transition phase of hypertrophy to HF suggests that phosphorylation of various myocardial proteins may be an important step during this process (unpublished observation).

5.2. NF-κB Signaling Cascade

NF-κB is a ubiquitous inducible transcription factor that activates a number of genes, including inflammatory cytokines. Another key role of NF-κB has been identified in the pathophysiology of myocardial infarction, ischemia, ischemia-reperfusion injury, ischemia preconditioning, and unstable angina *(27–30)*. However, although recent evidence suggests that NF-κB plays a pivotal role in HF in humans, no suitable model had been used for studying in detail the progression of the disease at its molecular level. To investigate whether myotrophin overexpression activates NF-κB binding activity in Myo-Tg mice during the progression to HF, EMSA was performed. In our Myo-Tg model, we observed a significant increase in NF-κB binding activity throughout the progression of the disease and were more pronounced during the transition to HF. In addition, we also tested the other signaling components associated with NF-κB. We observed the upregulation of IκBα (both at protein and mRNA levels) and the cascade was mediated through IKKβ. We have therefore concluded that the NF-κB signaling cascade is necessary for the initiation of hypertrophy and that it also plays an important role in the progression of hypertrophy to HF (unpublished observation).

Earlier in the chapter, we described one HF model in which myotrophin was overexpressed specifically in the heart. There are other animal models that have been reported in the literature with different methods of induction. The following is a brief summary of such HF models.

6. Genetically Altered Heart Failure Tg Mouse Models

6.1. Transgenic Mouse Model Overexpressing TNF-α

Cytokines, such as TNFα, are produced by many different cell types, including T cells and B lymphocytes, granulocytes, smooth muscle cells, eosinophils, chondrocytes, osteoblasts, mast cells, glial cells, and keratinocytes. TNF-α is also observed in high amount in the plasma of HF patients. Tg mice in which we observed only modest overexpression of TNF-α using an α-MHC promoter experienced a marked decline in cardiac function, associated with lymphocytic inflammatory infiltrates, ventricular dilation, and hypertrophy, that eventually led to HF *(20,21)*. The phenotype of this model closely mimics human HF, and it has been suggested that this molecule should be tested in a clinical trial. But preliminary clinical trials based on using either high levels of antibody against TNF-α or its receptor antagonist have failed to produce any beneficial effect.

6.2. Genes Related to Calcium Regulation

Cardiac muscle contraction is mainly initiated by a transient increase in intracellular Ca^{2+} triggered by depolarization of the sarcolemmal membrane during action potential. Ca^{2+} signaling is mediated by a sequential activation of various Ca^{2+}-regulated gene expression. These include opening the L-type Ca^{2+} channel, activating the Ca^{2+} current, causing the Ca^{2+} influx to release the ryanodine receptors, and finally getting the receptors sequestered into the sarcoplasmic reticulum. The genes involved in the activation and removal of calcium are sarco/endoplasmic reticulum Ca^{2+} adenosine triphosphatase (ATPase) (SERCA), phospholamban (PLN), and Na^+-Ca^{2+} exchanger. It is also noted that imbalance in Ca^{2+} homeostasis is a hallmark in HF, but the underlying mechanism is not well understood.

Overexpression of human cardiac L-type Ca^{2+} channel pores [hCa(v)1.2] in mice causes HF because of poor translation of hCa(v)1.2 and of its accessory subunits, altered sarcolemmal insertion of functional channels, and lower single-channel activity of overexpressed channels *(31)*.

6.3. Calsequestrin

Calsequestrin is located in the junctional sarcoplasmic reticulum (SR) and is a crucial molecule for Ca^{2+} binding. Cardiac-specific overexpression of murine cardiac calsequestrin results in depressed contractile parameters and in hypertrophy in Tg mice that progressed to HF *(32–34)*.

6.4. SERCA2

It is evident that reduction in SERCA2 levels in combination with pressure overload accelerates the HF process. SERCA2 is located in the free SR and is partly responsible for the release of Ca^{2+} into the SR. The SERCA pump promotes muscle relaxation by lowering cytosolic Ca^{2+} transport restores the intracellular Ca^{2+} stores, thus providing Ca^{2+} needed for the next contraction. It has been shown by Ito et al. *(35)* that creating pressure overload by aortic stenosis in Tg mice overexpressing SERCA leads to HF. Deficiency in SERCA2 is lethal in the embryonic phase *(36)*. Another Tg mouse model, with a single allele of SERCA2 (*Serca2*$^{+/-}$), showed impaired contractile function; with pressure overload imposed, the condition rapidly accelerated to HF *(37)*.

6.5. Phospholamban

PLN, another SR protein located in the free SR, has a high affinity to SERCA2 for Ca^{2+}. PLN is a small phosphoprotein regulator of the Ca^{2+} pump of cardiac sarcoplasmic reticulum. Dephosphorylated PLN inhibits the Ca^{2+} pump and depresses contractility, whereas phosphorylation of PLN by cAMP-activated mechanisms relieves this inhibition and increases contractility. Several reports have shown that increases in PLN activity may depress SR function and contractility in failing hearts *(38)*. Targeted overexpression of PLN into mouse atrium showed depressed Ca^{2+} transport and contractility *(39)*. Tg mice overexpressing PLN showed increased adrenergic drive and reduced ventricular contractility *(40)*. But during the aging process, these mice develop congestive HF. Recently Schmitt et al. *(41)* showed that a mutation in PLN (PLN[R9C]) caused HF in humans because of SERCA inhibition. Furthermore, Tg mice overexpressing PLN[R9C] showed a phenotype similar to that of human HF, suggesting that PLN may be a potential target for therapeutic intervention.

6.6. Calcineurin

Calcineurin, a serine-threonine phosphatase activated by calmodulin, has been shown to play an important role in HF. A general paradigm of calcineurin as a regulator of intracellular signaling through the transcription factor called nuclear factor of activated T cells (NF-AT) has been well established *(42)*. Calcineurin Tg mice that express activated forms of calcineurin or NF-AT3 in the heart develop cardiac hypertrophy and HF that mimic those of human heart disease. Pharmacological inhibition of calcineurin showed inhibition of hypertrophy, suggesting that this method may be a novel therapeutic approach to preventing cardiac hypertrophy and HF *(43)*. Overexpression of calcineurin in Tg mice results in cardiac hypertrophy and unexpected deaths *(44)*. Extensive work has been done to study calcineurin by using various models of Tg mice that either overexpress calcineurin or knockout models in which the calcineurin gene has been deleted to establish a cause-and-effect relationship of Ca^{2+} signaling and HF *(45)*.

The previously mentioned Ca^{2+}-regulated genes are known to play an important role in HF. In our Tg mouse model, we also observed a gradual upregulation of Ca^{2+}-regulated genes during the progression of hypertrophy. Interestingly, all are downregulated at the transition of hypertrophy to HF. Therefore, through the Tg approach, it is possible to determine the role of various Ca^{2+}-regulated genes and their function during HF. It is also noted that Ca^{2+}-regulated genes, especially *SERCA2*, have been reported to be involved in abnormal calcium handling and altered myocardial relaxation. Therefore, it is possible that suppression of any of the Ca^{2+}-regulated genes, in the myotrophin overexpressed Tg mice, could have contributed to cardiac dysfunction.

7. Nongenetically Altered Mouse Models

In addition to those mentioned previously, there are other models of HF that have been described in the literature and by which we can understand the pathophysiology of HF. The following sections will summarize both genetically altered and nongenetically altered models and their etiology, as well as the methods used for understanding the mechanism of action for transition to hypertrophy to HF.

7.1. Pressure Overload/Aortic Banding

One of the most commonly used surgical interventions for pressure-overload induced hypertrophy is coarctation of the ascending aorta, i.e., aortic banding. Over the years, this system has been very well characterized and has proven to be highly reproducible, with a low mortality rate of 10–20% or less in experienced hands. In mice, transverse aortic constriction (TAC) is used to create mechanically induced (LV) cardiac pressure overload, ultimately leading to cardiac hypertrophy and HF. TAC is generally induced by a traditional thoracotomy approach by minimally invasive aortic banding through a small incision in the proximal sternum *(46–48)*. This TAC model is used to study the profiles of various genes expressed during the onset of hypertrophy, although it does not completely mimic human cardiac remodeling. Aortic banding is a good model system with which to evaluate the development of LV hypertrophy in response to hemodynamic overload. After several months, a subset of animals progresses to HF.

7.2. Cardiac Volume Overload

CHF occurs when the heart can no longer meet the metabolic demands of the body at normal physiological venous pressures. Ventricular volume overload occurs in intracardial shunting of blood or in valvular incompetence with back-flow of blood. Volume overload, as observed in chronic aortic and/or mitral valvular regurgitant disease, shifts the entire diastolic pressure-volume curve to the right, indicating increased chamber stiffness and concentric LV hypertrophy (as occurs in aortic stenosis, hypertension, and hypertrophic cardiomyopathy) *(49)*. In general, the volume-overload HF model can be induced by aortocaval shunt. In brief, the vena cava and the abdominal aorta are dissected above the renal arteries. A clamp is made on the aorta proximal to the renal arteries; a needle of 0.6 mm is used to puncture the aorta distally and is then advanced into the vena cava to connect both vessels. The needle is removed afterward and the wound is sealed. The aortocaval shunt is visually seen by a swelling and a mixture of both arterial and venous blood in the vena cava. Cardiac hypertrophy develops within 4–5 wk with compromised LV contractility and enhanced end-diastolic pressure *(50)*.

8. Conclusion

This review of the types of animal models most used in research on hypertrophy and HF has necessarily been brief. The key to successful productive investigation is to choose an animal model most appropriate to the human disease condition that one is studying. The ideal model would give us animals in which disease progression replicates the course in human disease, could be reproduced for confirmation of data by other investigators, and would be cost-effective, yielding truly meaningful results that would justify the use of the animals for this purpose.

The use of Tg models has almost unlimited possibilities. Most exciting is the increasing number of publications showing the successful targeting of genes and their receptors. With this growing ability in genetic targets, there is a greater hope than ever that new therapies ("designer drugs" and genetic interventions) can be more swiftly developed to help solve the widespread occurrence of the hypertrophy/HF disease process in patients worldwide.

References

1. Cleland, J. G., Khand, A., and Clark, A. L. (2001) The HF epidemic: exactly how big is it? *Eur. Heart J.* **22**, 623–626.
2. Mann, D. L. and Bristow, M. R. (2005) Mechanisms and models in HF: the biomechanical model and beyond. *Circulation* **111**, 2837–2849.
3. Hoshijima, M. and Chien, K. R. (2002) Mixed signals in HF: cancer rules. *J. Clin. Invest.* **109**, 849–855.
4. McMurray, J. and Pfeffer, M. A. (2002) New therapeutic options in congestive HF: Part I. *Circulation* **105**, 2099–2106.
5. McMurray, J. and Pfeffer, M. A. (2002) New therapeutic options in congestive HF: Part II. *Circulation* **105**, 2223–2228.

6. Dignam, J. D., Martin, P. L., Shastry, B. S., and Roeder, R. G. (1983) Eukaryotic gene transcription with purified components. *Methods Enzymol.* **101,** 582–598.

7. Iwaki, K., Sukhatme, V. P., Shubeita, H. E., and Chien, K. R. (1990) Alpha- and beta-adrenergic stimulation induces distinct patterns of immediate early gene expression in neonatal rat myocardial cells. fos/jun expression is associated with sarcomere assembly; Egr-1 induction is primarily an alpha 1-mediated response. *J. Biol. Chem.* **265,** 13,809–13,817.

8. Tamayo, P., Slonim, D. Mesirov, J., et al. (1999) Interpreting patterns of gene expression with self-organizing maps: methods and application to hematopoietic differentiation. *Proc. Natl. Acad. Sci. USA* **96,** 2907–2912.

9. Sen, S., Kundu, G., Mekhail, N., Castel, J., Misono, K., and Healy, B. (1990) Myotrophin: purification of a novel peptide from spontaneously hypertensive rat heart that influences myocardial growth. *J. Biol. Chem.* **265,** 16,635–16,643.

10. Sil, P., Misono, K., and Sen, S. (1993) Myotrophin in human cardiomyopathic heart. *Circ. Res.* **73,** 98–108.

11. Mukherjee, D. P., McTiernan, C. F., and Sen, S. (1993) Myotrophin induces early response genes and enhances cardiac gene expression. *Hypertension* **21,** 142–148.

12. Sil, P., Kandaswamy, V., and Sen, S. (1998) Increased protein kinase C activity in myotrophin-induced myocyte growth. *Circ. Res.* **82,** 1173–1188.

13. Sivasubramanian, N., Adhikary, G., Sil, P. C., and Sen, S. (1996) Cardiac myotrophin exhibits rel/NF-kappa B interacting activity *in vitro. J. Biol. Chem.* **271,** 2812–2816.

14. Anderson, K. M., Berrebi-Bertrand, I., Kirkpatrick, R. B., et al. (1999) cDNA sequence and characterization of the gene that encodes human myotrophin/V-1 protein, a mediator of cardiac hypertrophy. *J. Mol. Cell. Cardiol.* **31,** 705–719.

15. Gupta, S. and Sen, S. (2002) Myotrophin-kappaB DNA interaction in the initiation process of cardiac hypertrophy. *Biochim. Biophys. Acta* **1589,** 247–260.

16. Gupta, S., Purcell, N. H., Lin, A., and Sen, S. (2002) Activation of nuclear factor-kappaB is necessary for myotrophin-induced cardiac hypertrophy. *J. Cell Biol.* **159,** 1019–1028.

17. Adhikary, G., Gupta, S., Sil, P., Saad, Y., and Sen, S. (2005) Characterization and functional significance of myotrophin: a gene with multiple transcripts. *Gene* **353,** 31–40.

18. Subramaniam, A., Jones, W. K., Gulick, J., Wert, S., Neumann, J., and Robbins, J. (1991) Tissue-specific regulation of the alpha-myosin heavy chain gene promoter in transgenic mice. *J. Biol. Chem.* **266,** 24,613–24,620.

19. Sarkar, S., Leaman, D. W., Gupta, S., et al. (2004) Cardiac overexpression of myotrophin triggers myocardial hypertrophy and HF in transgenic mice. *J. Biol. Chem.* **279,** 20,422–20,434.

20. Kubota, T., McTiernan, C. F., Frye, C. S., Demetris, A. J., and Feldman, A. M. (1997) Cardiac-specific overexpression of tumor necrosis factor-alpha causes lethal myocarditis in transgenic mice. *J. Card. Fail.* **3,** 117–124.

21. Kubota, T., McTiernan, C. F., Frye, C. S., et al. (1997) Dilated cardiomyopathy in transgenic mice with cardiac-specific overexpression of tumor necrosis factor-alpha. *Circ. Res.* **81,** 627–635.

22. Nishizuka, Y. (1986) Studies and perspectives of protein kinase C. *Science* **233,** 305–312.

23. Bowling, N., Walsh, R. A., Song, G., et al. (1999) Increased protein kinase C activity and expression of Ca^{2+}-sensitive isoforms in the failing human heart. *Circulation* **99,** 384–391.

24. Wakasaki, H., Koya, D., Schoen, F. J., et al. (1997) Targeted overexpression of protein kinase C beta2 isoform in myocardium causes cardiomyopathy. *Proc. Natl. Acad. Sci. USA* **94,** 9320–9325.

25. Bowman, J. C., Steinberg, S. F., Jiang, T., Geenen, D. L., Fishman, G. I., and Buttrick, P. M. (1997) Expression of protein kinase C beta in the heart causes hypertrophy in adult mice and sudden death in neonates. *J. Clin. Invest.* **100,** 2189–2195.

26. Roman, B. B., Geenen, D. L., Leitges, M., and Buttrick, P. M. (2001) PKC-beta is not necessary for cardiac hypertrophy. *Am. J. Physiol. Heart Circ. Physiol.* **280,** H2264–H2270.

27. Xuan, Y. T., Tang, X. L., Banerjee, S., et al. (1999) Nuclear factor-kappaB plays an essential role in the late phase of ischemic preconditioning in conscious rabbits. *Circ. Res.* **84,** 1095–1109.

28. Morgan, E. N., Boyle, E. M., Jr., Yun, W., et al. (1999) An essential role for NF-kappaB in the cardioadaptive response to ischemia. *Ann. Thorac. Surg.* **68,** 377–382.

29. Ritchie, M. E. (1998) Nuclear factor-kappaB is selectively and markedly activated in humans with unstable angina pectoris. *Circulation* **98,** 1707–1713.

30. Wong, S. C., Fukuchi, M., Melnyk, P., Rodger, I., and Giaid, A. (1998) Induction of cyclooxygenase-2 and activation of nuclear factor-kappaB in myocardium of patients with congestive HF. *Circulation* **98,** 100–103.

31. Groner, F., Rubio, M., Schulte-Euler, P., et al. (2004) Single-channel gating and regulation of human L-type calcium channels in cardiomyocytes of transgenic mice. *Biochem. Biophys. Res. Commun.* **314,** 878–884.

32. Sato, Y., Ferguson, D. G., Sako, H., et al. (1998) Cardiac-specific overexpression of mouse cardiac calsequestrin is associated with depressed cardiovascular function and hypertrophy in transgenic mice. *J. Biol. Chem.* **273,** 28,470–28,477.

33. Jones, L. R., Suzuki, Y. J., Wang, W., et al. (1998) Regulation of Ca^{2+} signaling in transgenic mouse cardiac myocytes overexpressing calsequestrin. *J. Clin. Invest.* **101,** 1385–1393.

34. Linck, B., Boknik, P., Huke, S., et al. (2000) Functional properties of transgenic mouse hearts overexpressing both calsequestrin and the Na^+-Ca^{2+} exchanger. *J. Pharmacol. Exp. Ther.* **294,** 648–657.

35. Ito, K., Yan, X., Feng, X., Manning, W. J., Dillmann, W. H., and Lorell, B. H. (2001) Transgenic expression of sarcoplasmic reticulum Ca^{2+} ATPase modifies the transition from hypertrophy to early HF. *Circ. Res.* **89,** 422–429.

36. Periasamy, M., Reed, T. D., Liu, L. H., et al. (1999) Impaired cardiac performance in heterozygous mice with a null mutation in the sarco(endo)plasmic reticulum Ca^{2+}-ATPase isoform 2 (SERCA2) gene. *J. Biol. Chem.* **274,** 2556–2562.

37. Schultz Jel, J., Glascock, B. J., Witt, S. A., et al. (2004) Accelerated onset of HF in mice during pressure overload with chronically decreased SERCA2 calcium pump activity. *Am. J. Physiol. Heart. Circ. Physiol.* **286,** H1146–H1153.
38. Meyer, M., Schillinger, W., Pieske, B., et al. (1995) Alterations of sarcoplasmic reticulum proteins in failing human dilated cardiomyopathy. *Circulation* **92,** 778–784.
39. Neumann, J., Boknik, P., DePaoli-Roach, A. A., et al. (1998) Targeted overexpression of phospholamban to mouse atrium depresses Ca^{2+} transport and contractility. *J. Mol. Cell. Cardiol.* **30,** 1991–2002.
40. Dash, R., Kadambi, V., Schmidt, A. G., et al. (2001) Interactions between phospholamban and beta-adrenergic drive may lead to cardiomyopathy and early mortality. *Circulation* **103,** 889–896.
41. Schmitt, J. P., Kamisago, M., Asahi, M., et al. (2003) Dilated cardiomyopathy and HF caused by a mutation in phospholamban. *Science* **299,** 1410–1413.
42. Crabtree, G. R. (1999) Generic signals and specific outcomes: signaling through calcium^{2+}, calcineurin and NF-AT. *Cell* **96,** 611–614.
43. Molkentin, J. D., Lu, J. R., Antos, C. L., et al. (1998) A calcineurin-dependent transcriptional pathway for cardiac hypertrophy. *Cell* **93,** 215–228.
44. Dong, D., Duan, Y., Guo, J., et al. (2003) Overexpression of calcineurin in mouse causes sudden cardiac death associated with decreased density of K^+ channels. *Cardiovasc. Res.* **57,** 320–332.
45. Molkentin, J. D. and Dorn, G. W. II. (2001) Cytoplasmic signaling pathways that regulate cardiac hypertrophy. *Annu. Rev. Physiol.* **63,** 391–426.
46. Rockman, H. A., Ross, R. S., Harris, A. N., et al. (1991) Segregation of atrial-specific and inducible expression of an atrial natriuretic factor transgene in an *in vivo* murine model of cardiac hypertrophy. *Proc. Natl. Acad. Sci. USA* **88,** 8277–8281. [Erratum re Fig. 2B is noted in *Proc. Natl. Acad. Sci. USA* **88,** 9907.]
47. Boluyt, M. O., Robinson, K. G., Meredith, A. L., et al. (2005) Heart failure after long-term supravalvular aortic constriction in rats. *Am. J. Hypertens.* **18(2 Pt 1),** 202–212.
48. Esposito, G., Rapacciuolo, A., Naga Prasad, S. V., et al. (2002) Genetic alterations that inhibit *in vivo* pressure-overload hypertrophy prevent cardiac dysfunction despite increased wall stress. *Circulation* **105,** 85–92.
49. Carabello, B. A. (1996) Models of volume overload hypertrophy. *J. Card. Fail.* **2,** 55–64.
50. Scheuermann-Freestone, M., Freestone, N. S., Langenickel, T., Hohnel, K., Dietz, R., and Willenbrock, R. (2001) A new model of congestive HF in the mouse due to chronic volume overload. *Eur. J. Heart Fail.* **5,** 535–543.

8

Animal Models for Hypertension/Blood Pressure Recording

Ralph Plehm, Marcos E. Barbosa, and Michael Bader

Summary

Hypertension is an important disease with polygenic inheritance. In order to identify the genes involved in blood pressure regulation, hypertensive rat and mouse models have been developed either by selective breeding or by transgenic technology. The most essential technological prerequisite in these studies is a reliable assessment of the blood pressure in rodents. Three methods are used most frequently for this purpose: tail cuff plethysmography, intra-arterial catheters, and radiotelemetry. Plethysmography is noninvasive, relatively simple, and suitable for a large number of animals, but also imprecise. Intra-arterial catheters are more precise, but require surgery. And both methods restrain and thereby stress the animals, which leads to alterations in blood pressure. Therefore, the telemetric blood pressure measurement, which allows the study of conscious, freely moving animals, has become the gold standard for measuring blood pressure in rodents. However, this method is extremely expensive. Thus, for each experiment the costs have to be put in relation to the quality of data required. This chapter will describe blood pressure measurement methods in technical detail.

Key Words: Blood pressure; heart rate; tail cuff plethysmography; radiotelemetry; tip catheter.

1. Introduction

Hypertension is a major health problem, contributing to stroke and myocardial infarction as well as heart and renal failure, and thereby causing the highest mortality worldwide. Blood pressure is, to a large extent, genetically determined, but the genes involved are only partially known. It is clear that hypertension is a polygenic trait, i.e., in most cases, not only one gene is involved in the development of high blood pressure but several. If these genes could be identified, therapy for hypertension could become more rational: at the moment, it is based on a few

From: *Methods in Molecular Medicine, vol. 129:*
Cardiovascular Disease: Methods and Protocols, Volume 2: Molecular Medicine
Edited by: Q. K. Wang © Humana Press Inc., Totowa, NJ

classes of drugs that are used in a trial-and-error fashion to treat patients. In order to discover the genes implicated in blood pressure regulation, animal models have been used for several decades. The classic method of creating such models has been to inbreed rats in order to select the animals with the highest blood pressure in each generation. This strategy has led to several genetically hypertensive models such as the spontaneously hypertensive rat (SHR), the spontaneously hypertensive stroke-prone rat (SHR-SP), the Dahl-S rat, and the Milan and Lyon hypertensive rats *(1)*. However, in these animals, hypertension is also polygenically inherited, and just now, on the basis of the progress made in rat genetics, the genes involved may be close to being elucidated *(2,3)*. In order to understand the contribution of single genes in the regulation of blood pressure, several transgenic rat and mouse strains have been developed, most of them targeting the renin–angiotensin system *(4)*. Two models are used most frequently. The TGR(mREN2)27 rat carries a mouse renin transgene, becomes extremely hypertensive, and shows all signs of hypertensive end-organ damage such as cardiac hypertrophy and fibrosis as well as renal damage *(5,6)*. The double transgenic rats carrying both a human renin and a human angiotensinogen transgene are even more hypertensive, being based on a humanized renin–angiotensin system, and die from end-organ damage at 7 wk of age *(7,8)*. They are ideal models by which to study human renin inhibitors, because this novel class of antihypertensive drugs acts species-specifically *(9)*.

For the phenotypical analysis of these animal models, methods for blood pressure measurements are essential. In the past, a variety of invasive and noninvasive methods have been developed to determine blood pressure in conscious rats and mice *(10,11)*. The most commonly employed techniques for the monitoring of blood pressure in these species are the use of a tail cuff device and the use of an exteriorized, fluid-filled catheter connected to a transducer near the animal. The plethysmographic tail cuff technique is noninvasive, does not require surgery, and also makes it possible to obtain repeated measurements of systolic blood pressure in conscious or slightly narcotized animals in studies with short or long duration *(12,13)*. Compared with direct, invasive methods of blood pressure determination, it has relative low costs but it is also less precise. A mercury sphygmomanometer is used in this method. The convex meniscus of the mercury level in an open-ended manometer is recorded. The rodent tail artery is compressed over a sufficiently long segment by means of an inflatable cuff. Once the artery wall's transmural pressure (pressure differences between the inside and outside of the artery) is zero, the cuff pressure corresponds to the intra-arterial blood pressure. With inflation of the cuff, the external pressure on the artery rises, and, hence, the artery is increasingly compressed. At pressures exceeding the systolic blood pressure, the artery will be occluded. When the cuff is slowly deflated, the cuff pressure, and hence the external pressure on the

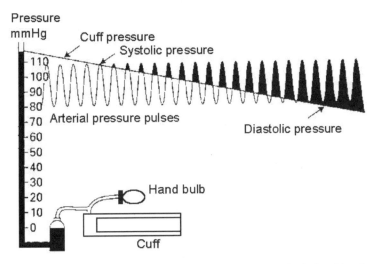

Fig. 1. The principle of tail cuff plethysmography method for blood pressure measurement.

artery, will be lowered to that of the systolic blood pressure. At this moment, small amounts of blood pass through the compressed artery segment and cause changes in artery volume conducted to the cuff. The blood flowing through the tail artery, between systolic and diastolic pressures, causes vibrations in the arterial wall (**Fig. 1**). At suprasystolic cuff pressures, small oscillations are produced. They rapidly increase in amplitude when the cuff pressure falls below systolic pressure. The point at which the amplitude of oscillations increases is generally taken to be the systolic pressure. The cuff pressure at the point of maximal amplitude corresponds to the mean arterial pressure. Pressure oscillations in the cuff related to changes in blood flow occur during occlusion or release, and this point can be sensed and measured by an aneroid manometer. Expansion of a small metal bellows is detected by a lever mechanism, which amplifies the movement and drives a pointer on a scale. Additionally, the photoelectric, oscillometric, Doppler, chamber volume, and acoustic sensors in different equipment on the market can be used to document the systolic blood pressure and diastolic blood pressure.

Continuous monitoring of arterial blood pressure using intra-arterial cannulation is a particularly useful and direct method by which to assess, with high fidelity, mean arterial blood pressure and heart hemodynamics. This procedure can be effectively used for acute studies in anesthetized and conscious animals and is more precise than tail cuff plethysmography. In this method, either a fluid-filled catheter with a pressure transducer on its distal end or a catheter containing a pressure transducer in the tip is inserted into an artery. A transducer is a device that converts energy from one form to another and, in this case, generates an electrical signal for processing and display. This voltage signal is proportional to the applied pressure and is transmitted to a signal conditioning unit, which processes it by amplification, filtering, and conversion of analog to digital. The information is then displayed or stored.

The most important problem with the methods described previously is that the animals must be restrained and sometimes anesthetized. Restraint stress and anesthesia can affect the animal's blood pressure *(14)*. Moreover, continuous recording of arterial pressure cannot be accomplished with the tail cuff method, and the duration of measurements using exteriorized catheters is limited to a maximum of 3 wk as a result of catheter problems. As a consequence of continued advances in miniaturization, telemetry systems for chronic implantation into rodents have been developed *(15)*. Pressure telemetry units small enough in size to be implanted in the aorta of mice and rats are now available. The easy-to-use wireless technology represents a significant advance in hypertension research. This system has been extensively validated in the rat, the species most frequently used in hypertension research. The availability of new mouse models based on knockout technology forced the development of smaller transmitters for this species *(16,17)*.

We describe the setup of the equipment, the surgical procedures, and the acquisition and processing of blood pressure data for tail cuff plethysmography, tip catheters, and radiotelemetry.

2. Materials

2.1. Tail Plethysmography and Intra-Arterial Blood Pressure Measurement

1. Standard surgical instruments.
2. Standard surgical suture.
3. Commercial blood pressure system equipment with table, cuff, sphygmomanometer, and oscilloscope.
4. Rodent ventilator.
5. Commercial tip catheter system/transducer/amplifier/software.
6. Rat incubator (37°C).
7. NaCl 0.9% saline solution.
8. Sodium pentobarbital.
9. Xylazine.
10. Ketamine.

2.2. Blood Pressure Telemetry

2.2.1. Hardware (Dataquest A.R.T. System)

The Dataquest A.R.T. radiotelemetry system (**Fig. 2**) consists of:

1. Ambient pressure reference (APR)-1: this device obtains the absolute value of the barometric pressure. The implantable transmitter measures the absolute pressure

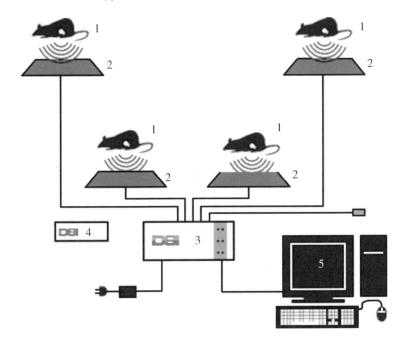

Fig. 2. Dataquest A.R.T. radiotelemetry system. (**1**) Animals containing implants; (**2**) receiver; (**3**) data exchange matrix (DEM); (**4**) ambient pressure reference (APR-1); (**5**) computer system including software and acquisition card.

so that the atmospheric must be subtracted from the overall pressure. This procedure is performed automatically by the Dataquest system. The recorded values are the blood pressure in millimeters of mercury.

2. Dataquest PCI card, the aquisition card located in the computer that is connected to the data exchange matrix (DEM).
3. Receiver (i.e., RPC-1 for rats and mice in plastic cages): the receiver amplifies and detects the signal from the transmitter and converts it to a digital signal, which can be decoded from the acquisition computer.
4. DEM: the DEM provides a link between the receiver and the Dataquest system and allows the telemetry receivers and the DEM to be located within the animal room and the computer in a remote location.
5. Personal computer, Pentium 4 (Windows 2000 or Windows XP).

2.2.2. Software

Dataquest A.R.T. 3.1.

2.2.3. Animal Implants

1. TA11PA-C40 for rats (**Fig. 3**).
2. TA11PA-C20 or TA11PA-C10 for mice.

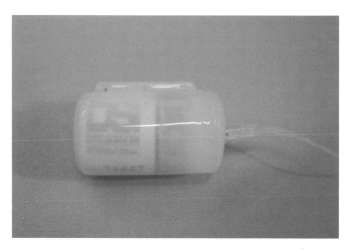

Fig. 3. TA11 PA-C40 rat blood pressure implant.

These devices consist of a catheter, which is inserted into the blood vessel, a pressure transducer to convert the blood pressure into an electrical signal, a temperature compensation, and a radio transmitter that sends the signal to the receiver. A reasonable number of animal implants (at least double the animals that one plans to use in the experiment) is necessary to provide continuous experimental work. These implants are the most expensive part of the telemetry system in purchase and maintenance.

2.2.4. Anesthesia Unit

Univentor 400 from Univentor High Precision Instruments, Malta. This unit is designed to control the anesthesia of animals weighing from 20 to 500 g and is calibrated for isoflurane.

An air-conditioned, sound-absorbent room, equipped with a flexible light regime to provide a day–night cycle (*see* **Note 1**), is required.

3. Methods
3.1. Tail Cuff Plethysmography

1. Select the animals (*see* **Note 2**).
2. Prepare the equipment as described in the instructions of the manufacturer.
3. Calibrate the equipment as required.
4. Determine the body weight of the rat.
5. Inject 30 mg/kg sodium pentobarbital intraperitoneally (*see* **Note 3**).
6. Prewarm the animals in an incubator 37°C for 10 min prior to the measurements.
7. Place the rat on the equipment table.
8. Fit the cuff around the tail of the rat (*see* **Note 4**).

9. Inflate the cuff with a hand-bulb sphygmomanometer until it reaches a pressure of approx 30 mmHg above systolic pressure.
10. Slowly deflate the cuff at a rate of 3–4 mmHg/s, watching the pulse display on the oscilloscope.
11. Note the reading on the oscilloscope when the pulsations reappear during deflation. Register the value as the systolic pressure (**Fig. 1**).
12. Repeat the process at least three times at 3-min intervals.
13. Let the animal recover.

3.2. Tip Catheter

1. Select the animals.
2. Prepare the surgical instruments.
3. Prepare and calibrate the equipment and software as required per the manufacturer's instructions.
4. Follow basic institutional guidelines to perform animal handling.
5. Determine the body weight of the rat.
6. Anesthetise the rat with 10 mg/kg xylazine and 50 mg/kg ketamine intraperitoneally (*see* **Note 5**).
7. Fix the animal in supine position on a 37°C surgery table.
8. Retract the tongue of the rat, cannulate the trachea, and connect a rodent ventilator.
9. Isolate and expose the carotid artery through a midline incision over the trachea and throat of the rat (*see* **Note 6**).
10. Three sutures are required before the introduction of the catheter:
    a. The first suture is placed distal and just proximal to carotid sinus and ligated.
    b. A proximal suture is placed close to the chest area and it is not closed.
    c. Just in the middle, a suture is placed between the proximal and distal sutures; do not close until the catheter is introduced.
11. Make a small incision on the carotid, just enough to introduce the catheter.
12. Close the middle suture to prevent or reduce blood flow when introducing the catheter.
13. Introduce and advance the catheter in the carotid.
14. The introduced catheter is able to record the mean blood pressure.
15. Advance the catheter to the heart's left ventricle.
16. Record the hemodynamics and cardiac parameters.
17. Retract the catheter and take it carefully out of the artery.
18. Prepare the animal for blood and tissue collection.

3.3. Blood Pressure Telemetry

3.3.1. System Installation (Use the Manual)

1. System installation according to the manufacturer's (DSI's) instruction.
2. Connect the DEM to the PCI card, connect all of the matrices together, and connect the receivers and the APR to a matrix (*see* **Note 7**).

3. Configure the hardware.
4. Prepare your study and create a study folder.

3.3.2. Transmitter Implantation

1. Transmitter calibration. The blood pressure implants are supplied with three calibration values. Test the true zero line on a receiver prior to implantation. Switch on the transmitter some hours before. Put the sterile package containing the transmitter flat on a receiver, enter the calibration data into the system, and choose the "Continuous Sampling Trace" function. The deviation should be within the range of +/– 4 mmHg. Otherwise, contact the company.
   Note the value of deviation. You can enter this offset value into the acquisition program to correct the blood pressure data.
2. Preparation of the transmitter. Place the transmitter in a beaker of sterile saline. Chill it to about 6–10°C in a freezer. The chilling will stiffen the catheter to make it easier to insert into the vessel. The saline is required in order to fill the hydrophilic catheter and transmitter material prior to implantation.
3. Anesthesia. Do not feed the animals for 12–24 h prior to implantation. Use an isoflurane anesthesia unit (e.g., Univentor 400 from Univentor LTD, Malta).
   Initial phase:

   Put the animal (especially rats) in a chamber until the animal is asleep.
   Flow: Mice: approx 400–500 mL/min
         Rats: approx 700–800 mL/min
         Concentration: approx 4.5%

   During implantation:

   Once the animal is asleep, turn the stopcock, route the gas to the mask, and decrease concentration and airflow:
   Flow: Mice: approx 150–250 mL/min
         Rats: approx 400–500 mL/min
         Concentration: 1.7–2.5%

4. Shave the abdomen of the animal and fix the animal on the desk. Place a stack of gauze pads at the left side of the animal near the tail root to a height even with the abdomen. This will support the transmitter body during the insertion of the catheter.
5. Make an incision 4–5 cm (2–3 cm for mice) long in the skin along the midline.
6. Expose the descending aorta. Use sterile, warm, saline-soaked gauze pads and retractor to retain the intestines aside of the aorta.
7. Expose the descending aorta below the renal arteries.
8. Isolate the lower abdominal aorta from the vena cava.
9. Insert a ligature (Perma-Hand Seide 5-0 [6-0 for mice], Ethicon) around the abdominal aorta caudal to the renal artery. Use this suture to temporarily occlude the blood flow in the aorta for the implantation of the transmitter catheter. Alternatively, the blood flow can be stopped by pressing on the aorta with a sterile cotton swab. We have used both techniques successfully.

10. Catheter insertion. Curve the distal 1 cm of a sterile 20 G (mice 29 G) needle at a 45° angle with the beveled surface of the needle on the outside radius. If you implant the transmitter in a mouse, rinse the vessel before the implantation with 2% lidocaine in order to relax the muscular vessel walls. Place the mouse on a heated table during and after the surgery. After vessel occlusion, use the curved needle to puncture the vessel 1–2 mm anterior to the bifurcation and insert the transmitter catheter through the small hole (*see* **Note 8**).

Insert the catheter so that all of the thin-walled section is within the vessel (*see* **Note 9**).

Then, dry the catheter entry area with cotton swabs and seal the catheter in place with Vetbond tissue adhesive.

Apply a patch of paper fiber over the entry point and fix this also with tissue adhesive.

Carefully replace the intestine, and fix the body of the catheter on the abdominal musculature with a 4-0 nonabsorbable suture by passing the suture through the muscle and the tab located along the length of transmitter body. Keep the intestines moist during the surgery by rinsing the cavity with prewarmed 0.9% saline. Close the wound by suture. The skin can be closed by suture or wound clips. The clips are preferred only if the suture is eaten up by the animal in the recovery period (*see* **Note 10**).

11. Recovery. Administer a small dose of ampicillin (i.e., Binotal, Bayer Leverkusen) as a safeguard against infection. After implantation, keep the animal warm on a heated table or under a red light lamp. The animals should be allowed to recover from surgery for 10 d before starting any measurement.

3.3.3. Data Acquisition and Analysis

The process of data acquisition and analysis is described detailed in the DSI manual.

1. Parameters derived from the waveform:
   a. Systolic blood pressure (SBP).
   b. Mean arterial pressure (MAP).
   c. Diastolic blood pressure (DBP).
   d. Heart rate (HR).
   e. Respiration inter-breath interval. This is a special option called RespiRATE.
   f. Pulse pressure.
2. Parameters not derived from the waveform:
   a. Motor activity.
   b. Signal strength (only for technical reasons).
3. Two different types of data acquisition are distinguished:
   a. Discontinuous recording of one data set for every animal (i.e., every 5 min). This is the usual way to record the data from a large number of animals. One can investigate the parameter itself and the time course of the data (for instance,

the day–night rhythm, long-term fluctuations, and the effect of drugs). The amount of data is limited.

b. Continuous recording of the blood pressure waveform. This data recording mode allows a more sophisticated analysis and is necessary for short-term spectral analysis, for beat-to-beat analysis, and to investigate the interaction between heart rate and blood pressure (baroreflex). The amount of data is very high and the number of simultaneous registrations is restricted to only four animals per DEM. The waveform registration is an additional tool for a registration length of few hours (*see* **Note 11**).

3.3.4. Data Backup

1. Avoid loss of the data obtained in telemetry studies, as they are unique and valuable. Copy the data daily on a medium that is stored outside the computer room.
2. Use a battery backup system for your acquisition computer (i.e., UPS RS 1000 from APC). A break in the power supply or a voltage fluctuation could stop the acquisition and lead to a gap in the data (*see* **Note 12**).

3.3.5. Transmitter Reuse

The costs are the major disadvantage of blood pressure telemetry, not only the cost of acquiring the initial equipment, but also that of the periodic refurbishment of the transmitters (*see* **Note 13**). We have successfully reused telemetry transmitters up to three times before returning them to the manufacturer for refurbishment. The number of times depends on the implantation time of prior experiments.

1. Switch off the transmitter.
2. Sacrifice the animal and explant the transmitter.
3. Clean the transmitter.
4. Sterilize the transmitters in 2% lysoformin (Lysoform, Berlin, Germany) for 24 h.
5. Wash the transmitters in clear water.
6. Refill the catheter tip carefully according to the manufacturer's instructions.
7. Control the zero line.
8. Write down the deviation value. Enter this value into the acquisition program when configuring the next experiment using this transmitter. This is one additional step after entering the calibration values. Click "Advanced" in the "Signal Properties" window. The last value is "Offset." Enter the earlier measured zero line deviation here.

4. Notes

1. The computer should not be placed in this room.
2. It is very important that a single technician perform the measurements each day at the same time. It is recommended that the technician be experienced and trained to notice the instance pulsations when they reappear during deflation.

3. Ethylic ether can be an alternative to sodium pentobarbital injection for the light anesthesthetizing of the animals, but it is no longer in use in the United States and some other countries.

4. The cuff size is very important because this component differs for animals in different ages. Its width should be 20% greater than the diameter of the tail. The use of noncoherent cuffs for the measurement leads to imprecise results, or strong difficulty in determining and acquiring signals during repeat measurements. A smaller cuff overestimates blood pressure and a larger one underestimates it.

5. Isofluran can also be used as narcotic (*see* **Subheading 3.3.2.**).

6. To expose the carotid, dissect carefully to avoid damage to the vagal nerve, which may affect cardiac hemodynamics.

7. The distance between two receivers should not be less than 40 cm because of cross-talking.

8. As visibility is poor during bleeding, it is useful to mark the end of the thin-walled section by a waterproof pencil so as to ensure that the catheter is inserted deeply enough.

9. Use an AM radio. After insertion of the catheter, open the blood flow for a short moment. If you hear the modulation of the blood pressure wave, then the catheter position is right. Then, stop the blood flow again.

10. Control the suture daily in the first week. Rarely, the animals chew the suture and open the cavity.

11. Sampling rate: rat, 250–500 Hz; mouse, 500–1000 Hz.

12. The price of the backup system is lower than that of refurbishing one transmitter.

13. Save battery power by switching off the transmitters as often as possible, e.g., during the recovery period and immediately after the end of the study.

References

1. Horie, R., Kihara, M., Lovenberg, W., et al. (1986) Comparison of various genetic hypertensive rat strains. *J. Hypertens. Suppl.* **4,** S11–S14.

2. Hübner, N., Wallace, C. A., Zimdahl, H., et al. (2005) Integrated transcriptional profiling and linkage analysis for identification of genes underlying disease. *Nat. Genet.* **37,** 243–253.

3. The Rat Genome Sequencing Consortium. (2004) Genome sequence of the Brown Norway rat yields insights into mammalian evolution. *Nature* **428,** 493–521.

4. Bader, M. and Ganten, D. (2004) Transgenics of the RAS, in *Handbook of Experimental Pharmacology: Angiotensin,* (Unger, T. and Schölkens, B. A., eds.), Springer Verlag, Heidelberg, Germany: pp. 229–249.

5. Mullins, J. J., Peters, J., and Ganten, D. (1990) Fulminant hypertension in transgenic rats harbouring the mouse Ren-2 gene. *Nature* **344,** 541–544.

6. Lee, M. A., Böhm, M., Paul, M., Bader, M., Ganten, U., and Ganten, D. (1996) Physiological characterization of the hypertensive transgenic rat TGR(mREN2)27. *Am. J. Physiol.* **270,** E919–E929.

7. Ganten, D., Wagner, J., Zeh, K., et al. (1992) Species specificity of renin kinetics in transgenic rats harboring the human renin and angiotensinogen genes. *Proc. Natl. Acad. Sci. USA* **89,** 7806–7810.

8. Luft, F. C., Mervaala, E., Müller, D. N., et al. (1999) Hypertension-induced end-organ damage: a new transgenic approach to an old problem. *Hypertension* **33,** 212–218.

9. Bohlender, J., Fukamizu, A., Lippoldt, A., et al. (1997) High human renin hypertension in transgenic rats. *Hypertension* **29,** 428–434.

10. Pickering, T. G. (2002) Principles and techniques of blood pressure measurement. *Cardiol. Clin.* **20,** 207–223.

11. Kurtz, T. W., Griffin, K. A., Bidani, A. K., Davisson, R. L., and Hall, J. E. (2005) American Heart Association: recommendations for blood pressure measurement in humans and experimental animals. Part 2: blood pressure measurement in experimental animals: a statement for professionals from the subcommittee of professional and public education of the American Heart Association council on high blood pressure research. *Hypertension* **45,** 299–310.

12. Beevers, G., Lip, G. Y. H., and O'Brien, E. (2001) Blood pressure measurement. Conventional sphygmomanometry: Technique of auscultatory blood pressure measurement: Part II. *Brit. Med. J.* **322,** 1043–1047.

13. Lee, R. P., Wang, D., Lin, N. T., Chou, Y. W., and Chen, H. I. (2002) A modified technique for tail cuff pressure measurement in unrestrained conscious rats. *J. Biomed. Sci.* **9,** 424–427.

14. Vatner, S. F. (1976) Effects of anesthesia on cardiovascular control mechanisms. *Environ. Health Perspect.* **26,** 193–206.

15. Brockway, B., Mills, P., and Azar, S. (1991) A new method for continuous chronic measurement and recording of blood pressure, heart rate and activity in the rat via radiotelemetry. *Clin. Exp. Hypertens. A.* **13,** 885–895.

16. Gross, V., Milia, A. F., Plehm, R., Inagami, T., and Luft, F. C. (2000) Long-term blood pressure telemetry in AT2 receptor-disrupted mice. *J. Hypertens.* **18,** 955–961.

17. Bader, M. (2005) Mouse knockout models for hypertension, in *Hypertension: Methods and Protocols,* (Fennell, J. and Baker, A. H., eds.), Humana Press, Totowa, NJ: pp. 17–32.

9

Animal Models for Cardiac Arrhythmias

Sandro L. Yong and Qing K. Wang

Summary

Transgenic and gene-targeted mice are now frequently used to expand the study of cardiac physiology and pathophysiology owing to the ease with which the mouse genome can be manipulated. There are many measures by which an assessment of the phenotypical expression of the transgenic mouse can be made. In the case of cardiac channelopathies and how they relate to cardiac function, telemetry is a technology that utilizes transmitters that are surgically implanted in animals for the purpose of acquiring biopotentials or physioloigical parameters. Electrophysiological techniques have also been used to assess cardiac function at the cellular level, by measuring whole-cell ionic currents and/or transmembrane potentials. This chapter will discuss the surgical procedures involved in successfully implanting the transmitter device in a mouse, as well as highlight the recording of and analysis of electrocardiograms. This chapter will also outline the procedures involved in isolating single-ventricular myocytes from a mouse heart. It is a protocol that was developed in our laboratory for which we have routinely and successfully isolated myocytes from both transgenic and nontransgenic mouse hearts. Although no one isolation protocol is alike, we also present our own observations that have assisted in maximizing myocyte bioavailability and yield.

Key Words: Arrhythmia; cardiac; electrophysiology; isolated myocytes; perfusion; SCN5A; telemetry; transgenic.

1. Introduction

In cardiac research, telemetry is often used as a noninvasive form of recording electrocardiograms (ECGs) from the animal of interest. This technology and its application will be discussed in the mouse whose genomic sequence has been modified with a cardiac sodium channel mutation (*1*). Unlike isolated hearts or myocyte preparations, telemetry affords researchers the means to evaluate the effects of genetic modifications on the heart as it exists in the animal as a whole. The required supplies and guidelines for selecting an implant site, administrating anesthesia, a brief description of the surgical procedures, and postsurgical

From: *Methods in Molecular Medicine, vol. 129:*
Cardiovascular Disease: Methods and Protocols, Volume 2: Molecular Medicine
Edited by: Q. K. Wang © Humana Press Inc., Totowa, NJ

antibiotics/analgesia will be discussed. Much of the details are in accordance to Data Sciences International, the leading vendor of this technology.

When a more in-depth assessment of cardiac function is required, an examination at the level of the single cell may be warranted. The techniques for isolating mammalian, nonhuman, cardiac myocytes have evolved considerably. The heterogeneous animals that are available and the different experimental purposes for their isolation have made myocyte isolation an often "elaborate" and nonuniversal technique. In principle, the process is simple. It is a technique that relies on the ability to perfuse the heart with different buffer and enzyme solutions to degrade and loosen the intracellular and collagen matrixes that connect the myocytes to each other in the myocardium. However, there is no universal consensus on a standardized protocol for isolating myocytes from one particular animal species. Often, it is one laboratory that adapts one method from several other laboratories and incorporates their own nuances and variations to develop their own distinct isolation protocol. It is the reproducibility and success of one method that sets it apart from other isolation procedures. And, over time, such isolation methods will become increasingly more refined. This chapter represents a step toward contributing to that refinement. Briefly, this protocol entails removing the heart, cannulating the aorta on a perfusion system, arresting the heart with a retrograde perfusion of calcium-free buffer, dissociating myocytes using a collagenase-based enzymatic solution, and reintroducing calcium to successfully isolate single, quiescent, rod-shaped myocytes.

With such advancements in transgenesis, particularly involving the mouse genome, characterizing phenotypical expression along with the investigation of single cardiac myocytes both stand to be invaluable arsenals in cardiovascular research. However, the utility of the mouse as a model to study human diseases remains controversial and should be interpreted and extrapolated with caution given the marked electrophysiological differences between mouse and human hearts. The inherent possibilities and advantages of nonhuman models often outweigh such limitations. As such, this chapter is targeted at new researchers in this field, with particular emphasis on several aspects in the isolation procedure that are important for optimizing acute myocyte isolation and bioavailability. General electrophysiological techniques for recording ion currents or transmembrane voltage changes from single myocytes will also be discussed.

2. Materials

2.1. Telemetry

2.1.1. Hardware

1. ETA/EA-F20: an implantable mouse transmitter device (**Fig. 1**).
2. RPC-1 receivers: platforms onto which a housing cage can be placed to monitor mice housed in their basin cages.

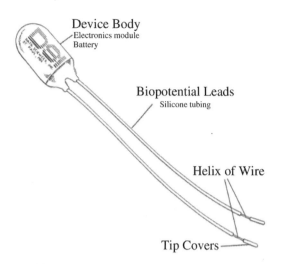

Fig. 1. The implantable mouse transmitter device (ETA/EA-F20), which consists of a body that houses the electronics and battery supply. Two biopotential leads extend from this body and are used to receive and transmit surface biopontentials to the transmitter body.

3. Dataquest A.R.T. Data Acquisition System: software package used to collect and analyze electrical signals from one or several receivers and graphically represent these signals as waveforms.
4. A standard Pentium desktop computer with sufficient processing and memory capabilities, as recommended by the software manufacturer, to collect, display, and store data.

2.1.2. Surgical Instruments and Supplies

1. One small dissecting scissor (cat. no. 14393-G, straight, 10 cm; World Precision Instruments).
2. One medium surgical scissor (cat. no. 501754, sharp/sharp, 11.5 cm; World Precision Instruments).
3. One large surgical forceps (cat. no. 500178-G, 1 × 2 teeth, 12 cm; World Precision Instruments).
4. Scalpel and blade.
5. Large trocar (D70).
6. 2 × 2 sterile gauze.
7. Sterile cotton-tip applicators.
8. Sterile drape.
9. 70% ethanol.
10. Surgical gloves.
11. Mask and cap (if desired).
12. Heating pad or lamp.

Table 1
Myocyte Isolation Buffers

	Incubation buffer (mM)	Perfusion buffer (mM)
NaCl	118	118
KCl	4.8	4.8
MgCl$_2$	2.5	2.5
KH$_2$PO$_4$	1.2	1.2
CaCl$_2$	1.2	–
Glucose	11	11
HEPES	25	–
Pyruvic Acid	4.9	4.9
NaHCO$_3$	–	13.8
pH	–	7.2 with 95%O$_2$/5%CO$_2$

2.2. Isolation of Single Cardiac Myocytes and Electrophysiological Recordings

2.2.1. Myocyte Isolation Buffers

Please refer to **Table 1**. Incubation buffer is made in advance, alliquoted in 50-mL tubes, and stored at –4°C, whereas the perfusion buffer is prepared at the day of isolation. Buffer solutions should be made with double-distilled water. Used glassware should be thoroughly washed with a mild, organically based detergent (e.g., Sparkleen, Fisher) along with the help of a flexible bottle brush, and rinsed with double distilled water.

2.2.2. Perfusion Materials and Collagenase

The following are the "dry" materials that are prepared at the day of isolation.

1. Take five empty 15-mL test tubes and label them 1, 2, 3, 4, and 5.
2. Weigh out 200 mg of bovine serum albumin (BSA;, Fraction V, Sigma) into tubes 4 and 5.
3. Weigh out 20 mg of BSA into tube 1.
4. Weigh out 0.04 mg/mL protease (10.5 U/mg, Type XXIV, Sigma) into tube 2 (*see* **Note 1**).
5. Weigh out 0.07 mg/mL trypsin (1000–2000 BAEE U/mg; Type II, Sigma) into tube 3 (*see* **Note 1**).
6. Collagenase (*see* **Note 2**). From our most recent batch (Type II, 205 U/mg, 4.06 U/mg Clostripain, Worthington), 40–45 mg is weighed out.

Table 2
Whole-Cell Action Potential Recordings

	External (mM)	Internal (mM)
NaCl	140	–
KCl	4	135
CaCl$_2$	1.8	–
MgCl$_2$	2	2
EGTA	–	10
HEPES	10	10
Glucose	10	5
pH	7.2 (with 5 N NaOH)	7.2 (with 5 N KOH)
mOsm	approx 308	approx 308

Table 3
Inward Sodium Current (I_{Na}) Recordings

	External (mM)	Internal (mM)
NaCl	20	–
CsCl	110	130
KCl	–	–
CaCl$_2$	1.8	0.5
CoCl$_2$	2	–
MgCl$_2$	2 mM	2
Na$_2$ATP	–	5
GTP	–	0.5
EGTA	–	5
HEPES	10	10
Glucose	10	10
pH	7.2 (with 1 N CsOH)	7.2 (with 1 N CsOH)
mOsm	approx 303	approx 304

2.2.3. Electrophysiological Recording Solutions

Tables 2–5 list the chemical ingredients and concentrations for the recording solutions. Each is listed for the recording of whole-cell action potentials, I_{Na}, I_{TO}, and $I_{Ca,L}$.

Table 4
Transient Outward Potassium Current (I$_{TO}$) Recordings

	External (mM)	Internal (mM)
NaCl	140	–
KCl	4	135
CaCl$_2$	1.8	–
MgCl$_2$	2	2
CoCl$_2$	5	–
EGTA	–	10
HEPES	10	10
Glucose	10	5
Tetrodotoxin	0.02	–
pH	7.2	7.2
	(with 5 N NaOH)	(with 5 N KOH)
mOsm	approx 310	approx 308

Table 5
L-Type Inward Calcium Current (I$_{Ca,L}$) Recordings

	External (mM)	Internal (mM)
NaCl	140	–
CsCl	10	120
CaCl$_2$	2	–
MgCl$_2$	1.2	1.2
Mg$_2$ATP	–	5
HEPES	10	10
Glucose	10	5
Tetrodotoxin	0.02	–
pH	7.2	7.2
	(with 5 N NaOH)	(with 1 N CsOH)
mOsm	approx 308	approx 308

2.2.4. Isolation Glassware and Hardware

The glassware and hardware required to perfuse mouse hearts are assembled and illustrated in **Fig. 2**. This schematic depicts a typical assembly of the essential components. Variations of this assembly and its components exist among many laboratories, but the underlying framework is the same. In the following, the main components are enumerated and discussed.

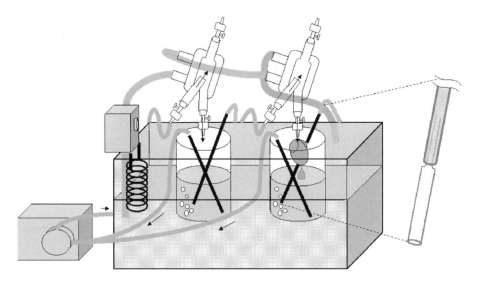

Fig. 2. The perfusion apparatus. This diagram highlights the main components that are essential in its assembly; *see* **Subheading 2.2.4.** for details. The inset shows a magnified view of how the glass pipets are inserted (narrow-tip first) into the perfusion tube lines.

1. Two standard Pyrex glass beakers are required, preferably in volumes of 100 and 125 mL; the different volume sizes help to distinguish between the two perfusates. These beakers will contain the perfusate buffer solutions such that the beakers will be submersed just below the level of the buffer in the large, water-filled heating chamber **(Fig. 2)**. The submersion will help maintain the temperature in the perfusate solutions at a constant 37°C.
2. Integral components in the perfusion system include two water-filled heating bubble-trap jackets (cat. no. 120150, Radnoti) just above the beaker chambers. The design of the bubble traps helps remove gas bubbles that may be introduced during aeration or perfusate flow. Removing air bubbles in the perfusate reduces the risk of coronary embolization. The internal chamber is water-jacketed to prevent cooling of the perfusate.
3. A lab stand from Radnoti (cat. no. 159953-2) is a heavy-duty steel base with support rods that is specially designed to support all the glassware and perfusion accessories into a compact assembly.
4. The transference and recirculation of buffer solutions is performed using a variable-flow peristaltic pump. An ideal feature of the pump is a digital flow rate control for fine-tuning capability. The flow rate range of the pump should be broad for adaptability with a minimum range of 0.5 to 2 mL/min to accommodate the perfusion requirements of the mouse hearts. It should be noted that flow rate is also proportional tubing diameter.
5. Tubing made from a flexible, silicone composite (e.g., Tygon) offers the best durability and resiliency for peristaltic pumps. Two continuous but separate perfusing

lines will be required—one dedicated to the Ca^{2+}-free perfusate and the other to the Ca^{2+}-containing perfusate.

6. For heating the large, open water-filled chamber, a thermostatically controlled immersion heater with water circulation capability is ideal (e.g., cat. no. 13-873-44A, Fisher). The preferred style is one in which it can be clamped to the edge of the chamber with the stainless steel coil immersed in the water. Most models have a temperature range of up to 100°C and are equipped with an automatic shut-off feature for maintaining a constant temperature.

7. Hardware for securing the beakers over the open water-filled chamber includes three-prong clamps (e.g., cat. no. 21570-127, VWR or cat. no. 05-769-8, Fisher). To reduce perfusate splatter, standard funnels (plastic or Pyrex) are held in position above the beakers by support rings (e.g., cat. no. 60130-004, VWR) to direct perfusate flow from the bubble-jackets to their respective beakers below.

8. For measuring the pH and temperature of the buffer solutions, a standard digital bench-top pH/temperature meter (e.g., Mettler, Orion, Beckman Coulter) is sufficient. Different models require separate pH and temperature electrode probes. To minimize space requirements in and around the work area during perfusion, one recommendation would be the use of a combination pH/temperature electrode probe (e.g., InLab* 1010 Open Junction Combination pH Electrode, Mettler Toledo).

9. The perfusion procedure requires accurate time keeping. As such, a multichannel digital timer with countdown capability is an essential requirement.

10. To minimize the introduction of foreign particles (e.g., dust) into the filtered perfusate when transferring the solubilized solutions from tubes 1 and 2, a sterilized syringe (~5 cc, Becton Dickinson) and syringe filter (25 mm, 0.22 μm, Whatman) assembly are used. This step is in accordance to reducing the risk of developing coronary embolism.

11. In keeping with the reduction of foreign particle contamination, plastic and disposable transfer pipets (cat. no. 202, Samco) are also used when handling solutions.

12. To reduce foreign particle contamination from the plastic tubing that is used in the transference of solutions throughout the perfusion system, disposable Pyrex Pasteur pipets are used to make the contact between the tubes and the buffer solutions (*see* **Subheading 3.3.**).

13. Surgical instruments used in the heart isolation procedure are enumerated:

    a. One dissecting microscope (cat. no. 43300-516, VWR) with a zoom range of ×0.65 to ×4.5 and a working distance of 89 mm.

    b. One fiber optics light source illuminator (cat. no. 43300-740, VWR) and bifurcated light guide (cat. no. 4330-738, VWR).

    c. One small dissecting scissor (cat. no. 14393-G, straight, 10 cm, World Precision Instruments).

    d. One medium surgical scissor (cat. no. 501754, sharp/sharp, 11.5 cm, World Precision Instruments).

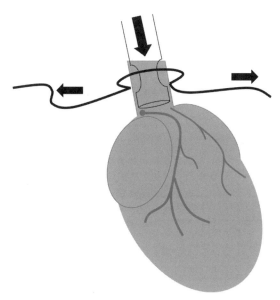

Fig. 3. The proper cannulation of a mouse heart. The aorta is slipped just above the beveled section of the buffer-filled needle and the aorta and heart are secured with a suture line along this beveled section.

    e. Two fine surgical forceps (cat. no. 555229F, tips bent at 45°, 11 cm, World Precision Instruments).

    f. One large surgical forceps (cat. no. 500178-G, 1 × 2 teeth, 12 cm, World Precision Instruments).

    g. A single 1-cc syringe and a 20-G syringe needle (Becton Dickinson); the needle is modified with tapered sides along the outside of the blunt-ended tip (**Fig. 3**; *see* **Note 3**).

2.2.5. Electrophysiological Hardware

1. Nikon ECLIPSE TE300 Inverted Microscope.
2. Burleigh PCS-500 Micromanipulator with SSH Steep/Shallow Headstage Adapter.
3. Burleigh PCS-500-19 Mounting Bracket.
4. Kinetic System Vibration Isolation Table (cat. no. 9101-01-85).
5. Bioptech Delta T Open Dish System (cat. no. 0420-4-03): a temperature-controlled heating stage with 35 mm OD and 23-mm central aperture dishes.
6. Narishge Vertical Pipet Puller (cat. no. PP-830).
7. Narishige Microforge (cat. no. MF-830) for fire-polishing microelectrode tips.
8. Axon Instruments MultiClamp 700A-2.
9. Axon Instruments Digidata 1322A.
10. Axon Instruments pClamp 9.0 Acquisition and Analysis Software.
11. Standard desktop Pentium computer.

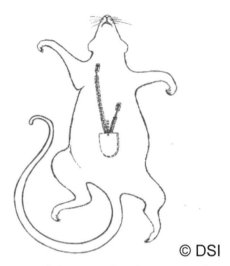

© DSI

Fig. 4. The ideal placement of the transmitter in a mouse, in accordance with the manufacturer's specifications for optimal capture of biopotential signals. The lead placement is also in accordance with the lead II configuration for electrocardiograms.

3. Methods

3.1. Surgical Procedure

The following steps describe procedures for implanting an intraperiotneal transmitter **(Fig. 4)**.

1. Administer the desired anesthesia.
2. Remove the hair from the ventral abdomen and at the sites of lead placement.
3. Disinfect the area with 70% alcohol.
4. Position the sterile drape.
5. Make an incision large enough to accommodate the implant along the abdominal midline immediately caudal to the xyphoid space.
6. Place the device body into the abdominal cavity with the suture rib up.
7. Make a small incision at the site of the negative lead placement.
8. Tunnel subcutaneously from the abdominal incision to approx 1 cm beyond the lead incision using a trocar.
9. Slide the plastic sleeve over the end of the trocar and use the trocar to guide the sleeve into the prepared tunnel.
10. Remove the trocar, leaving the sleeve in place.
11. Shorten the leads to the appropriate length by placing the leads in their approximate position. As shown in **Fig. 4**, the leads are placed in a Lead II configuration (*see* **Note 4**).
12. Pass the 14-G needle through the abdominal wall lateral to the cranial aspect of the incision, going from the outside into the abdominal cavity.
13. Pass one of the leads through the needle and out of the abdomen.

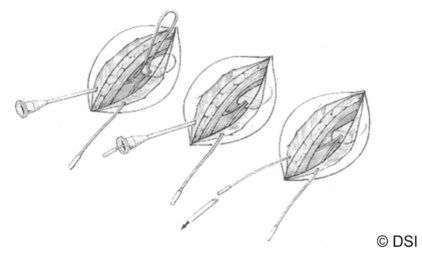

© DSI

Fig. 5. The surgical placement of the transmitter device into the abdominal cavity; *see* **Subheading 3.1.** for details. In brief, the transmitter body is inserted inside the abdominal cavity while the two biopotential leads are inserted through the abdominal wall.

14. Withdraw the needle leaving the lead externalized.
15. Once externalized, pass the lead through the waiting plastic sleeve to the desired site and remove the sleeve.
16. Cut around the silicone tubing on the tip of the lead using a sharp sterile blade and remove 1.5 cm of the silicone to expose the stainless steel wire.
17. Bluntly dissect the muscle fibers at the desired site to provide a shallow area in which to place the electrode. Place the lead within the muscle tissue and secure the lead by suturing to the muscle tissue up over the lead using a 4-0 nonabsorbable suture.
18. Secure the transmitter body by closing the abdominal incision and incorporating the suture rib of the implant into the closure using suture in a simple interrupted pattern (**Fig. 5**).
19. Close the skin incisions using suture.
20. Place the animal into a warm environment.
21. Monitor the animal's recovery until it is fully awake.
22. Administer postsurgical antibiotics and/or analgesics.
23. After recovery (2–3 d after surgery), place the cage with the animal on the telemetry monitoring platform (the receiver), and start to collect data with the Dataquest A.R.T. Data Acquisition System following the detailed instructions from the manufacturer. The data are stored and analyzed in a computer with the Acquisition System software.

3.2. Sample ECG Traces

Following the manufacture's instructions for the telemetry system, electrocardiographic activity of the animal is recorded. The following ECG traces were chosen to illustrate the benefits of telemetry in detecting cardiac abnormalities.

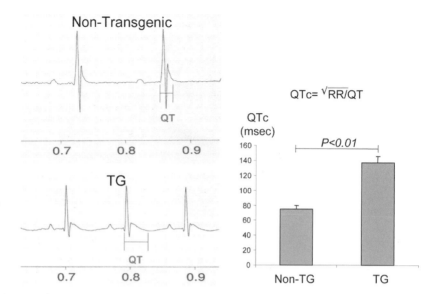

Fig. 6. ECGs from a nontransgenic and transgenic (TG) mouse. The QT interval is shown from the start of the Q wave to the end of the T wave. The QT intervals for both mouse groups were corrected for heart rate with Bazette's formula and the averaged corrected values for each group are graphically represented. The QTc interval for TG mice was significantly longer than for non-TG mice. (Reproduced from **ref.** *1*, with permission.)

Figure 6 shows the phenotypical expression as a consequence of the gain-of-function sodium channel SCN5A mutation, $N_{1325}S$ *(1)*. The $N_{1325}S$ mutation results in the long QT phenotype that is most commonly found in humans. More specifically, the QT interval (*see* **Note 5**) in TG mice was significantly prolonged compared with non-TG mice and this was corrected for heart rate using Bazette's formula (*see* **Note 6**).

Other traces (**Figs. 7–9**) illustrate other cardiac dysrhythmias from the transgenic mouse model that would not otherwise be apparent at the cellular level. As such, these traces are a testament to the power that is afforded by telemetry in increasing the detection tools in cardiac research and, thus, the knowledge-base for identifying and characterizing genetically based cardiac diseases.

3.3. Preparation of Perfusion Apparatus

1. Run distilled water through the perfusion system and bring the large heating water chamber to 37°C.
2. Two incubation buffer (50 mL) tubes are made available from the freezer; one tube is brought to 37°C by immersing it in the large, heating water bath chamber while the second is thawed to liquid between –5 and 0°C at room temperature.

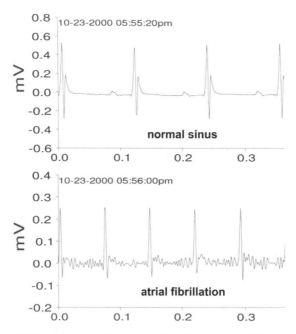

Fig. 7. Mouse ECG with normal sinus that is subsequently followed by atrial fibrillation. Note the shorter RR interval in the lower trace.

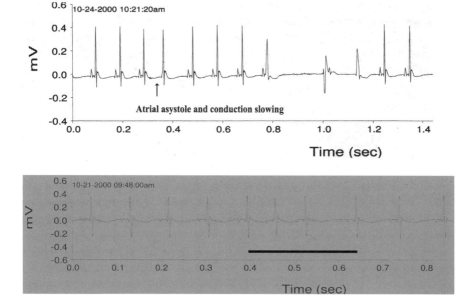

Fig. 8. Sample of ECG traces showing atrial dysrhythmias and conduction abnormalities.

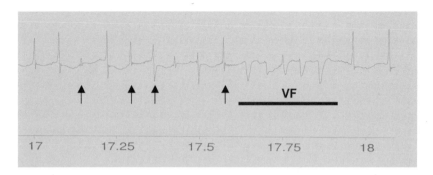

Fig. 9. Representative ECG trace from a transgenic mouse in normal sinus (upper trace) followed by premature ventricular contractions (arrows) and a brief episode of ventricular fibrillation (VF). The lower trace is the continuation of the trace that shows a sustained episode of VF.

3. The perfusion buffer is prepared at the day of isolation and, once in solution, it is filtered using a 500-mL vacuum receiver with a filter holder (cat. no. 28199-440, Nalgene) that holds a 47-mm, 0.45-µm cellulose nitrate membrane (cat. no. 7184-004, Whatman).

4. Volumes of 80 and 100 mL of the filtered perfusate are transferred into the 100- and 125-mL glass beakers, respectively.

5. Into the 80- and 100-mL perfusate solutions, respectively, add 0.0375 mM EGTA and 1.2 mM $CaCl_2$. The perfusate-filled beakers are immersed in the large heating chamber to the level of the perfusate as shown in **Fig. 1**.

6. Disposable Pyrex Pasteur pipets are inserted (pointed tips first; *see* **Fig. 1**) into the perfusing tube lines. The wider open ends of the pipets are then placed inside the perfusate solutions (*see* **Fig. 1**, right inset).

7. The peristaltic pump is turned on and the perfusate is allowed to flow through the tubing system.

8. A second set of disposable Pyrex Pasteur pipets are inserted into the carbogen tube lines in the same configuration as described in **step 5**; adjust perfusate pH by adjusting carbogen flow.

9. When perfusate first enters the bubble jackets, fill the inner chamber of both bubble-jackets up to the mid-line of the chamber and seal off the inner chamber to atmospheric pressure using the upper valve.

10. Open the outlet valve directly above the beakers and the perfusate should recirculate throughout the system without changes in the mid-line levels of perfusate within the inner chambers of the jackets.

11. Adjust perfusion rate or perfusate flow rate to approx 2–3 mL/min.

12. Insert pH and temperature probes into the 125-mL beaker and verify that the pH and temperature values are approx 7.2 and 37°C, respectively.

13. At the end of the isolation procedure, cleaning the perfusion system involves filling and running the system (tubes and chambers) with 70% ethanol followed by distilled water (*see* **Note 7**).

3.4. Preparation of the Animal and Heart Isolation

1. Mice (C57BL, male, 6–8 wk old) were injected with heparin (1000 U/kg, ip; *see* **Note 8**) 20 min prior the start of the experimental protocol. Intraperitoneal injection of ketamine/xylazine (0.1 mL/100 g) was the euthanasia of choice (*see* **Note 9**), and this anesthetic combination has little direct cardiac toxicity.

2. Prior to the start of the surgical procedure, the following checklist should be observed and established:
   a. Ensure that tubes 1–5 all contain their respective contents (*see* **Subheading 2.**).
   b. Run oxygenated perfusion buffers through the perfusion system and ensure that the system has been primed for at least 10–15 min.
   c. Ensure that the perfusion rate is approx 2–3 mL/min.
   d. Ensure that the pH (~7.2) and temperature (~32°C) of the perfusion buffers are within normal parameters.
   e. Remove any air bubbles in the perfusion system, i.e., particularly in the tubing and the 20-G needle–syringe assembly used for attaching the heart (*see* **Note 10**).
   f. Prepare the surgical area:
      i. Fill culture dishes 1 and 2 (e.g., 60 × 15 mm, BD Falcon) with ice-cold incubation buffer (~20 mL).
      ii. Fill 20-G needle–syringe assembly with ice-cold incubation buffer.
      iii. Position the needle–syringe assembly at a fixed 45° angle (e.g., with a vertically mounted three-prong clamp) over culture dish 2 with 2–3 mm of the 20-G needle tip submerged under the surface of the incubation buffer.
      iv. Cut a 10–15 cm length of 6-0 surgical thread, knot loosely, and place along the shaft of the needle.

3. Once the animal is anesthetized (i.e., there is an absence of withdrawal reflex), a surgical incision is made posterior to the xiphoid process.

4. Lateral cuts are made down the chest cavity on either side along the rib cage from the xiphoid process until the diaphragm is evident.

5. Starting from the diaphragm, incisions on either side of the sternum are made toward the scapula taking care to avoid damaging the heart.

6. Using forceps, peel back the rib cage to expose the heart.

7. Using forceps, carefully remove or pull away the thin layer of pericardium from the heart. The heart should be gently lifted up using the index finger and thumb and an incision is made across the aorta from below.

8. The heart is immediately placed in culture dish 1 within ice-cold incubation buffer where all remnant tissue (i.e., thymus and lungs) around the heart is subsequently and delicately removed to expose the aorta (*see* **Note 11**).

9. The heart was transferred to culture dish 2 for fine surgical manipulation with the aid of a surgical microscope.

10. Ensure that there is sufficient aortic stem length for proper cannulation, i.e., incision is made to the carotid bifurcation.

11. Using fine forceps, the aortic stem was carefully fitted over the blunt-end of stationary 20-G needle that is itself attached to an incubation buffer-filled syringe.

12. Depending on the length of the aortic stem, insertion of the needle end into the aortic stem should not penetrate the aortic valves or exceed a significant distance to cause obstruction of the coronary openings, just before the aortic valves (**Fig. 3**). This is a critical step to ensure adequate perfusion of perfusate to the circulatory system heart.

13. The aorta was secured to the perfusion needle (*see* **Note 12**) with surgical thread.

14. A slight delivery of incubation buffer from the syringe was introduced into the heart as an initial wash (to flush blood from the vasculature) and to assess the needle placement. This was passed through the heart as a single time without recirculation. Extension of the ventricular cavity or discoloration of the heart tissue following the delivery of the buffer is indicative of improper needle placement, presence of foreign material or air bubble, or a combination of all three; carefully adjust the needle accordingly and reassess the situation before proceeding.

15. Once proper needle placement has been made and adequate perfusion has been established, the heart and needle assembly is transferred to and mounted to the waiting air-bubble trap of the Ca^{2+}-containing perfusate as shown in **Fig. 1**, being careful not to introduce air bubbles by way of the open, syringe-end of the needle.

16. To reduce the effects of ischemia, the time between the removal of the heart and proper perfusion of the heart should not exceed 5–7 min.

3.5. Heart Perfusion and Isolation of Myocytes

1. The isolated heart is initially mounted onto the air-bubble trap that is directly over the Ca^{2+}-containing perfusate. This phase of the perfusion protocol allows the heart to recover and dispel the remaining blood constituents as it contracts rhythmically.

2. If the procedure is performed successfully, the coronary arteries will fill with buffer solution and the heart will begin to contract rhythmically. A good perfusion rate or perfusate flow rate for mouse hearts (6 mo old) is 2–3 mL/min.

3. The heart is allowed to recover during this wash-out period for approx 10 min before the heart and needle assembly is transferred to the adjoining air-bubble trap that is directly over the Ca^{2+}-free, EGTA-containing perfusate.

4. Once the heart has been transferred to the Ca^{2+}-free perfusate flow assembly, the heart should slowly cease to contract.

5. A collection container is immediately placed under the heart to collect 20 mL perfusate; this is an ideal step in the protocol to check and adjust the perfusion rate.

6. Once 20 mL of perfusate has been collected, transfer approx 4 mL of the Ca^{2+}-free perfusate using disposable Pasteur pipets into tube 1 and dissolve its contents. A standard bench-top mini vortexer (e.g., cat. no. 58816-121, VWR) facilitates this process.

7. Transfer the dissolved collagenase solution from tube 1 into the syringe-filter assembly. Carefully depress the plunger and add the filtered solution to the Ca^{2+}-free perfusate. Using a disposable Pasteur pipet, aspirate the beaker solution

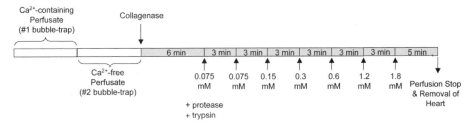

Fig. 10. The perfusion timeline. Perfusion begins with the Ca^{2+}-containing perfusate, followed by a series of incremental increases in Ca^{2+} concentrations in the Ca^{2+}-free perfusate, and ends after a total enzyme digestion time of 30 min.

several times to ensure adequate mixing. Let the perfusate flow for 6 min. Timer should be started with a count-down or count-up setting (*see* **Fig. 10**).

8. At the end of 6 min, begin adding CaCl$_2$ (1 *M*) into the collagenase-containing perfusate starting with 0.125 m*M*. Continue with incremental increases in CaCl$_2$ every 3 min, thereafter.

9. After the 0.25 m*M* CaCl$_2$ addition, transfer approx 4 mL of the collagenase-containing perfusate to tubes 2 and 3 and dissolve its contents. Transfer the dissolved protease- and trypsin-containing solutions from tubes 2 and 3 into separate syringe-filter assemblies and carefully add the filtered solutions into the collagenase-containing perfusate. Aspirate the beaker solution with a disposable Pasteur pipet to mix.

10. During the perfusion period, dissolve contents in tubes 4 and 5 with approx 14 mL of 37°C incubation buffer (i.e., the incubation buffer in the 50-mL tube that was immersed in the large, heating water bath at the start of the experiment). Immerse tubes 4 and 5 into the large heating chamber to maintain the dissolved solutions at 37°C.

11. During perfusion with collagenase, the heart will become swollen and turn slightly pale.

12. At the end of the perfusion period, disconnect the heart-and-needle assembly and transfer it to an incubation buffer-filled 35 × 10 mm Petri dish. Using the dissecting microscope, carefully disconnect the 20-G needle from the aorta. Visually, the heart tissue should be flaccid with a consistency of a liquid gel that is uniform in a light pink texture. Using fine forceps and scissors, carefully dissect out the atrial appendages and remnants of the aortic branch, leaving only the left and right ventricular sections.

13. Place the entire ventricular section into a small, 50-mL Pyrex Erlenmeyer flask filled with 10 mL incubation buffer (37°C).

14. Insert the cutting ends of a small surgical scissors into the flask and cut the ventricular tissue in half in a lengthwise fashion. A small and fine "cloud-like" dispersion of tissue segments immediately following the incision serves as a visual cue that the heart tissue was adequately digested. Another cue is that upon incision, the

tissue should exhibit a yielding and "soft" quality. A rigid or inflexible consistency often indicates inadequate perfusion, collagenase perfusion time, or collagenase quantity (*see* **Note 13**).

15. Using a sufficient section of Parafilm wax paper, cover the top of the flask and immerse the flask in the large, heating chamber. Incubate the ventricular tissue at 37°C for 20 min.

16. At the end of 20 min, remove and discard the incubation buffer with a disposable Pasteur pipet without disturbing the ventricular tissue.

17. Transfer the dissolved BSA solution from tube 4 into the flask; the serum also serves to inactivate any remaining proteases.

18. Attach a flexible latex rubber bulb (e.g., cat. no. 56311-060, VWR) on the thin end of a disposable Pyrex Pasteur pipet and place the larger and rounded end inside the flask. With minimal and slow pressures on the bulb, triturate the ventricular tissue up and down the pipette until it completely disperses into very fine pieces. When triturating, place the pipet end a few millimeters above the bottom of the flask so that the ventricular tissue is gently "forced" through and, thereby, facilitate the dispersion process.

19. When the ventricular tissue is adequately dispersed into smaller pieces, transfer several drops of the cell suspension to a (inverted) microscope stage with ×10–20 objective lens to visually inspect the myocytes. Myocytes should be single, quiescent, and rod-shaped with clear striations and well-defined outer membrane edges. Cell features other than those described are indicative of overdigestion or underdigestion with collagenase.

20. Transfer the cell suspension through a 4 × 4-cm nylon mesh (200 μm, Spectrum Laboratories) into a new 15-mL tube using a disposable Pasteur pipet. Leave any undispersed tissue pieces in the flask.

21. Transfer the second BSA-containing solution from tube 5 into the flask with the remaining undispersed tissue pieces.

22. Triturate the remaining tissue pieces with the inverted Pyrex Pasteur pipet as before and transfer the cell suspension into a second 15-mL tube through the nylon mesh. At the end of isolation, a total of 2 × 14 mL (28 mL) of cell suspension should be collected.

23. Allow both cell suspensions in the tubes to collect as pellets by gravity sedimentation.

24. If desired, the number of viable cells can be determined using a hemacytometer.

25. Carefully aspirate the supernatant and resuspend cell pellets in recording bath solution as required by the experiment.

3.6. Electrophysiological Recordings

A representative sample of myocyte suspension (~100–200 μL) is transferred to the Bioptech Delta T Open Dish System with external bathing solution required by the experiment. Ionic currents and transmembrane voltage changes were recorded using the ruptured-patch technique under the whole-cell configuration.

Voltage- and current-clamp command pulses were generated using the computer-interfaced amplifier, MultiClamp 700A-2, and pClamp 9.0 software. Recordings were acquired using a Pentium computer that controlled data acquisition hardware and software from which the recordings were filtered (online) at 2 kHz and sampled at 10 kHz (4-pole Bessel); the sampling rate was set at 50 kHz (12-bit resolution). Glass pipets (cat. no. 30-31-0, Borosil 1.2 mm OD × 0.9 mm ID, FHC Inc.) were pulled and their tips were heat polished to establish an electrode resistance of 2–3 MΩ for voltage-clamp and 0.8–1.5 MΩ for current-clamp protocols when pipets were filled with internal solution. Series resistance was 4–8 MΩ, and this was 60–80% electronically compensated. Capacitative transients were nulled by analog compensation and whole-cell capacitance was calculated by the ratio of the total amount of charge by the amplitude of the voltage step; cell capacitance was estimated by integrating the area under the capacity transients. All recordings were made 5 min after membrane rupture to minimize time-dependent changes. Leak currents were typically <100 pA and were not corrected.

For sodium currents, myocytes are held at −80 or −100 mV and depolarized with 10 ms steps to 0 or −20 mV. Inward L-type Ca^{2+} currents are produced by depolarizing myocytes with 200 ms steps to +10 mV from a holding potential of −40 mV. Transient outward potassium currents are elicited by 400 ms depolarizing steps to +60 mV from a holding potential of −60 or −70 mV. In the current-clamp mode, action potentials are elicited by 25–50 ms pulse widths of 1500–2000 pA amplitudes at a starting stimulation frequency of 1 Hz (1000 ms). Cell resting membrane potential was between −65 and −70 mV and, if necessary, this was maintained by applying a maximum of (and often not exceeding) 100 pA of holding current.

4. Notes

1. The variability between collagenase batches is the greatest source of variability in myocyte isolation. Moreover, crude collagenase when used alone to digest heart tissue almost always yields little or no viable isolated myocytes *(2)*. Consequently, collagenases have often been used in combination with other enzymes, like protease and trypsin *(2–4)*. In our laboratory, we have had good results when collagenase is supplemented with both protease and trypsin.
2. Commercially available collagenase is produced from bacterial strains, primarily from *Clostridium histolyticum*. Bacterial collagenase is a crude complex that contains collagenase, more specifically, clostridiopeptidaase A, which is a protease with a specificity for the X-Gly bond in the sequence, Pro-X-Gly-Pro (where X is a neutral amino acid). Generally, however, crude collagenase extracts are contaminated by proteases whose activities are generally very high and uncontrolled. For this reason, the variability between enzyme batches is high and, thus, is a great source of variability. And, this lends itself to the many and varying theories by

many researchers on "optimizing" myocyte isolation conditions. One important factor when selecting digesting enzymes is to consider the fractions of the proteases present in crude collagenase. Clostripain is one protease that has been identified to be important in the isolation of viable cells *(3)*. Type 2 is a collagenase profile offered by Worthington that contains a greater clostripain (a trypsin-like enzyme) activity and is generally recommended for dissociating heart tissue.

3. The sharp tip of the 20-G needle should be made blunt and tapered. This can be accomplished by cutting off the sharp tip and filing the remaining end to a flat, dull edge being careful to maintain the needle opening. To facilitate the attachment of the aorta to the needle, the sides near the tip-end should be notched or filed in to achieve a tapered, concave-like surface (*see* **Fig. 3**). This tapered end serves to: (1) prevent snagging the aorta when cannulating, (2) reduce slippage when attaching aorta, (3) facilitate the fastening of the surgical thread, and (4) act as a visual "depth"-marker when attaching the aorta to the needle.

4. Lead placement requires a particular arrangement of the positive and negative electrodes so that a particular ECG pattern will be produced. To have a monitoring lead, a minimum of two electrodes (positive and negative) is required. The objective for *limb* lead placement is to look at the heart along the right and left frontal (vertical) planes from the top to the bottom right and left. The primary lead placement most coxonly used is the Lead II configuration—the positive electrode on the lower extreme right side of the right chest and the negative electrode on the second intercostals space in the midline of the upper left chest. For additional reference, please refer to any standard electrocardiogram analysis textbook.

5. Recording a high signal-to-noise ratio ECG trace is ideal. One of the primary reasons is to be able to discern the different peaks and waveforms associated with one heart beat and to be able to distinguish between motion artifacts or "noise" from an arrhythmia. In rodents, it is often difficult to accurately interpret the QT interval owing to their high basal heart rates and often negative isoelectric potentials. For these reasons it is critical to minimize motion artifacts and optimize the signal-to-noise ratio when recording via telemetric transmitters. Another consideration to reduce variability in the QT measurement is to establish a dedicated and experienced observer and analyst to record and measure the QT interval and other parameters in a highly repeatable and reproducible manner. There should also be a clearly defined definition of the QT interval.

6. Although it is relatively easy to measure both PR and QRS, measurement of the QT interval is complicated for the reasons stated in **Note 5**, but also for the variations in QT owing to variations in heart rate. Various corrections factors (e.g., Bazette's formula) have been used and such corrections were originally devised for humans and many have limited applicability in other species. In rodents, such corrections factors have not been shown to change appreciably with heart rate *(5)*. Others have shown that with a slight modification to Bazette's formula to account for the high resting heart rates of rodents, the relationship between the QT interval and RR interval can be reasonably approximated by the square root function of the RR interval *(6)*. All in all, greater precision in the measurement of the QT

interval as well as caution when correction factors are implemented should be exercised in the mouse ECG.

7. Enzyme, proteins, and other particles may slowly adhere to the glassware and tubing with continual use of the perfusion system. To help maintain optimal isolation conditions, it is critical to properly clean the perfusion system before and after each use.

8. Adequate heparinization is essential to reduce or limit blood clotting in the coronary arteries during heart extraction.

9. Anesthetics such as ketamine have long onset period and a high risk of depressing the respirator rate. As a consequence, respiratory depression leads to a higher risk for ischemia, which can reduce myocyte yield. An alternative anesthetic is isoflurane, an inhalation anesthetic, which has a faster pharmacokinetic properties and, as such, a lower risk for developing ischemia. Delivery of isoflurane requires an atomizer with a scale range of 1 to 5% and is often combined with 100% O_2.

10. The presence of air bubbles in the cannulation needle and within the perfusion will increase the risk of occluding the coronary arteries. Careful attention to such details and an air bubble trap (*see* **Fig. 2**) will limit and prevent air bubbles in the perfusion system.

11. The researcher should familiarize himself/herself with the general anatomy of the heart. To help identify the aorta when dissecting out extraneous, noncardiac tissues, one visual cue is to observe the vessel orifice from which the blood is expelled when the heart spontaneously contracts.

12. Prior to connecting the aorta to the 20-G needle, ensure that the perfusate is continuous from syringe, needle, and perfusate in the dish.

13. Ventricular tissue that has bee adequately digested with collagenase should exhibit a "soft" and "tender" quality when it is cut using the surgical scissors. Often, a small and fine "cloud-like" dispersion of tissue segments can be observed. Evidence of this often serves as a visual cue that there is a high degree of fragility and brittleness—both precursors that the tissue will disperse with high probability and ease. On the contrary, it could also represent a state of over-digestion, i.e., excessive exposure time and/or quantity of collagenase. A magnified visual inspection of the cells from a small aliquot sample of the incubation buffer using a microscope can be conducted to confirm this. If, however, the tissue exhibits a rigid or inflexible consistency following the cut, this may be a sign of inadequate collagenase digestion or inadequate perfusion procedure. If this is the case, cell yield and bioavailability will be low and a decision may be made as to continue with the preparation or to start over.

14. Although myocyte isolation techniques vary among researchers, there is a shared understanding that the amount of Ca^{2+} ions after the Ca^{2+}-free period is critical for yielding sufficient numbers of Ca^{2+}-tolerant cells. In contrast, others have noted that crude collagenase does not present any sensitivity to added Ca^{2+} ions (*3,4*). The general consensus is that the addition of Ca^{2+} ions during the isolation procedure will act as a collagenase "activator." More specifically, however, Ca^{2+} ions may be more of an activator of proteolytic activities (*3,4*). In any case, we have

found that "optimal" conditions consist of a Ca^{2+}-free perfusion period with collagenase of approx 6 min, followed by incremental or step-wise increases in Ca^{2+} concentration up to a final concentration of 1.8 mM. A timeline of the perfusion protocol is illustrated in **Fig. 10**. For the reasons previously stated, it is also imperative that management of extracellular Ca^{2+} should take on special attention in transgenic mice. Regardless of the cardiac-specific mutation that is of interest, there is a high probability that cardiac remodeling of some degree may be present from a developing fetus to adult. Thus, it is highly likely that changes in intracellular Ca^{2+} and the way the cardiac cell "handles" its Ca^{2+} ions may have also been altered. If that is the case, the removal and re-introduction of extracellular Ca^{2+} may have some unidentifiable untoward affect to the Ca^{2+}-tolerance state of the cell during its recovery from digestion. This may be an added source of variability that must be considered for the purposes of optimizing cell bioavailability and yield.

References

1. Tian, X. L., Yong, S. L., Wan, X., et al. (2004) Mechanisms by which SCN5A mutation N1325S causes cardiac arrhythmias and sudden death in vivo. *Cardiovasc. Res.* **61,** 256–267.
2. Mitra, R. and Morad, M. (1985) A uniform enzymatic method for dissociation of myocytes from hearts and stomachs of vertebrates. *Am. J. Physiol.* **249,** H1056–H1060.
3. Le Guennec, J. Y., Peineau, N., Esnard, F., et al. (1993) A simple method for calibrating collagenase/pronase E ratio to optimize heart cell isolation. *Biol. Cell* **79,** 161–165.
4. Yagisawa, S., Morita, F., Nagai, Y., Noda, H., and Ogura, Y. (1965) Kinetic studies on the actions of collagenase. *J. Biochem. (Tokyo)* **58,** 407–416.
5. Hayes, E., Pugsley, M. K., Penz, W. P., Adaikan, G., and Walker, M. J. (1994) Relationships between QaT and RR intervals in rats, guinea pigs, rabbits, and primates. *J. Pharmacol. Toxicol. Methods* **4,** 201–207.
6. Mitchell, G. F., Jeron, A., and Koren, G. (1998) Measurement of heart rate and Q-T interval in the conscious mouse. *Am. J. Physiol.* **274,** H747–H751.

10

Optical Mapping of Shock-Induced Arrhythmogenesis in the Rabbit Heart With Healed Myocardial Infarction

Fluorescent Imaging With a Photodiode Array

Yuanna Cheng

Summary

Optical mapping of electrical activity in the heart employs digital imaging and voltage-sensitive dyes. These methods have become an increasingly common research tools in basic cardiac electrophysiology. Significant advantages of this approach include simultaneous noncontact recording of entire action potentials free of electrical stimulus-induced artifacts from multiple closely adjacent sites, and adjustable spatial and temporal resolutions. In this way, the activation pattern as well as the repolarization pattern can be monitored by dynamic registration of transmembrane potential changes. As a result, the success of these techniques is most evident in the investigation of the mechanisms of pacing, vulnerability, and defibrillation, in which conventional electrical recordings are hampered by stimulus-induced artifacts. Using optical mapping technology and instrumentation driven by LabVIEW software, we mapped changes in transmembrane voltage during defibrillation shocks and identified the mechanisms of vulnerability and defibrillation in rabbit hearts with healed myocardial infarction (≥ 4 wk postinfarction).

Key Words: Optical mapping; voltage-sensitive dye; healed myocardial infarction; infarction border zone; cardiac vulnerability; and defibrillation.

1. Introduction

Application of strong electric shocks is the only effective therapy to terminate life-threatening ventricular tachycardia/fibrillation in patients. Little has been known about processes occurring in cardiac cells during defibrillation shocks as a result of a lack of appropriate experimental techniques, as any electrode-based instrumentation used to record electrical activity is always overwhelmed by the

From: *Methods in Molecular Medicine, vol. 129:*
Cardiovascular Disease: Methods and Protocols, Volume 2: Molecular Medicine
Edited by: Q. K. Wang © Humana Press Inc., Totowa, NJ

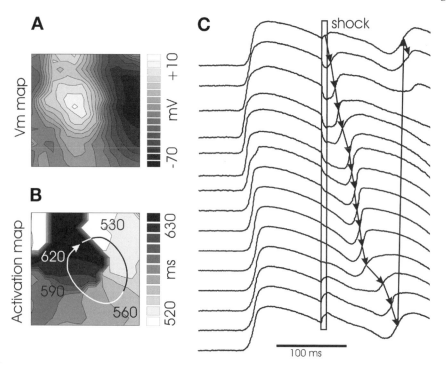

Fig. 1. Virtual electrode-induced phase singularity in a structurally normal heart. (**A**) Virtual electrode polarization developed at the end of monophasic cathodal shock (–100 V, 8 ms). (**B**) Isochronal map of postshock activation. (**C**) Optical recordings collected around the virtual electrode-induced phase singularity. Recording sites were sequentially selected along the circle in **B**.

strong electric shock. Introduction of voltage-sensitive dyes and imaging techniques has finally delivered technology that is capable of mapping electrical activity in the heart during shocks and that is free of the overwhelming artifacts present in any conventional electrode recordings. Experimental findings resulting from this technology advancement have facilitated the formulation of Virtual Electrode Polarization Hypothesis of Defibrillation *(1)*. According to this hypothesis, an electric shock simultaneously produces both areas of depolarized (positive) and hyperpolarized (negative) changes in transmembrane potential. The success or failure of the shock is determined by this shock-induced polarization pattern, called a virtual electrode polarization pattern. This new concept has advanced our understanding of mechanisms of vulnerability and defibrillation. **Figure 1** presents experimental evidence of a virtual electrode-induced phase singularity mechanism of shock-induced arrhythmogenesis in a structurally normal rabbit heart. **Figure 1A** illustrates the typical pattern of virtual electrode polarization mapped as a distribution of transmembrane potential seen immediately after the application of a shock. As a result, a shock-induced wavefront of break excitation can form a reentrant pattern around the virtual electrode-induced phase singularity *(1–3)*.

However, many of these findings have been limited to studies on structurally normal hearts. Most patients who receive implantable cardioverter defibrillators suffer from coronary artery disease, which creates discontinuities in the myocardium due to areas of regional ischemia, and zones of infarction. The infarction border zone (surviving tissue abutting the infarct) is known to have an altered electrophysiological substrate and to host sources of arrhythmia in the setting of chronic/healed myocardial infarction (MI; ≥4 wk). However, cardiac vulnerability and defibrillation under this condition has not been well studied. In this chapter, we present detailed procedures for optical imaging and voltage-sensitive dye technique to identify the mechanisms of shock-induced arrhythmias vulnerability in the setting of healed MI in rabbit hearts.

2. Materials

1. Heart preparation: New Zealand white rabbits of either sex weighing 2–4 kg were used in the study. The Langendorff-perfused intact heart from normal and healed myocardial infarcted rabbits were used for an optical mapping study to compare incidence of shock-induced arrhythmia and to elucidate the mechanism of initiation of shock-induced arrhythmia under these settings (*see* **Note 1**).

2. Voltage-sensitive dye: voltage-sensitive dye is light-sensitive dye. Thus, caution should be taken to avoid dye exposure to the light. A stock solution of 5 mg voltage-sensitive dye di-4-ANEPPS (Molecular Probes Inc.) is prepared in 4 mL dimethylsulfoxide (DMSO) (Fisher Scientific) at a concentration of 1.25 mg/mL and kept frozen at $-20°C$. At this condition, the dissolved dye can be kept for at least 10 mo without losing its potency. The final dye solution is prepared immediately prior to staining. Following gentle warming, a syringe is filled with 500 µL of the stock dye solution. During staining, 100–200 µL of the dye is gradually injected into an injection port above the bubble trap of the perfusion system by means of an infusion pump. The slow aorta perfusion of the dye usually lasts for 5–10 min. As a result of washout of the dye during the experiment, restaining the heart with dye is routinely performed (*see* **Note 2**).

3. Modified tyrode solution: the isolated intact rabbit heart is retrogradely perfused via aorta with oxygenated (95% O_2/5% CO_2) modified Tyrode's solution of the following composition: NaCl 128.2 mM, $CaCl_2$ 1.3 mM, KCl 4.7 mM, $MgCl_2$ 1.05 mM, NaH_2PO_4 1.19 mM, $NaHCO_3$ 25 mM, and glucose 11 mM. The solution is freshly prepared prior to the experiment from pre-prepared stock solutions. Stock solution I contains 25X concentrated solution of NaCl, $CaCl_2$, KCl, $MgCl_2$, and NaH_2PO_4, and stock solution II contains 25X concentrated solution of $NaHCO_3$. Final perfusion solution is prepared by taking desired amount of stock solution I and diluting it with distilled water before adding the same amount of

stock solution II to avoid precipitations. After adding glucose and shaking the solution to completely dissolve the glucose, additional distilled water is added to achieve the final concentration of perfusion solution.

4. Excitation-contraction uncoupler: it is necessary to avoid motion artifact caused by cardiac muscle contraction in order to faithfully record entire action potential optically. Fifteen millimolar 2,3-butanedione monoxime (BDM) (Fisher Scientific), an excitation-contraction uncoupler, is freshly prepared prior to the experiment and added to the perfusate (*see* **Note 1**).

3. Methods

3.1. Survival Surgery

The study contains two groups of samples: structurally normal hearts as a control and healed myocardial infarcted hearts. Rabbits are anesthetized with ketamine (35 mg/kg) and xylazine (5 mg/kg) intramuscularly. A 22-G intravenous catheter is inserted into the marginal ear vein for continuous infusion of normal saline solution and for injection of antiarrhythmic agent (lidocaine) during the surgery. Rabbits are intubated with an endotracheal tube (3.0 mm ID) and mechanically ventilated (rate: 76 breaths/min, tidal volume 8 mL) with a mixture of isoflurane (1.0–2.0%) and oxygen. The rabbits are placed on a water blanket maintained at 38°C. The electrocardiogram (ECG) is monitored continuously.

The chest is opened through the fourth left intercostal space. The heart is exposed via incision of the pericardium. Lidocaine (1 mg/kg) is intravenously administered to minimize potential ventricular arrhythmias prior to coronary artery ligation. The infarction is created by ligation of the lateral division or posterolateral division of the left coronary artery at a level of 40–70% from the apex. Following the ligation, a chest tube is inserted into the thoracic cavity. The lungs are inflated, the ribs on both sides of the incision are approximated by three evenly placed loops of heavy-duty thread, and the thoracic cavity is then sealed via multiple suture layers. The negative pressure in the chest is created by applying negative pressure via chest tube. Then the chest tube is withdrawn while negative pressure is applied. Long-lasting antibiotic (ambi-pen, 300,000 U/mL, intramuscular injection) is given just prior to the surgery and analgesic (buprenex, 0.05 mg/Kg, subcutaneous injection) is provided for 3 d postoperatively. Rabbits are allowed to heal for more than 4 wk before the acute experiments. No survival surgery is performed on the control hearts.

3.2. Experimental Preparation

Acute experiments are performed in vitro on Langendorff-perfused intact hearts obtained from normal controls and infarcted rabbits. Rabbits are anesthetized by

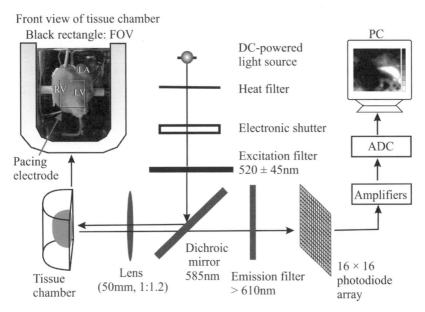

Fig. 2. Schematics of an optical mapping system. ADC, analog-to-digital converter; FOV, field of view; LV, left ventricle; RV, right ventricle; LA, left atria.

a combination injection of sodium pentobarbital (50 mg/kg) and heparin (1000 U/kg) via an ear vein. Following opening the chest, the heart is removed and placed on a Langendorff apparatus, where it is retrogradely perfused with oxygenated (95% O_2/5% CO_2) modified Tyrode's solution. A pacing bipolar Ag/AgCl electrode with 1-mm interelectrode distance is placed at the apex of the right ventricle. Three 12-mm Ag/AgCl pellets positioned on the right and left sides and at the bottom of the chamber are used to monitor ECG. A modified 10-mm coil electrode is inserted into the right ventricular cavity through the pulmonary artery for shock delivery. The modified 5-cm shock delivery reference coil electrode is positioned in the bath 1 cm above and 1 cm behind the heart (4007L, Angeion). Temperature and pH are continuously maintained at $37 \pm 0.5°C$ and 7.35 ± 0.05, respectively.

The heart is positioned in a temperature-controlled water-jacketed glass chamber with the anterior wall facing the optical apparatus **(Fig. 2)**. The chamber is filled with the modified Tyrode's solution. The solution level is adjusted to cover the heart and the active areas of the shock electrode. The cylindrical tissue chamber (7 cm internal diameter, 10 cm height) is water-jacketed everywhere around the heart except for the flat surface facing the optical apparatus. The heart is gently held against this surface by three pistons positioned on posterior, left, and right lateral sides of the heart, which is adjustable from outside of the chamber. The aortic pressure is monitored and maintained at a level of 45 mmHg by adjusting the rate of perfusion with a peristaltic pump. After equilibration of the heart in the chamber for 15–20 min under modified Tyrode solution, 15 mM BDM is added to the perfusate to eliminate motion artifact. The heart is further equilibrated under BDM for 20 min, and then stained with di-4-ANEPPS. Optical recording starts 10–15 min following the staining procedure.

3.3. Experimental Protocol

We use an S1-S2 protocol to measure the shock-induced arrhythmia vulnerability of control and infarcted hearts. The heart is paced at a basic cycle length of 300 ms at twice the diastolic pacing threshold with a stimulus isolator (A385, World Precision Instruments). After 20 basic stimuli (S1), a truncated exponential monophasic shock (S2, 8-ms duration, 61% tilt, both polarities) is delivered from a 150-μF capacitor clinical defibrillator (HVS-02, Ventritex, CA) at the preset coupling interval (the time interval between the last S1 stimulus and S2 stimulus). The leading edge voltages of the shocks are ±100 V, ±130 V, ±160 V, ±190 V, and ±220 V. Shocks are delivered at a phase defined as the percentage of action potential duration, (coupling interval – conduction delay)/APD × 100%. Conduction delay is defined as the time interval between the pacing stimulus and average activation time in the field of view. The action potential duration (APD) is calculated using an APD90 definition. In every acute experiment, shocks are applied at 25, 50, and 75% APD.

3.4. Optical Recording System

A schematic drawing of the system is shown in **Fig. 2**. Fluorescence in cardiac preparation stained with the voltage-sensitive dye di-4-ANEPPS is excited by light produced by a 250-W DC-powered tungsten halogen light source (Oriel Corp.). After passing a heat filter and an electric shutter controlling the light beam, the beam is passed through 520 ± 45 nm excitation filter. It is then deflected by means of a dichroic mirror and focused on the surface of a heart by the imaging lens. The fluorescence emitted from the heart is collected by a 50-mm lens (1:1.2, AF Nikkor), passed through a 610-nm-ong emission filter, and focused an image of a chosen region of the heart on sensing area of the 16 × 16 photodiode array (C4675, Hamamatsu). The optical apparatus and photodiode array are mounted on a ball-bearing boomstand. This design permitted easy readjustment of focusing on desired areas of the preparation. Excitation and emission lights are separated by a 585-nm dichroic mirror. After collecting emitted light by photodiode array, the current produced by each photodiode is passed through a separate current-to-voltage converter (first stage operational amplifiers with 10-MΩ feedback resistors). The outputs of the first-stage amplifiers are connected to 256 second-stage amplifiers, AC coupled with a time constant of 30 s. Automatic resetting of the second-stage amplifiers prior to data acquisition is used in order to remove the DC offset of the optical signals caused by background fluorescence. Signals were filtered by Bessell filters. After amplification, the signals are fed to a multiplexer and an A/D converter (DAP 3200/415e, Microstar Laboratories). Each frame includes 256 optical channels and 8 instrumentation channels, and is stored for off-line analysis. Instrumentation channels recorded ECG, stimulation and defibrillation triggers, and aortic pressure *(4)* (*see* **Note 3**).

3.5. Data Acquisition and Analysis

Custom-developed data acquisition and analysis software is used. The software is designed using the LabVIEW visual data acquisition and analysis language (National Instruments) and the data acquisition driver DAPL 2000 (MicroStar Laboratories). The computer program controls experimental pacing, shock application, light sources, and data acquisition. The computer-controlled shutter is opened 2 s prior to data acquisition and closed 500 ms after its completion. Each scan contains 1–2 s of data, including the last basic beat action potential, the action potential altered by a shock, and two or more subsequent action potentials (**Fig. 3**, upper panel). Software for data analysis automatically calculates maps of activation, repolarization, action potential duration, transmembrane voltage, and the gradient of the transmembrane potential and its derivative. Activation maps are reconstructed using $-(dF/dt)_{max}$ algorithm *(5)*. It is based on calculating the first derivative of the inverted fluorescence intensity ($-dF/dt$) and finding its maximum. Timing of the maximum $-(dF/dt)_{max}$ is considered the activation time point at the recording site from which the signal is acquired. Repolarization is calculated based on calculating of the second derivative of the inverted fluorescent signal intensity and locating the local maximum peak $-(d2F/dt2)_{max}$, which corresponds to the repolarization time point at the recording site *(6)*. APD is calculated as the difference between repolarization and depolarization times. Because the fluorescent signal cannot be absolutely calibrated with respect to millivolt value of transmembrane voltage, we use pseudo-millivolts calibration. Transmembrane voltage maps are reconstructed from optical recordings based on the assumptions *(7)* that the resting potential is –85 mV and the action potential amplitude is 100 mV in all sites. The gradient of the transmembrane potential and its derivative (dV/dt) was calculated using a five-point algorithm *(5)*. Activation, action potential, repolarization, and transmembrane polarization data are usually presented as isochronal maps (*see* **Fig. 3**) allowing quantitative assessment of

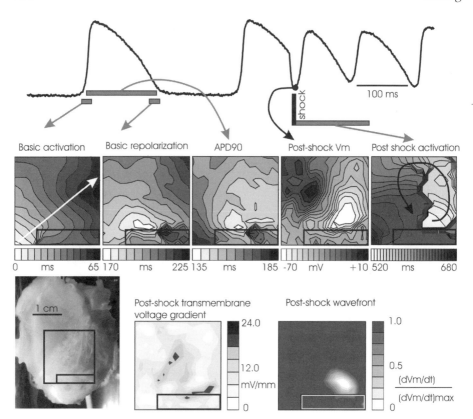

Fig. 3. Wavefront of shock-induced re-excitation originates at site of maximum transmembrane voltage gradient at the border zone of a heart 6 wk postinfarction. The upper panel shows an example of raw optical recordings taken by one of 256 photodiodes. It typically contains a last basic beat action potential (AP) and another AP terminated by a shock (−100 V, 8 ms). In this case, a shock-induced arrhythmia was observed. Bars and dot indicate the time scales and location used to reconstruct maps below. The middle panel shows (left to right): maps of basic beat activation, basic beat repolarization, APD90, postshock transmembrane voltage, postshock activation. The lower panel shows: the photograph of the heart with the field of view and area of infarction inside the field of view, map of transmembrane voltage gradient at the end of shock, and the map of the postshock wavefront (marked with high value of the first temporal derivative of the transmembrane potential) 12 ms following shock withdrawal. (Reproduced with permission from **ref. 8**.)

spread of activation and repolarization and distribution of APD and Vm in highly anisotropic heart muscle under normal and pathological conditions.

Publication-quality plots are built using the following computer programs: Origin (OriginLab Corp.) and CorelDraw (Corel Corp.).

3.6. Shock-Induced Arrhythmogenesis in Structurally Normal Hearts and in Chronically Infarcted Hearts

Optical imaging studies are performed on structurally normal hearts ($n = 8$) and healed MI hearts ($n = 8$) to assess shock-induced arrhythmia vulnerability. By grouping each shock polarity applied at 25, 50, and 75% of APD together in each of the control group and the infarcted group, we calculate the incidence of arrhythmia (≥ 1 extra beats), sustained arrhythmia (≥ 6 extra beats), and long-lasting arrhythmia (>30 s), which required a rescue shock to terminate. For anodal shock application, 28% postshock arrhythmia occurs in the control group vs 52% in the infarcted group ($p < 0.01$). Sustained arrhythmia is 7.5% in the control vs 33 % in the infarcted group ($p < 0.01$), whereas long-lasting arrhythmia is 1.7 vs 30% ($p < 0.01$). For cathodal shock application, 68% postshock arrhythmia occurs in the control group vs 78% in the infarcted group ($p = 0.08$). Sustained arrhythmia is 45% in the control vs 59% in the infarcted group ($p < 0.01$), while long-lasting arrhythmia was 25 vs 59% ($p < 0.01$) *(8)*. To explore the mechanisms of this increased shock-induced arrhythmia vulnerability in the infarcted hearts, we compare the initiation of shock-induced arrhythmias in the control and infarcted hearts. **Figure 3** shows one typical example. In this case, a shock of -100 V is applied during the plateau phase of APD. The shock produces a virtual electrode polarization pattern with depolarized/excited area (red) near the shock lead and an adjacent hyperpolarized/de-excited area (blue) as shown in the postshock transmembrane potential (Vm) map. The maximum transmembrane voltage gradient (dark blue areas, middle of the third row) is located at the border zone (the boundary between infarcted area and adjacent noninfarct area) as well as at the boundary between the depolarized and hyperpolarized areas (virtual electrode polarization boundary). However, the resulting break-excitation wavefront (pink area, right panel of the third row) is only originated at the border zone gradient and propagated toward the base, forming a long-lasting reentrant arrhythmia (postshock activation map). On the contrary, in structurally normal heart, postshock break-excitation wavefront usually initiates from virtual electrode polarization boundary as shown in **Fig. 1**.

We can further systematically examine all arrhythmias in the control and infarcted hearts to evaluate the general patterns of postshock arrhythmia initiation. The primary mechanism of shock-induced arrhythmia initiation in the control hearts is via virtual electrode-induced phase singularity **(Fig. 1)** initiatiating from the virtual electrode polarization boundary. In the infarcted hearts, for anodal shock applications, at early shock delivery phase, postshock arrhythmias predominantly initiate from the infarct border zone. At the later shock delivery phase, both the infarct border zone and the virtual electrode polarization play important roles in postshock arrhythmia initiation. For cathodal shock applications, virtual electrode polarization becomes less important and most of the postshock arrhythmias are initiated from the border zone area.

We conclude that a significant increase of shock-induced arrhythmia vulnerability is observed in infarcted heart compared with control hearts. Regional myocardial infarction modulates shock-induced virtual electrode polarization patterns in a different way than in structurally normal hearts. The infarction border zone is responsible for initiation of increased shock-induced arrhythmias.

4. Notes

1. Experimental preparation. Aside from intact heart preparation, optical mapping has been used to investigate cardiac electrical activity in a variety of other preparations such as single myocytes, cell cultures, and isolated tissue preparation *(9)*. The repolarization phase of optical action potential is often distorted by motion artifacts caused by muscle contractions whereas action potential upstrokes are generally well preserved. There are three basic ways to overcome motion artifacts: (1) mechanical immobilization of preparation if contractions are weak; (2) use of motion-artifact insensitive signal analysis algorithms; and (3) pharmacological immobilization of the preparation. Pharmacological intervention is the most commonly used means to produce mechanically quiescent preparations. A frequently used pharmacological agent is an electrical-mechanical uncoupler, BDM (Fisher Scientific) *(4,10–13)*. However, it is known that BDM alters electrical properties of cardiac tissue *(14–17)*, which should be taken into account in interpretation of experimental data. Another agent used in optical mapping studies is cytochalasin D (Cyto D; Sigma), which appears to affect electrical properties to a lesser degree than BDM in some species, including in canine *(17)* and rabbit *(18)* cardiac preparations. However, Cyto D is toxic and is much more costly than that of BDM.

2. Staining the cardiac preparation with voltage-sensitive dye. Voltage-sensitive dyes bind to the cell membrane. The fluorescence is changed when transmembrane potential is altered. The fluorescent dyes are by far the most sensitive sensors of transmembrane potential, providing highest signal-to-noise (S/N) ratio. These dyes are very fast, responding to transmembrane potential changes with microsecond resolution, and linear, within a range of at least ±400 mV. The two most popular dyes in cardiac mapping are di-4-ANEPPS and RH-237 (Molecular Probes Inc.). Another dye, di-8-ANEPPS, provides more stable optical recordings but it is more difficult to load and its application is limited to single myocytes and cell cultures.

   Di-4-ANEPPS and RH-237 are only weakly soluble in water and should be dissolved in an organic solvent such as DMSO or ethanol. It is convenient to prepare a 2–5 mM stock solution of dye in DMSO in advance and store it in a –20°C freezer. At this condition, the dissolved dye can be kept for at least 10 mo without losing its potency. Immediately before an experiment, the stock solution is thawed and dissolved in the perfusion solution at a concentration determined by the method of staining.

There are three main methods for dye staining: (1) by bolus injection, (2) by slow coronary perfusion, and (3) by superfusion. The first two methods are employed in experiments in which a whole heart or an isolated tissue preparation is perfused via a coronary artery. In the bolus injection method, stock solution is dissolved and 1–2 mL are injected directly into the perfusion system, most often into the bubble trap. The dye solution should be filtered to avoid blockage of capillaries with small nondissolved particles. This method is very quick: once the dye solution has passed through the heart, it is ready for optical measurements. However, the drawback is that it may damage the tissue preparation as a result of the toxicity of the dye if a high dose of dye is injected. In the coronary perfusion method, a lower-concentration dye solution is perfused through the heart for 5–10 min. This is the safest and most efficient way to stain the heart. In the third method, the dye is added to the superfusion solution at a higher concentration and staining lasts longer (up to 30 min) to allow for dye diffusion across the tissue surface. This is normally used in the preparation when coronary artery perfusion is not available, such as in atrial-ventricular node preparation. However, even in this preparation, the preferable way of the dye staining is first through coronary perfusion and then through superfusion.

After staining, levels of optical signals and S/N ratios decrease during the course of an experiment because dye molecules gradually leak out of the cell membrane into extracellular and intracellular spaces. To offset washout of the dye, periodic additional dye staining or a continuous dye infusion at a submicromolar concentration can be performed.

3. Optical mapping system. **Figure 1** shows the structure of a typical single-lens optical mapping system. The main elements of any optical imaging system consist of light source, a set of optical filters, focusing optics, a two-dimensional optical sensor accompanied by signal conditioning instrument, and specialized data-acquisition hardware and software. All existing systems are custom built, because complete optical systems suitable for cardiac mapping are not yet commercially available. Review articles/chapters have described the details of design of an optical mapping system *(19,20)*.

Acknowledgment

This study was supported by National American Heart Association grant 0235172N to Dr. Cheng.

References

1. Efimov, I. R., Gray, E. A., and Roth, B. J. (2000) Virtual Electrodes and De-excitation: New Insights into Fibrillation Induction and Defibrillation. *J. Cardiovasc. Electrophysiol.* **11,** 339–353.
2. Efimov, I. R., Cheng, Y., Van Wagoner, D. R., Mazgalev, T., and Tchou, P. J. (1998) Virtual electrode-induced phase singularity: a basic mechanism of failure to defibrillate. *Circ. Res.* **82,** 918–925.

3. Lin, S. -F., Roth, B. J., and Wikswo, J. P. (1999) Quatrefoil reentry in myocardium: an optical imaging study of the induction mechanism. *J. Cardiovasc. Electrophysiol.* **10,** 574–586.
4. Efimov, I. R., Cheng, Y. N., Biermann, M., Van Wagoner, D. R., Mazgalev, T., and Tchou, P. J. (1997) Transmembrane voltage changes produced by real and virtual electrodes during monophasic defibrillation shock delivered by an implantable electrode. *J. Cardiovasc. Electrophysiol.* **8,** 1031–1045.
5. Salama, G., Kanai, A., and Efimov, I. R. (1994) Subthreshold stimulation of Purkinje fibers interrupts ventricular tachycardia in intact hearts. Experimental study with voltage-sensitive dyes and imaging techniques. *Circ. Res.* **74,** 604–619.
6. Efimov, I. R., Huang, D. T., Rendt, J. M., and Salama, G. (1994) Optical mapping of repolarization and refractoriness from intact hearts. *Circulation* **90,** 1469–1480.
7. Cheng, Y., Mowrey, K. A., Van Wagoner, D. R., Tchou, P. J., and Efimov, I. R. (1999) Virtual electrode induced re-excitation: a basic mechanism of defibrillation. *Circ. Res.* **85,** 1056–1066.
8. Li, L., Nikolski, V., Wallick, D. W., Efimov, I. R., and Cheng, Y. (2005) Mechanisms of enhanced shock-induced arrhythmogenesis in the rabbit heart with healed myocardial infarction. *Am. J. Physiol. Heart Circ. Physiol.* **289(3),** H1054–H1068.
9. Rosenbaum, D. S. and Jalife, J. (2002) *Optical mapping of cardiac excitation and arrythmias.* Futura Publishing, Armonk, NY.
10. Banville, I., Gray, R. A., Ideker, R. E., and Smith, W. M. (1999) Shock-induced figure-of-eight reentry in the isolated rabbit heart. *Circ. Res.* **85,** 742–752.
11. Davidenko, J. M., Pertsov, A. V., Salomonsz, R., Baxter, W., and Jalife, J. (1992) Stationary and drifting spiral waves of excitation in isolated cardiac muscle. *Nature* **355,** 349–351.
12. Gray, R. A., Jalife, J., Panfilov, A., et al. (1995) Nonstationary vortexlike reentrant activity as a mechanism of polymorphic ventricular tachycardia in the isolated rabbit heart. *Circulation* **91,** 2454–2469.
13. Knisley, S. B., Hill, B. C., and Ideker, R. E. (1994) Virtual electrode effects in myocardial fibers. *Biophys. J.* **66,** 719–728.
14. Liu, Y. C., Cabo, C., Salomonsz, R., Delmar, M., Davidenko, J., and Jalife, J. (1993) Effects of diacetyl monoxime on the electrical properties of sheep and guinea pig ventricular muscle. *Cardiovasc. Res.* **27,** 1991–1997.
15. Lee, M. H., Lin, S. F., Ohara, T., et al. (2001) Effects of diacetyl monoxime and cytochalasin D on ventricular fibrillation in swine right ventricles. *Am. J. Physiol. Heart Circ. Physiol.* **280,** H2689–H2696.
16. Biermann, M., Rubart, M., Wu, J., Moreno, A., Josiah-Durant, A., and Zipes, D. P. (1998) Effect of cytochalasin D and 2,3-butanedione monoxime on isometric twitch force and transmembrane action potentials in isolated canine right ventricular trabecular fibers. *J. Cardiovasc. Electrophysiol.* **9,** 1336–1347.
17. Wu, J., Biermann, M., Rubart, M., and Zipes, D. P. (1998) Cytochalasin D as excitation-contraction uncoupler for optically mapping action potentials in wedges of ventricular myocardium. *J. Cardiovasc. Electrophysiol.* **9,** 1336–1347.

18. Cheng, Y., Li, L., Nikolski, V., Wallick, D. W., and Efimov, I. R. (2004) Shock-induced arrhythmogenesis is enhanced by 2,3-butanedione monoxime compared with cytochalasin D. *Am. J. Physiol. Heart Circ. Physiol.* **286,** H310–H318.
19. Efimov, I. R. and Cheng, Y. (2002) Optical mapping of cardiac stimulation: fluorescent imaging with a photodiode array, in *Quantitative Cardiac Electrophysiology,* (Carbo, C., Rosenbaum, D. S., eds.), Marcel Dekker, Inc., New York.
20. Efimov, I. R., Nikolski, V. P., and Salama, G. (2004) Optical imaging of the heart. *Circ. Res.* **95,** 21–33.
21. Fast, V. G. (2004) Recording action potentials using voltage-sensitive dyes, in *Practical Methods in Cardiovascular Research,* (Dhein, S., Mohr, F. W., and Delmar, M., eds.), Springer, Heidelberg.

11

Methods for Studying Voltage-Gated Sodium Channels in Heterologous Expression Systems

Margaret S. Dice, Tyce Kearl, and Peter C. Ruben

Summary

The discovery that oocytes of the frog *Xenopus laevis* can be induced to express working membrane ion channels by introducing channel mRNA into their cytoplasm (heterologous expression) has greatly impacted the field of ion channel physiology. With the addition of site-directed mutagenesis techniques, the functional consequences of virtually any mutation can now be specifically and easily assessed. Here, we describe an effective procedure for investigating cardiac sodium channel gating (hNa$_V$1.5) both in *Xenopus* oocytes, and in a mammalian expression system, human embryonic kidney (HEK) 293 cells. We describe cell attached patch clamp for oocytes, and whole cell voltage clamp in HEK 293 cells.

Key Words: Electrophysiology; patch-clamp; voltage-clamp; heterologous expression; ion channel.

1. Introduction

Heterologous expression of ion channel proteins in the immature oocytes of *Xenopus laevis,* first reported in 1981 *(1)*, was a major advance in the study of protein structure and function. The technique has permitted a level of control that, when combined with molecular biological techniques (e.g., site-directed mutagenesis), makes possible the functional assay of virtually any channel protein and mutation thereof.

The achievement of heterologous expression was reported the same year as the publication of another landmark in ion channel physiology—a method for creating a very high-resistance seal between a polished micropipet tip and an adjoining cell membrane. By applying a small amount of suction to the pipet, a giga-ohmic seal (a "gigaseal") is created, effectively isolating a small patch of membrane and its imbedded ion channels *(2)*. Voltage in the membrane patch

From: *Methods in Molecular Medicine, vol. 129:*
Cardiovascular Disease: Methods and Protocols, Volume 2: Molecular Medicine
Edited by: Q. K. Wang © Humana Press Inc., Totowa, NJ

can be regulated by a specialized technique that includes a high-resistance feedback circuit. Thus, the whole process is called "patch-clamping."

Here, we describe an effective procedure for using patch-clamp to investigate cardiac sodium channel ($hNa_V1.5$) gating, both in *Xenopus* oocytes and in a mammalian expression system, human embryonic kidney (HEK) 293 cells. We describe cell-attached patch clamp for oocytes, and whole-cell voltage clamp in HEK 293 cells. Although each part of the procedure is itself not complex, many steps are involved. The major sections for oocyte macropatch are (1) *X. laevis* and their care, (2) harvest, separation, and maintenance of *Xenopus* oocytes, (3) mRNA injection, (4) micropipet fabrication, (5) electrophysiological equipment setup, and (6) obtaining a gigaseal and making recordings. Whole-cell voltage clamp in HEK cells involves (1) HEK cell culture, (2) transfection, and (3) electrophysiological recording.

2. Materials

2.1. Oocytes/Macropatch

2.1.1. X. laevis and Their Care

1. Complete systems for maintaining frogs can be obtained from specialized sources (e.g., www.stranco.com, or www.marinebiotech.com).
2. Gravid *X. laevis* are available from Xenopus I, Dexter, Michigan (www.xenopusone.com) or other supplier. An approved Institutional Animal Care and Use Committee (IACUC) procedure is required prior to ordering frogs (www.iacuc.org).
3. Tank for maintaining frogs (**Fig. 1**). If possible, use more than one tank and treat each separately. The separation works to minimize research delays by providing a backup in the event of tank contamination. Our tanks were purchased from Red Ewald (Karnes City, TX) and put together on site (*see* **Note 1**).
4. Chlorine removal system. As chlorine is toxic to frogs, all fresh (municipal) water entering the tank passes through a dechlorinating reservoir containing a carbon filter (*see* **Note 2**).
5. Water filtration. To remove waste and uneaten food, tank water is recirculated in a separate closed system for each tank (**Fig. 1**). The water is continuously pumped through a 20-gallon side tank containing an array of seven bio-filters in series. Flow is slow (a trickle back into the frog tank) to avoid "gas bubble disease" (www.xlaevis.com/system.html).
6. Siphon for cleaning debris from the tank floor (one for each tank; *see* **Note 3**).
7. Shelter. The frogs will naturally hide from view. Provide them with hiding places, such as halved terracotta flowerpots laid flat.
8. Net of fine mesh, one for each tank, large enough for scooping frogs (about 15 × 20 cm).
9. Temperature control system. Our water temperature is controlled via room temperature, and is maintained at approx 70°F (*see* **Note 4**).

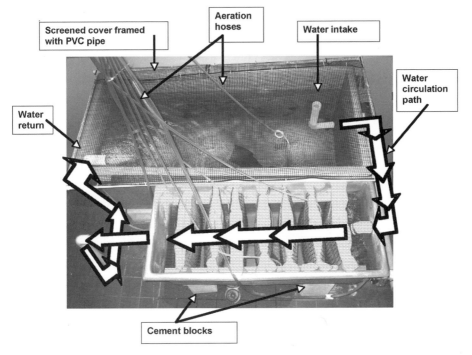

Fig. 1. Illustration of re-circulating frog tank.

10. Light cycle control system for maintaining the frogs on a 12 h light/dark cycle.
11. Air pump and aquarium "stones" for water oxygenation (our system utilizes six for each tank).
12. Frog Brittle (Nasco) food for frogs (*see* **Note 5**).
13. Small "hospital" tank, if desired (*see* **Note 6**).

2.1.2. Oocyte Harvest and Incubation

1. Tricaine anesthetic: 1.7% w/vol 3-aminobenzoic acid ethyl ester methanesulfonate salt, 2 g/L sodium bicarbonate (or more to approximate physiological pH) (*see* **Note 7**).
2. Magnesium oocyte ringer 2 (MgOR2): 96 mM NaCl, 2 mM KCl, 20 mM MgCl$_2$, 5 mM HEPES (pH 7.4). A ringer's solution in which Mg^{2+} is substituted for Ca^{2+}. MgOR2 is used during oocyte separation, during injection of mRNA, and as a basis for solutions listed next (*see* **Note 8**).
3. Sorting solution: unmodified MgOR2. Oocytes removed from the frog are placed immediately in a 50-mL conical tube (Falcon, cat. no. 352070) of MgOR2. Following surgery, MgOR2 serves as the solution for culling of damaged oocytes (sorting).
4. Dissociation solution for dissociation of oocytes from Theca and follicle cells: 2 mg/mL collagenase (metalloproteinase-1; Sigma , cat. no. C-9891 type 1A) in MgOR2.

5. Standard oocyte solution minus serum (SOS–): 2.5 mM pyruvic acid in MgOR2 (pH 7.4). This is the basis for the oocyte incubation medium. Sterilize by autoclave or filtering (0.2 μ). Store at 4°C until needed to make SOS+, described later.

6. Standard oocyte solution plus serum and gentamicin (SOS+): 1–5% horse serum (v/v) and 100 mg/L gentamicin sulfate added to SOS–. Can be stored at 4°C until supply is exhausted.

7. Dissecting microscope. Two dissecting microscopes are strongly recommended. Use one microscope to sort the oocytes, to inject the oocytes with mRNA, and to remove the vitelline membrane just prior to an experiment. The other microscope can then be permanently located and grounded on the patch-clamping apparatus.

8. Fiber-optic illumination. Two unit are needed, one each for the dissecting microscopes.

9. Surgical instruments. All of a small size from Fine Science Tools (FST) (http://www.finescience.com) or other source—at minimum, a small pair of forceps (Dumont no. 5 World Precision Instrument, Inc., cat. no. 500342) for removing oocytes and handling tissue, straight hemostats or needle holders (such as FST, cat. no. 91308-12), scissors for cutting skin and muscle (such as FST iris scissors, cat. no. 91460-11, or FST student surgical scissors, cat. no. 91402-12), 3-0 sutures. Especially fine forceps are usually required for removing the vitelline membrane. Many lab members prefer the finest Dumont tip: FST, cat. no. 11254-20 (*see* **Note 9**).

10. Incubator capable of maintaining temperatures of 18–20°C (VWR).

11. Orbiting mixer (Vibramax) set inside the incubator to gently swirl the oocytes during incubation (*see* **Note 10**).

12. Assorted Petri dishes: 100-mm dishes for oocyte sorting; 60-mm dishes for oocyte incubation; 33-mm tissue culture-coated (Corning, cat. no. 430165) dishes for use as a bath chamber during experiments.

13. Modified pipetors for handling oocytes (**Fig. 2**). The Pipette Pump (Bel-Art products, cat. no. F37898) holds a 5.75-in. Pasteur pipet (Fisher, cat. no. 13-6788-2B for a box of 360) that has been bent at about a 45° angle by heating over a flame from a lab burner (**Fig. 2**). If the tip diameter is too small, the pipet can be cut at a wider portion more proximal to the pipet base: score the circumference with a sharp instrument such as a whetstone, and break. The rough edges can then be fire-polished so as to avoid damaging the cell membrane.

2.1.3. mRNA Injection

1. Automatic injector (Drummond "Nanoject," cat. no. 3-000-203-XV) mounted on a mechanical micromanipulator. In our setup, the bench top is covered by 1-in. thick steel plate approx 3 ft square. The weight of the steel stabilizes the working surface and permits the use of movable magnetic base (MK-B) for the injector/micromanipulator complex.

2. Injection pipet/patch electrode puller. Flaming Brown type (Sutter Instruments) model P-97, with box filament (Sutter, cat. no. FB330B).

3. Injection needles: glass capillary tubes from World Precision Instruments (cat. no. 4878).

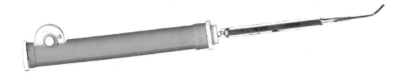

Fig. 2. Oocyte harvest and incubation: modified pipetor.

4. Microforge (Narishige MF-83).
5. Mineral oil.
6. Flexible needle (World Precision Instruments, cat. no. MF34G): use to fill injection needle with mineral oil.
7. Injection Petri dish: a 60-mm or larger Petri dish, the interior bottom of which has been roughened to prevent the oocytes from sliding when impaled by the injection needle. Roughening can be accomplished using sandpaper or by repeated scratching with a needle or other sharp instrument (*see* **Note 11**).

2.2. HEK 293 Heterologous Expression

2.2.1. HEK Cell Culture

1. Full HEK solution: 10% (v/v) fetal bovine serum (FBS), and 50 µg/L gentamicin in Dulbecco's modified Eagle's medium (DMEM) (*see* **Note 12**). Store at 4°C.
2. Calcium-magnesium-free rodent ringer (CaMgFRR): 145 m*M* NaCl, 5 m*M* KCl, 10 m*M* HEPES (*N*-[2-hydrocyethyl]piperaxine-*N'*-[2-ethanesulfonic acid], FW 238.3).
3. Trypsin solution: 0.5 g/L trypsin (bovine pancreas) in CaMgFRR.
4. Petri dishes: 100 mm for cell culture (Falcon, cat. no. 1029).
5. Microscope cover glass: 22 × 50 mm, 16–25 mm thick.
6. Tissue culture incubator and secured CO_2 tank with regulator.
7. Bench centrifuge for tissue culture.
8. Laminar flow hood.

2.2.2. Transfection

1. Polyfect Transfection Reagent (Qiagen, Valencia, CA; *see* **Note 13**).
2. cDNA for the channel under study.
3. cDNA cocktail: cDNA, 4% (v/v) polyfect transfection reagent, 15% DMEM in full HEK solution.

2.3. Pipet (Electrode) Fabrication

1. Electrode puller: Flaming Brown type (Sutter Instruments model P-97), with box filament (Sutter, cat. no. FB330B).
2. Electrode glass. For oocytes: aluminosilicate, O.D. 1.5 mm, I.D. 1.0 mm, 10 cm long (Sutter Instruments, cat. no. AF150-100-10) (*see* **Note 14**).
3. Dental wax for coating electrode tips to reduce capacitance (Patterson Dental Company, MN).

4. Electrode storage. A convenient storage container (consisting of a glass jar ringed inside with foam slots for the microelectrodes) is available from World Precision Instruments, cat. no. E215.

2.4. Electrophysiology Recording Equipment

In addition to the dissecting microscope already listed under **Subheading 2.1.2., item 7**, electrophysiological recording requires the following (*see* **Note 15**):

1. Air table (also called flotation table) and secured nitrogen tank with regulator.
2. Circular level: the air table top must be level for best operation.
3. A Faraday cage, which surrounds the microscope and head stage, protecting them from low-frequency noise. Several commercial Faraday cages are available. An inexpensive but effective cage may be constructed of wood and ordinary metal screening.
4. Amplifier, head stage, analog to digital board, and pipet holder: several suppliers manufacture patch clamp amplifiers, including Axon Instruments, Dagan, Warner Instruments, and HEKA Instruments. All come with comprehensive instruction manuals that describe the theory, design, and use of patch-clamp amplifiers (*see* **Note 16**).
5. Silver chlorided wire for converting the ionic current to electrical current within the micropipet, and for completing the electrical circuit via a ground inserted in the bath solution (*see* **Note 17**).
6. Micromanipulator: several types are available; a steady mechanical manipulator is sufficient for cell-attached patch clamping.
7. Data collection software: several suppliers manufacture data acquisition and analysis software, including Axon Instruments and HEKA, Inc. All are supplied with extensive manuals that detail the correct use of the programs.
8. Windows PC or Macintosh computer to run the data acquisition and analysis software.
9. Temperature controller, and temperature control block: we use a Dagan (cat. no. HCC100-A) temperature controller for both oocytes and HEK 293 cells. For oocytes, the temperature control block (Dagan, cat. no. HE-101D) serves as a microscope stage and holds the recording culture dish (Corning, cat. no. 430165 as listed previously). The temperature control block for whole-cell patch (Dagan, cat. no. HE-104R) is a separate unit placed on the microscope stage and holds the small volume recording chamber (Dagan, cat. no. RCP-6T).
10. Temperature probes. The Dagan controller requires two temperature probes, one within the temperature control block and, for oocytes, one inserted not far from the oocyte in the ISOP bath or, for HEK cells, inserted in the bath solution.
11. Pump for circulating cool water through the temperature control block (e.g., Little Giant Pump Co, cat. no. 501003). The pump is immersed in a large, stiff-walled reservoir that serves as a heat sink (*see* **Note 18**).
12. Source of positive pressure. We use a small aquarium pump regulated by the pressure gauge illustrated in **Figs. 3** and **4**.

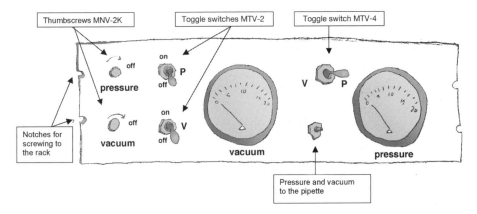

Fig. 3. Pressure/Suction control unit, front panel. http://www.dwyer-inst.com/

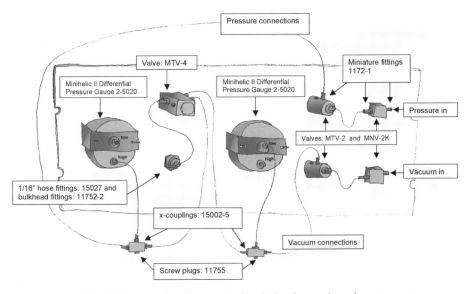

Fig. 4. Pressure/suction control unit, back panel, and parts.

2.4.1. Oocyte/Macropatch

1. Shrinking oocyte ringer 2 (SDOR2): 73g/L mannitol in MgOR2. The hypertonic solution shrinks intracellular contents to facilitate removal of the oocyte vitelline membrane. Made in small batches (500 mL or less) and stored at 4°C.
2. Inside-out patch (ISOP) bath: 9.6 mM NaCl, 88 mM KCl, 11 mM EGTA, 5 mM HEPES, pH 7.4 using 1 M N-methyl-D-glucamine pH 7.4. Store at 4°C.
3. Pipet solution: 96 mM NaCl, 4 mM KCl, 1 mM MgCl$_2$, 1.8 mM CaCl$_2$, 5 mM HEPES, pH 7.4. Store at 4°C. Source of suction. We use lab-supplied vacuum connected to a pressure gauge as illustrated in **Figs. 3** and **4**.

2.4.2. HEK 293/Whole-Cell Patch

1. Bath (extracellular) solution: 140 mM NaCl, 4 mM KCl, 10 mM CaCl$_2$, 1 mM MgCl$_2$, 10 mM HEPES, pH 7.4 with 1 M CsOH. Vacuum-filter (0.22 μm) and store at 4°C.
2. Pipet (intracellular) solution: 130 mM CsCl, 10 mM NaCl, 10 mM EGTA, 10 mM HEPES, 4 mM Mg-ATP, 0.38 mM Li-GTP, put on ice during addition of Mg-ATP and Li-GTP, pH 7.4 with 1 M CsOH, vacuum-filter (0.22 μm) under a laminar flow hood, and store in 1-mL aliquots at –20°C.
3. Source of suction. Two sources are used for HEK 293 cells: the lab suction described in **Figs. 3** and **4**, and mouth suction.

3. Methods

3.1. Oocyte Heterologous Expression

3.1.1. X. laevis and Their Care

1. Cleaning: clean the tank about three times a week, several hours after feeding. As much as one-third of the tank is removed during cleaning, and is replaced with fresh dechlorinated water. Cleaning this way accomplishes the additional task of replacing tank water (*see* **Note 19**).
2. Feeding: feed the frogs approximately three times a week, about three pellets of Frog Brittle per frog. According to IACUC rules, the frogs are observed daily, and their numbers and tank temperature is recorded.
3. Water chemistry. Assess water quality regularly by measuring pH, as well as ammonia, nitrate, nitrite contents.

3.1.2. Oocyte Harvest and Incubation

1. Tricaine. For 1 L: 1.7 g Tricaine , 0.890 g sodium bicarbonate (NaHC0$_3$), double-distilled (dd)H$_2$O up to 1 L (*see* **Note 20**).
2. MgOR2. For 2 L: 11.220 g NaCl, 0.298 g KCl, 3.808 g MgCl$_2$ anhydrous, 2.383 g HEPES, pH 7.4, ddH$_2$O up to 2 L.
3. Dissociation solution. For 25 mL: 50 mg collagenase(metaloproteinase1) (Sigma, cat. no. C-9891 type 1A, 25 mL MgOR2.
4. SOS–. For 1 L: 0.275 g Na pyruvic acid, MgOR2 up to 1 L.
5. SOS+. For 1 L: 1 L SOS–, 10 mL horse serum, 2 mL gentamicin (50 mg/mL in deionized water).
6. Frog selection. With the aquarium net scoop the frog from the tank and examine it for signs of recent surgery. If there are none identify the frog to ensure that there has been a sufficient interval since its last surgery (*see* **Note 21**).
7. Frog transportation. Place the frog with a little tank water (tap water may be too chlorinated) in a closed container for transport. We use a lunchbox-sized cooler for this purpose. Frogs will jump out of an open container and are not only extremely difficult to catch, but contact with dry surfaces will damage their protective mucus layer.

8. Anesthesia. Pour anesthesia solution over the frog in the cooler. Leave for about 15 min or until a firm toe-pinch with hemostats produces no response (*see* **Note 22**).

9. Surgical field. Fill a small box (just larger than the frog) with crushed ice and level the ice at the top edge. Cover with moist paper towels to prevent freezing damage to the frog at the points of contact with the ice. Place anesthetized supine frog on the moist towels.

10. Surgery. Make a small incision, grasping the skin with serrated forceps and using fine scissors to make the incision, approx 1 cm in length, in the lower abdomen approx 1 cm left or right of the midline. A second incision must be made through the fascia.

11. Remove oocytes. Reach into the incision with small forceps, and gently pull. Repeat until the forceps retrieve oocytes. Thereafter, tease oocytes out of the abdomen, trying to remove a follicle (an elongated lobe) at a time if possible, and leave in place while retrieving others. Lift and cut the follicle at the base frequently to enhance visibility and prevent oocytes from drying.

12. Place the oocytes in a 50-mL conical tube filled with MgOR2. They will sink to the bottom.

13. Rehydrate the frog's skin with sterile distilled water or isotonic saline as needed.

14. Close the incision. Suture the fascia using 3-0 Dextron and a curved needle with a single stitch. Using the same material, suture the skin closed with two to three stitches, as necessary. Ensure that no air is trapped as a bubble under the skin, as this can promote infection.

15. Allow the frog to recover. Replace frog in transport container in a small amount of distilled water, making sure that the nostrils reach the air (*see* **Note 23**).

16. Perform preliminary separation (optional). The oocytes now form a small "pellet" on the bottom of the tube. Pour off the excess MgOR2 (the "supernatant"), and transfer the oocytes into a large Petri dish and manually separated into smaller clumps before placing in the enzyme solution. Although some favor dividing the follicle into small pieces of about 20 cells or less before collagenase digestion, fewer damaged oocytes and a clearer solution can be obtained by either no precollagenase oocyte separation, or just a few tears to open up the ovarian follicle. The danger of too much enzymatic digestion appears to be similar between the two methods.

17. Separate oocytes. Place the tube containing oocytes and collagenase on a tube rocker and gently rock the oocytes until they appear 80–90% separated (about 20 min at room temperature). The extent of separation can be examined by gently swirling the tube and observing the proportion of individual oocytes.

18. Stop digestion. When oocytes appear separated, pour off as much of the collagenase as possible into another conical tube and set aside for potential re-collagenasing of residual clumps (in the event residual clumps require re-collagenasing). Stop the enzymatic activity by rinsing 6–10 times with MgOR2, filling the tube completely each time and pouring off the "supernatant."

19. Sort oocytes, stage 1. Decant oocytes into a large (100 mm or so) Petri dish, and under the dissecting microscope remove healthy stage V and VI oocytes (*see* **Fig. 5**) from among the dead and immature, placing them in 60-mm dishes of SOS+. Incubate the

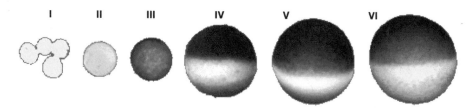

Fig. 5. Stages of oocyte development. http://www.luc.edu/depts/biology/dev/
xenoogen.gif

oocytes at 18–20°C on an orbiting mixer set on at low speed—enough to gently swirl
the oocytes (*see* **Note 24**).

20. Sort oocytes, stage 2. Three to six hours after separation, again examine the dish
    under the dissecting microscope and select out healthy oocytes for transfer to a
    clean dish of SOS+.
21. Change solutions daily. Each day, repeat the procedure for transferring healthy
    oocytes to a fresh dish of SOS+.

3.1.3. mRNA Injection

1. Injection usually takes place the day after surgery (*see* **Note 25**).
2. Construct the glass micropipet that serves as an injection needle. Wear gloves during this procedure to protect against RNAses. Using the glass capillaries listed
   under **Subheading 2.1.3.**, program the puller with the variables: heat, 622 (this
   setting changes with each filament); pull, 120; velocity, 100; time, 150. This gives
   a pipet with a very long, thin tip. Make the injection pipet by breaking the long tip
   with a flame-sterilized pair of small forceps. Practice will determine the appropriate place yield the diameter desired. For cytoplasmic oocyte injection, the tip
   should be approx 20–30 µm. Pipet size is a somewhat of a personal preference.
   Larger tips will be less easily obstructed by impurities in the mRNA. Too large of
   a tip, however, runs a greater risk of damaging the oocyte. To further sharpen the
   pipet, gently touch the longest side of the tip to the microforge heating element set
   at a temperature just high enough to melt the glass. The molten glass will form a
   sharp point as the pipet is withdrawn. Construct several more pipets than the
   minimum required for the injection. Pipet blockage or breakage is common, and
   having a readily available spare saves the mRNA from dessicating while a new
   pipet is made (*see* **Note 26**).
3. Fill the pipet with oil. Still wearing gloves, fill the injection pipet with mineral oil.
   Use a 1-mL syringe and a long, flexible needle (such as cat. no. MF34G from
   World Precision Instruments or one constructed by melting a disposable plastic
   pipetor [yellow] tip and cutting the elongated end with a razor blade and inserting
   the other end into a 1-mL syringe). Oil should completely fill the glass injection
   pipet and be absolutely free of air bubbles.
4. Insert pipet. Slide the oil-filled glass pipet over the plunger of the injection unit,
   making sure that the needle top goes past the first black rubber "O ring" (containing

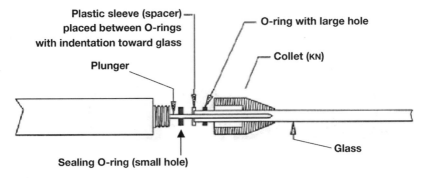

Fig. 6. Correct assembly of the Nanoject/micropipet complex.

the larger hole) and is seated on the white spacer, in the indentation or "shelf" (*see* **Fig. 6**). If the large and small holed "O" rings are not in the proper positions, the pipet will not go in easily and may leak. Likewise, the white spacer should be placed so that the indentation or "shelf" is facing the pipet tip.

5. Tighten the sleeve or "collet" (*see* **Fig. 6**) tightly and press "empty" on the control box to position the plunger as far toward the pipet tip as possible. Continue to press until the unit beeps. The fullest extension of the plunger will ensure maximal filling of the needle with mRNA. Move the entire assembly to the side and out of the way. In our setup this requires simply disengaging the MK-B magnet that secures it to the steel.

6. Fill the injector. Remove the mRNA from the freezer and combine or dilute as desired (*see* **Note 27**). Pipet 2–6 µL onto the inverted top of a 60-mm sterile Petri dish placed under the dissecting microscope. Reposition the injector next to the dish and with the microscope on high power maneuver the pipet tip into the mRNA droplet. Press the "FILL" button on the injector control to retract the plunger and fill the pipet with mRNA. Continue pressing the fill button until the injector beeps to indicate that the plunger is fully retracted. If all has gone well, all or most of the mRNA will have been drawn up into the pipet. This can be very difficult when the needle tip is small and the mRNA is highly viscous. Watch the oil/RNA interface as it travels up the glass pipet. Watch also for bubbles forming toward the top of the glass pipet; too many will displace the RNA and prevent complete filling of the needle. They will also compress during injection, resulting in an unreliable and irreproducible amount of mRNA injected into the oocytes. Bubbles can occur if the plunger is withdrawing faster than the liquid can enter the tip of the pipet. Alleviate this problem by pausing the fill process to allow the liquid to enter the tip releasing the pressure at the top.

7. Pipet oocytes into MgOR2. When the tone sounds indicating that the plunger has reached the top of its path, again move the assembly out of the way and fill the roughened injection Petri dish with MgOR2. Pipet as many oocytes into the dish as is estimated will be injected. Lining these up in a row and beginning the injecting at one end is an easy way to keep track of injected vs uninjected oocytes.

8. Set the injection volume. Set the volume of fluid injected on the Drummond injector using the "dip" switches. For example, the 50 nL that we inject requires switch settings of down-up-down-up.

9. Inject oocyte. With the microscope on medium power (so that three to five oocytes are in the visual field), begin injecting at one end of the row (the right end for the right-handed). Move the dish to position the needle above the oocyte at the equator between the animal and vegetal pole. Lower the needle into the oocyte and press the inject button. This specific placement is best for expression. Our volume is sufficient to produce a visible swelling of the oocyte. Thus, the absence of observable swelling is a sign that nothing has been injected.

10. Lift the pipet to the liquid/air interface. If the oocyte is still impaled, this will release it from the needle.

11. Transfer to SOS+. Following injection, transfer oocytes into a dish containing SOS+ and place in incubator. After 2–4 h, examine the oocytes and transfer the healthy oocytes into a fresh dish of SOS+. The presence of dead and dying oocytes adversely affects those remaining. Perhaps this is owing to lysosomal enzymes released into the medium. Consequently, we transfer healthy oocytes daily into fresh SOS+.

3.2. HEK 293 Heterologous Expression

3.2.1. HEK 293 Cell Passaging for Stock and Transfection Plates

The protocols explained here are for "weekend passaging"; Friday passaging usually enables us to transfect plates from the following Monday to about Thursday, depending on the confluence and the concentrations used. For "overnight passaging" (next-day transfection), the amount of resuspended cell solution placed in the 50-mL conical tube should be doubled.

1. Make full HEK solution: all work should be done under a laminar flow hood using sterile technique. To 180 mL DMEM, Add 20 mL FBS, 200 μL gentamicin solution (50 mg/mL in deionized water), and vacuum-filter (0.22 μm) to sterilize the solution. Store at 4°C (*see* **Notes 12** and **28**).

2. Make CaMgFRR: 975 mL ddH$_2$O, 8.47 g NaCl, 0.373 g of KCl, 2.38 g of HEPES. Place ddH$_2$O, NaCl, KCl, and HEPES into a 2-L beaker. pH to 7.4 using a 1 *M* NaOH solution. Add ddH$_2$O to bring the final volume to 1 L. Vacuum-filter into two sterile 500-mL bottles. One bottle can be stored at 4°C for later use; the other bottle will be used to make the trypsin solution.

3. Make trypsin solution: to 500 mL of CaMgFRR, add 0.5 g trypsin. Stir to dissolve. pH to 7.4 with 1 *M* NaOH. Vacuum-filter into a sterile 500-mL bottle. In a laminar flow hood, place 5-mL aliquots into sterile 15-mL conical tubes. Store at –20°C.

4. Prepare new stock and transfection tissue culture dishes (TCDs). In preparation for the next step, take one aliquot (5 mL) of trypsin solution from the –20°C freezer and let it thaw at 4°C for several hours. When thawed, take it, together with a bottle of full HEK solution from 4°C, and warm both up to room temperature (*see* **Note 29**). We have found that incompletely warmed full HEK and trypsin

solutions will still work, although the room temperature solutions appear to be slightly better for the cells. All remaining work (except centrifugation) should be done under a laminar flow hood. From the incubator, select a stock (100 mm) TCD of HEK 293 cells with a confluence of just under 100% (*see* **Note 30**). Pipet: 10 mL of full HEK solution into each of three fresh, sterile 100-mm TCDs; 12 mL of full HEK solution into a fresh, sterile 50-mL conical tube; and 3 mL of full HEK into a fresh, sterile 15-mL conical tube. This will allow the procedure to be completed quickly and minimizes cell death.

5. Discard spent medium. Using a sterile Pasteur pipet attached to a vacuum, aspirate the medium from the stock TCD.
6. Separate out cells. Immediately add the full 2 mL of trypsin solution and gently agitate the dish for 2 min. With a sterile 5-mL pipetor, transfer the trypsin/cell solution into the 15-mL conical tube containing 3 mL of full HEK solution. Centrifuge for 2 min (Centrific centrifuge, Fisher Scientific, speed setting 3). Attach a new sterile Pasteur pipet to the vacuum system and aspirate the medium from the cell pellet. Use a sterile, disposable bulb pipet to remove the last 2 mL (*see* **Note 31**).
7. Resuspend the cells by triturating with 6 mL of full HEK solution for 2 min with a sterile 10-mL pipetor (*see* **Note 32**).
8. Make stock cultures. Pipet 2.5, 1, and 0.5 mL of the resuspended cell solution into the three (stock) TCDs containing 10 mL of full HEK solution.
9. Make transfection dishes. Place 0.5 mL of the resuspended cell solution into the 50-mL conical tube containing 12 mL of full HEK solution and mix for 10 s.
10. From the 50-mL conical tube, add 4, 3, 2, and 1 mL of the solution to 4 mL of full HEK solution, respectively. The exact number of transfection (60 mm) TCDs depends on how many days one wants to record before the next passage. We use four TCDs to be able to patch for 3 d. As a rule of thumb, prepare $n + 1$ TCDs for n days sterile 60-mm (transfection) TCDs containing 1, 2, 3, and 4 mL of full HEK solution, respectively.
11. Incubate the TCDs in a humidified atmosphere at 37°C with 5% CO_2.

3.2.2. Transfection

1. Polyfect Transfection Reagent (Qiagen, Valencia, CA) (*see* **Note 13**).
2. cDNA cocktail: cDNA, 1.0 mL full HEK solution, 40 µL Polyfect Transfection Reagent (Qiagen), and approx 150 µL of DMEM.
3. Allow the full HEK solution and DMEM to warm to room temperature.
4. All remaining work (except vortexing, centrifugation, and selecting the appropriate TCD) should be done under a laminar flow hood.
5. Add the cDNA, DMEM, and polyfect transfection reagent to a sterile 1.5-mL reaction tube.
6. Vortex for 10 s (*see* **Note 33**), centrifuge for 5 s, and then incubate in the hood for 10 min.
7. During the incubation period, choose a transfection TCD with 40–60% confluency.
8. With 2 min remaining in the incubation period, aspirate the medium from the TCD and add 3 mL of full HEK solution.

9. At the end of the 10-min incubation period, gently add 1 mL of full HEK solution to the reaction tube and mix by pipetting up and down twice.
10. Gently add the cDNA solution to the TCD and swirl the TCD for a few seconds to allow the solutions to completely mix.
11. Incubate the TCD in a humidified atmosphere at 37°C with 5% CO_2 for 24 h.

3.2.3. Plating

1. All work (except centrifugation) should be done under a laminar flow hood.
2. With a sterile glass cutter, cut the cover glass into 4- to 5-mm squares, the exact size depending on the size of the well in the recording chamber.
3. Using sterile tweezers, dip each square into 70% ethanol and place as a single layer into two sterile 35-mm TCDs (about 13–17 squares per TCD).
4. Allow the ethanol to evaporate out of the dish (*see* **Note 34**).
5. Aspirate the solution from the transfection TCD (transfected the day before).
6. Immediately add the trypsin solution and let stand for 2 min (agitation is unnecessary owing to the low number of cells in the TCD).
7. During the 2 min, add 3 mL of full HEK to a sterile 15-mL conical tube.
8. Add the trypsin/cell solution to the tube.
9. Centrifuge for 2 min so that a pellet forms at the bottom of the tube.
10. Aspirate the medium from the solution using a sterile, disposable bulb pipet to remove the last 2 mL.
11. Resuspend the cells by triturating with 6 mL of full HEK solution for 2 min with a sterile 10-mL pipetor.
12. Add 2 mL of the resuspended cell solution to each 35-mm TCD.
13. Incubate the TCD overnight in a humidified atmosphere at 37°C with 5% CO_2 (*see* **Note 35**).

3.3. Pipet (Electrode) Fabrication

3.3.1. Macropatch Pipet (Electrode) Fabrication

1. Whole-cell and macropatch pipets are relatively short and stubby and have a large diameter tip (>0.7 μ). Methods of fabrication depend on the pipet puller and type of glass. Follow the procedure from the Sutter P-97 manual (*see* the appendix).
2. Apply dental wax to the outside of the patch pipets to reduce stray capacitive coupling between the solutions on the inside and the outside of the glass pipet. Coated pipets also have the advantage of protecting the fine glass tip from dirt and debris during storage. Melt dental wax (Patterson Dental Company, St. Paul, MN reorder, cat. no. 091-1503) in a small, heatproof container (such as a 20-mL Pyrex beaker) set on the low setting of a hot plate. We use dial number 2 or 3 on our hot plate (Fisher Scientific, cat. no. 11-500-4H). Coat electrodes by dipping into melted wax and flicking off excess over a waste container. Adjust temperature according to preference. At the low end of the melting temperature, wax will clump, which can reflect light and compromise visibility in the microscope field. On the higher end of the range, wax will coat thinly, but the higher temperature

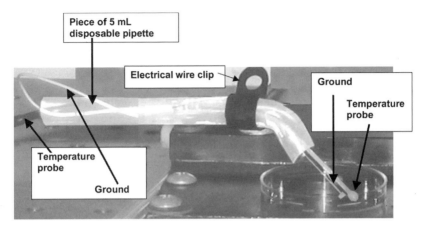

Fig. 7. Electrophysiology recording setup.

promotes faster wax breakdown, and thus uses more wax. Very thin wax may also compromise the ability to reduce capacitance.

3. Store coated electrodes until use. A convenient storage container consisting of a glass jar ringed inside with foam slots for the microelectrodes is available from World Precision Instruments (cat. no. E215 for 1.5 mm O.D. glass).

3.4. Electrophysiology Recording Setup

1. Air table setup: follow the manufacturer's instructions for air table setup. Ensure that the compressed nitrogen tank is securely fastened to a wall or other stable object in an approved manner. Connect the tank to the air table with high-pressure tubing and set the pressure to level recommended by air table manufacturer.

2. Microscope stage, temperature control block setup: for oocytes, secure the temperature control block to the air table in a level position. In our laboratory, the block is mounted on an open Plexiglas box, elevating it approx 5 in. above the table top. A finger-sized hole in the Plexiglas top permits reaching underneath to push out the culture dish. For HEK 293 cells, attach the block/recording chamber piece to the microscope stage. Place a temperature probe into the small hole at the back of the block (it can be secured to the block by a bit of dental wax). Connect the opposite end to the "block" temperature input on the controller.

3. Bath inserts: two wires go into the bath solution: the sensor for bath temperature, and a silver chloride wire that serves as ground, the other end of which inserts into the head stage. These two wires—bath temperature probe and ground—require some type of holder that will keep both stable and in repeatable locations in the dish. Our lab accomplishes this by enclosing both in a curved plastic tube fastened to the temperature block with the type of clip that usually holds electrical wiring (*see* **Fig. 7**).

4. Micromanipulator, head stage setup: attach the micromanipulator to the tabletop at a distance from the oocyte dish that allows the head stage, clamped to the micromanipulator, to point toward the recording dish at a 45° angle.

5. With all of the necessary equipment in place, the heating block and micromanipulator fastened to the tabletop, and all wires shielded and grounded, level the tabletop using the circular level.

3.5. Obtaining a "Gigaseal" and Making Recordings

Time to channel expression depends on channel isoform and perhaps several other (unknown) variables. After 2–3 d, begin to check for channel expression. Follow the procedures below for obtaining a "gigaseal" and monitor current amplitude. Currents of 100 pA or more are sufficiently above noise level to yield reliable data.

1. Set up the rig with the following steps:
   a. Start the water pump and make sure that the water is circulating through the temperature control block (holding the recording dish) and back into the water reservoir. Doing this first prevents possible overheating and burnout of the block.
   b. Insert a 35-mm Corning dish (these fit into the Dagan temperature control blocks, whereas Falcon Petri dishes do not; Fisher Scientific, cat. no. 0877220) into the temperature control block and fill with ISOP bath using a 10-mL syringe fitted with a 0.2-μ syringe filter. Filtering the bath solution is necessary to remove particulates that can interfere with seal formation.
   c. Insert the bath temperature probe (*see* **Subheading 2.**) together with the distal end of the head stage ground. It is crucial that the temperature probe be placed in the same position for all recordings. Channel kinetics are exquisitely sensitive to temperature, and the position of the temperature probe is critical to temperature maintenance. Temperature recorded with the probe at the dish sidewall will differ by more than 0.2°C from that with the probe in the center.
   d. Turn on the amplifier.
   e. Turn on the temperature controller (set to "standby").
   f. Turn on the source of positive pressure (small aquarium pump) (*see* **Note 36**).
   g. Finally, open the nitrogen supply and, if not already set, regulate the pressure to 80 psi, or whatever is recommended by the air table used.

2. Place one to four oocytes into a small dish of SDOR2 on the stage of the dissecting microscope. Although we usually try to select oocytes with uniform color and shape, it is also possible to obtain good recordings from those with uneven or patchy coloring of the animal pole. When swirls begin to develop, however, the oocytes should be discarded.

3. After a few minutes, set the microscope to highest magnification, or so that the oocyte fills about half the field. Grasp the vitelline membrane somewhat indirectly using the following technique, which minimizes punctures. Lay the open forceps sideways (at about a 45° angle) against the oocyte and close them so that the tip only grips the membrane. Lift up and hold the open second pair of forceps to either side of the first pair, pinch, and pull gently. The membrane will tear and part with the oocyte. If only part of the membrane is removed, hold the left forceps still

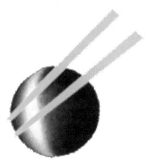

Fig. 8. Initial forceps placement for vitelline membrane removal.

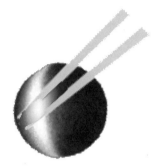

Fig. 9. First grasping of vitelline membrane.

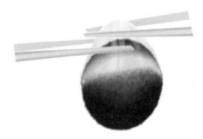

Fig. 10. Technique for securing membrane with second forceps.

and with the right, again pinch to either side. Repeat until the membrane is removed (*see* **Note 37**). As soon as the vitelline membrane is removed, transfer the oocyte to a dish of ISOP bath medium while peeling the remaining eggs (a convenient dish for this purpose is the top of the culture dish used as the recording chamber) (*see* **Figs. 8–10**).
4. Place the oocytes in the recording chamber in the center of the dish or wherever is most convenient given the setup between the head stage and the dish. Wait for the oocytes to resume normal size—10 min or more. Failure to allow full recovery from the shrinking solution seems to make sealing more difficult.

5. Polish a microelectrode: choose a microelectrode pipet and mount it in the micro-forge. With the microscope on high power, heat the wire and bring the tip close enough to produce visible rounding or "firepolishing" of the glass edges. Fire-polishing the tip facilitates seal formation and melts the dental wax from the tip of the pipet.

6. Fill the polished microelectrode about halfway with pipet solution. The same type of thin needle used to fill the injection pipet can be used, or a very inexpensive one can be constructed by heating the side of a plastic pipet tip and stretching it out to the right thickness. If the tip base does not already fit a syringe, it can easily be cut at the proper diameter.

7. On the computer, open the data acquisition software and create a folder for the day's experiments. Our file labeling system consists of a separate folder for each day, labeled with the date, channel, and other information such as the co-expression of β-subunits, temperature, a rig identifier, and the initials of the experimenter. Within the folder, data files are created, labeled similarly with the date and channel, and in addition, an oocyte and patch number. Thus, an experimental file using the human cardiac channel $hNa_V1.5$ might be labeled: "051005hNaV153b+ B1_22C." From the left side this reads: date; isoform (i.e., channel type or mutant); number of the oocyte (oocyte number 3 in this case); patch number (patch b in this case, indicating the second patch on this oocyte); co-expressed with the β1-subunit; recorded at 22°C.

8. Secure the micropipet onto the head stage: unscrew the head stage holder. Slide the filled tip onto the wire and all the way into electrode assembly and tighten the holder. Check the positive pressure to insure a small steady pressure flows into the pipet to keep out the bath liquid and keep the pipet tip clean. Lower the pipet into the bath until it is close to but not touching the egg. Use the data acquisition software to measure pipet resistance. For macropatching oocytes, we use pipets with resistances in the 0.8 to 1 MΩ range. For whole cell recordings, pipet resistances are in the 1 to 4 MΩ range.

9. Advance the microelectrode: turn the fine control to lower the pipet slowly toward the oocyte/HEK cell while monitoring pipet resistance. When the pipet touches the membrane, resistance will suddenly increase. Suction should be applied at this point to increase seal resistance. Once resistance begins to increase quickly, suction should be terminated to avoid rupturing the membrane.

10. When the seal resistance stabilizes, the holding potential should be set to an appropriate value (*see* **Note 38**). If using HEK cells, the whole-cell configuration should be attained by a brief application of strong suction. The whole-cell configuration is attained when the capacitance suddenly increases, reflecting the fact that the membrane capacitance is now part of the electrical circuit.

11. After a rest period of about 5 min, data collection can begin. Specific voltage protocols are determined by the biophysical processes to be observed. In all cases, however, we precede our voltage protocols with a prolonged hyperpolarization (–150 mV for 30 s in oocytes; –130 mV for 30 s in HEK cells) to recover all channels from any residual inactivation.

4. Notes

1. Our two fiberglass tanks are larger for the number of frogs we house (approx 10 frogs in a 100-gallon tank) than most recommendations for frog density, which can be as low as one gallon per frog (http://www.xlaevis.com/system.html).

2. The common procedure of dechlorinating water by letting it stand will be ineffective if the local water is treated with the longer-lasting chloramines instead of chlorine. In this case, water must be prefiltered with a carbon filter or neutralized by several products available at pet or aquarium supply stores.

3. Although in the wild *Xenopus* inhabit stagnant pools, research on captive frogs shows filtered, dechlorinated water is preferable *(3,4)*.

4. We chose this temperature because it has been reported to optimize the frog's food consumption (http://www.xenopus.com/husbandry.htm).

5. We have experimented with several different foods—beef liver, beef heart, as well as several pelleted foods. The frogs seem to relish the meat, but improvement in oocyte quality (i.e., expression), if any, was not sufficient to offset the additional time spent in food preparation. Currently, we feed the frogs a pelleted food (Frog Brittle from Nasco), with good results.

6. In the past, we have attempted to treat sick frogs. We have discontinued this practice because of a poor success rate (no cures out of approximately six frogs).

7. Addition of this amount brings the pH of the Tricane solution from about pH 3.0 to approximately pH 6.0. The more physiological pH relieves the burden of acid stress and also reduces the time to adequate surgical anesthesia.

8. Because collagenase activity requires Ca^{2+} as a co-factor, restricting calcium during oocyte separation serves to modulate enzymatic digestion. Low Ca^{2+} levels during mRNA injection and vitelline membrane removal protect the cell from a Ca^{2+} overload, and inhibit lysosymic enzymes. Make MgOR2 either fresh in batches of about 2 L, or as a 10X stock, filter-sterilized. Once constituted, both stock and final solution will keep for several months at 4°C.

9. We autoclave the instruments for surgery. Sterility, however, is not required for vitelline membrane removal.

10. Filling a dish too full of medium will inhibit swirling.

11. Some use a fine mesh to stabilize the oocytes for injection. When choosing the mesh size, ensure that it is small enough to exclude the smallest oocytes. Small oocytes escaping through the mesh is not the only difficulty, however; the oocyte tends to become wedged in the mesh and cannot be easily rotated. As best expression seems to result from injecting in a specific location (the equator between the animal and vegetal poles), inability to expose that location is a major drawback.

12. DMEM (1X), liquid, high glucose, with L-glutamine, 110 mg/L sodium pyruvate, and pyridoxine hydrochloride. Store from 2 to 8°C, protect from light—an easy way is to wrap the bottles in aluminum foil.

13. The total amount of cDNA used should be 4.0 μg. When we co-express $hNa_V1.5$ with enhanced green florescent protein (EGFP) we use 3.5 μg $hNa_V1.5$ and 0.5 μg EGFP cDNA. The ratio of cDNAs can be adjusted and optimized for specific needs. The amount of DMEM depends on the volume of cDNA. The total volume

of cDNA and DMEM should be 150 µL. In our experiments, the cDNA volume is generally 8 µL and the DMEM volume is 142 µL.

14. For oocyte macropatches use aluminosilicate, thick-walled glass (Sutter, cat. no. AF-150-100-10) because of its low noise properties and because its properties allow very high-resistance seals with oocyte membranes. For HEK 293 whole-cell recordings, we use borosilicate glass, O.D. 1.5 mm, I.D. 0.86 mm, 10 cm long, Sutter Instruments (Sutter, cat. no. B150-86-10).

15. A former graduate student, Dr. Dave Featherstone, constructed an apparatus that consolidates the many pieces to control and automate suction and pressure onto a single control board. Instructions and specifications for the setup can be found in **Figs. 3** and **4**.

16. The "head stage," also called the "head amplifier," is a small preamplifier that enhances signal strength and controls voltage across the cell membrane. This is a highly sensitive component that must be handled with extreme care, including the discharge of any static electricity that may have accumulated prior to touching the headstage.

17. Chloriding the silver wire to make an Ag/AgCl electrode can be accomplished several ways, including dipping in standard chlorine bleach. In our laboratory, chloride is applied quickly by passing a current through the silver wire immersed in potassium chloride solution. A battery provides the current, and a second silver wire completes the circuit.

18. During lengthy experiments, the pump motor will gradually heat the water, reducing its cooling effectiveness and potentially compromising temperature stability. Thermal stability can be improved by enlarging the water reservoir (to 5–10 gallons). The reservoir container must be strong enough to withstand the pressure exerted by a large water volume. A convenient choice is a large (about 8 gallons) sharps container. If the water becomes warm, add a frozen water bottle or a little ice. Do not allow the reservoir to become significantly cooler than "room temperature," as this may directly change block temperature. Any effect on temperature independent of the central control mechanism will upset regulation; the information fed back to the controller does not directly reflect the output. For reliable temperature control, it is essential that the cooling flow be adequate. In order to test this, the manufacturer suggests setting the bath temperature to a level low enough to require maximum output from the cooling mechanism. Flow is adequate if a hand on the block detects little or no change when the unit is maximally cooling.

19. For a siphon, we use about 3 ft of PVC pipe secured to a length of 1-in. tubing to vacuum the bottom and flush waste down the floor drain.

20. More $NaHCO_3$ can be added to raise the pH to 7.4 if desired.

21. IACUC-approved protocol requires that frogs be subjected to surgery only once in 2 mo—long enough for incisions to heal completely and make identification of individual frogs difficult. A convenient waterproof and swim-proof identifier is thus needed. We have had some success with recording strong identifying marks but have found that the best identification technique is to become familiar with the individual frogs. Various labeling methods exist in the literature, including toe

removal, and branding with acid. Although these methods have the advantage of being readily visible on free-swimming frogs, we have discontinued them as time-consuming and inhumane. We have tried photographing them with standard film but this does not provide a view detailed enough view for identification. Currently, we are experimenting with scanning images into Adobe Photoshop by placing the anesthetized frogs supine (face up) on the scanner bed. This provides a clear view of the frog's dorsal markings, and contains promise as a workable system.

22. The toe pinch is used because the righting response has led to incomplete anesthesia. Cold Tricaine solution from the refrigerator facilitates anesthesia, but room temperature solution is acceptable if made fresh.

23. Making sure that the frog's nostrils reach the air by either propping up the head (e.g., with folded paper towels) or by tipping the container to expose the nose. Allow the frog to recover fully (several hours) before releasing it into the home tank. In the past, we have kept the frog in a recovery tank, but have found this unnecessary in our hands.

24. Reported incubation temperature varies. We have had success with 18 and 19°C temperatures, but have not collected enough data to reveal an expression difference, if any.

25. Oocytes can be injected the same day of, and up to 2 d after, surgery. We have not attempted to inject longer than 3 d after harvest.

26. Oocytes can also be injected directly into the nucleus using a smaller pipet tip if DNA is used for injection rather than mRNA. We obtained good, rapid expression with this technique, but had difficulty co-expressing the β-subunit with the α-subunit, and so did not pursue the technique further.

27. We store RNA in 2-μL aliquots, as this makes a convenient volume for coexpressing two-channel subunits.

28. Make full HEK solution fresh every 2–3 wk. The solution will lighten in color even when stored at 4°C. We have not noticed any detrimental effects from the color change if the solution was made within 2–3 wk and was stored at 4°C.

29. If pressed for time, place the tube in a beaker of room temperature ddH$_2$O.

30. If all of the stock TCDs are 100% confluent, use the one with the smallest amount of resuspended cell solution and increase the amount of full HEK used to resuspend the cells by 1–3 mL. Confluence can be estimated by examining the TCD under an inverted light microscope.

31. Be careful not to aspirate the pellet when using a vacuum system. Take extra care not to place the tip of the Pasteur pipet near the "strings" of cells that come out from the pellet.

32. One to three milliliters more if the original TCD had a confluence of 100%.

33. We have noticed that vortexing for less than 10 s significantly diminishes the expression of channels in the cells.

34. This procedure generally takes an hour or more depending on the volume of ethanol on each square. A small amount (size of a pin head) will probably remain under the middle of each square; this does not impact the procedure, however, excess ethanol remaining near the edges or on top of the squares prevents a seal

from being formed between the TCD and the glass. The glass will float when the cell solution is added if an adequate seal is not present. If this occurs, use sterile tweezers to press the squares to the bottom of the dish.

35. We generally plate in the afternoon/early evening and find that the cells are ready to use throughout the next day. The cells seem most robust about 18 h after plating.

36. In our lab the suction is constantly enabled from the lab outlet, but is modulated at the rig by a valve. A similar system regulates the positive air flow.

37. Long duration exposure (>15 min) to SDOR2 will damage the oocytes.

38. We find that holding potential is a critical determinant of sodium channel availability. We thus hold the potential as negative as will be tolerated by the seal. In oocytes and HEK cells, this value is usually −100 mV.

Appendix: Step-by-Step Patch Pipet Programming

Run a Ramp Test with the glass you intend to use for your particular application. Refer to the manual to review the Ramp Test procedure if necessary. When the Ramp value (R) is known, use it in the following program.

1. Program one line of code as follows:

	HEAT	PULL	VELOCITY	TIME
for box filament:	R	0	40	200

Note: the VELOCITY value will need to be manipulated.

2. PRESSURE should be set to 500 for thick-walled glass and 300 for thin-walled glass.

3. Insert the glass and execute the above program. The program should "loop" a multiple number of times (i.e., the same line will be repeatedly executed). The display will report the number of loops at the end of the pull sequence. This "looping" is the key to forming patch pipets. For thin-walled glass, three to four loops are typically all that is required. For thick-walled glass, three to five loops are typically required.

4. Increase the VELOCITY in 5- to 10-U increments and pull a pipet after each adjustment. Note the change in the number of loops and note the geometry of the pipet (viewed with microscope). As the VELOCITY increases, the number of loops decreases.

5. Repeat **step 4**, but this time, decrease the VELOCITY. As the VELOCITY decreases, the number of loops increases.

6. By adjusting the VELOCITY as described, establish the number of loops required to approximately form a pipet with the desired characteristics.

   Set the VELOCITY value in the program to the number that falls midway between the values required to loop one more and one less times than the desired number. For example, suppose one is experimenting with VELOCITY values and finds that when the glass separates after three loops, the resulting pipet looks reasonable. Let Y be equal to the VELOCITY value that results with the glass separating after four loops. Let Z be equal to the VELOCITY value that results with the glass separating after two loops. Set the program VELOCITY to a value midway between Y and Z. This value will be a very stable VELOCITY value and will provide the most reproducible results.

7. The one-line program just established maybe sufficient for the application. However, changes made in a one-line program are amplified throughout the program and can produce gross changes in the pipet. If fine adjustments to the pipet geometry must be made, then use a multiline program. The multiline program is based on the one-line program just established. It is developed as in **step 8**.

8. Write the one-line looping program out into an equivalent multiline program with the number of lines equal to the number of loops. For example, a one-line, four-loop program with the following values:

	HEAT	PULL	VELOCITY	TIME
loops four times:	300	0	45	200

would be written into an equivalent four-line program:

	HEAT	PULL	VELOCITY	TIME
line 1	300	0	45	200
line 2	300	0	45	200
line 3	300	0	45	200
line 4	300	0	45	200

9. Now, adjustments can be made to the <u>last</u> or <u>next to last</u> line to fine-tune the program and the resulting pipet.

10. Recommended changes to fine-tune the multiline program:

For **larger** diameter tips   Decrease **HEAT** in **last line.**

For **smaller** diameter tips   Increase or decrease **VELOCITY** in the **next to last line** by 5 or 10 U.

or

Increase or decrease **VELOCITY** in the **last line** by 5 or 10 U.

or

Add a small amount of **PULL** (10 or 20) to the **last line.**

References

1. Sumikawa, K., Houghton, M., Emtage, J. S., Richards, B. M., and Barnard, E. A. (1981) Active multi-subunit ACh receptor assembled by translation of heterologous mRNA in Xenopus oocytes. *Nature* **292,** 862–864.
2. Hamill, O. P., Marty, A., Neher, E., Sakmann, B., and Sigworth, F. J. (1981) Improved patch-clamp techniques for high-resolution current recording from cells and cell-free membrane patches. *Pflugers Arch.* **391,** 85–100.
3. Hilken, G., Dimigen, J., and Iglauer, F. (1995) Growth of Xenopus laevis under different laboratory rearing conditions. *Laboratory Animals* **29,** 152–162.
4. Major, N. and Wassersug, R. J. (1998) Survey of current techniques in the care and maintenance of the African clawed frog (Xenopus laevis). *Laboratory Animals Science* **37,** 57–60.

12

Laser-Induced Thrombosis in Zebrafish Larvae
A Novel Genetic Screening Method for Thrombosis

Pudur Jagadeeswaran, Ryan Paris, and Prashanth Rao

Summary

Classical genetic approaches to study hemostasis and thrombosis have not been available until our recent introduction of the teleost, *Danio rerio* (the zebrafish), as an effective genetic model for in vivo coagulation assays. The genetic screen for this model is carried out using the genome saturation mutagenesis approach. The resulting mutants are screened for hemostatic or thrombotic defects. We developed a global physiological screening method for thrombosis by utilizing a laser to induce thrombosis in a specifically targeted area of the major artery and vein. Using this assay, we have screened many fish for abnormal hemostasis, and have isolated a number of mutants with abnormal coagulation parameters. These mutants can be grown, bred, and further evaluated for the genetic etiology of their abnormal hemostatic pathways.

Key Words: Zebrafish; hemostasis; thrombosis; laser; coagulation; in vivo screening assays; thrombocytes; mutagenesis.

1. Introduction

Hemostasis is the defense mechanism by which organisms with a circulatory system prevent external loss of circulatory fluid *(1)*. When this mechanism occurs within the circulatory system, it is pathological, and is called thrombosis. Despite several decades of biochemical research in hemostasis and thrombosis function, several pathways remain elusive, such as the mechanisms involved in the initiation of hemostasis. Therefore, classical genetic methods, as they have been applied to *Drosophila*, become useful and complementary to the biochemical analysis *(2)*. Such classical genetic

From: *Methods in Molecular Medicine, vol. 129:*
Cardiovascular Disease: Methods and Protocols, Volume 2: Molecular Medicine
Edited by: Q. K. Wang © Humana Press Inc., Totowa, NJ

approaches to study hemostasis and thrombosis have not been available until our recent introduction of the teleost, *Danio rerio* (the zebrafish), as an effective genetic model for in vivo coagulation assays *(3)*. The genetic screen for this model is carried out using the genome saturation mutagenesis approach. An adult male zebrafish is mutagenized by submersion in the alkylating agent, ethylnitrosourea (ENU), resulting in single-locus DNA mutations in spermatogonial stem cells *(4)*. This male fish is then crossed with a wild-type female, producing a heterozygous progeny that is subsequently interbred to produce homozygous mutants using the conventional three-generation recessive mutagenesis screen. Alternatively, homozygous mutant progeny can be generated directly from heterozygous females by parthenogenetic diploidization methods *(5)*. The resulting mutants are screened for hemostatic or thrombotic defects. As Virchow pointed out, thrombosis is owing to a triad of components: the vessel wall, blood constituents, and parameters affecting blood flow/stasis *(6)*. In order to effectively screen for these three components, we developed a global physiological screening method for thrombosis *(7)*. As zebrafish larvae are transparent with easily visualized, well-defined blood vessels, we utilize a laser to induce thrombosis in a specifically targeted area of the major artery and vein. This laser-thrombosis assay was also facilitated by the fact that the zebrafish thrombocytes and other blood cells are of sufficient size to visualize microscopically while hemostatic mechanisms take effect following vascular injury *(8)*. Using this assay, we have screened many fish for abnormal hemostasis, and have isolated a number of mutants *(1,9)*. The assay is quantified by three different time parameters: time to adherence (TTA) of the first cell, time to occlusion (TTO), and time to thrombus dissolution (TTD) for both the dorsal aorta and inferior vena cava. We now describe the detailed methodology of the laser-thrombosis assay using zebrafish larvae, to screen for hemostatic defects.

2. Materials

2.1. Zebrafish Larval Production

1. Adult heterozygous mutant zebrafish.
2. Stapleflakes (The Wardley Corporation, Secaucus, NJ), frozen brine shrimp (San Francisco Bay Brand, Newark, CA), and freshly hatched *Artemia franciscana* (GSL Brine Shrimp, Ogden, UT).
3. Breeding tanks.
4. A temperature-controlled fish room (28.5°C) with regulated light and dark cycles (14 h light, 10 h dark).
5. Brine shrimp net for embryo collection.
6. Petri dishes to contain and rinse collected eggs.

7. E3 medium: 5 mM NaCl, 0.17 mM KCl, 0.33 mM CaCl$_2$, 0.33 mM MgSO$_4$, 10^{-5}% methylene blue.
8. Plastic Pasteur pipet (with tip cut off to create a wide bore).

2.2. Preparation of Zebrafish Larvae for Laser Thrombosis

1. Glass microscopic slides.
2. Rubber gasket to contain agarose on the microscopic slide.
3. Petroleum jelly as a gasket sealant.
4. 1.0% low melting agarose solution prepared in a microwave oven.
5. Diluted Tricaine (10 mM).
6. Dissection scope.
7. A plastic micropipet tip.

2.3. Laser Setup

1. Nikon Optiphot microscope with camera attachment and fluorescent port for delivery of the laser beam.
2. A high-power nitrogen laser (Laser Science, Inc.).
3. MicroPoint laser ablation system (Photonic Instruments, Inc.).
4. Slide-shaped laser adjustment mirror.
5. Nikon Coolpix 995 digital camera with video output, mounted on microscope.
6. Video recorder and monitor.

3. Methods

After fertilization, the zebrafish embryos develop for 3 d before hatching from the chorion. At this stage, and for several days after hatching, the blood vessels are visible but become increasingly masked in certain areas by melanin granules. The major artery, called the dorsal aorta, receives oxygenated blood pumped from the two-chambered heart via the gills. From the dorsal aorta the blood enters the caudal artery and returns deoxygenated blood via the caudal vein to the inferior vena cava, and then to the sinus venosus of the heart. Other parts of the body receive blood through branches of these major vessels. Myotomes, which have relatively consistent patterns of distribution in zebrafish, are reliable markers for repeatedly selecting an exact location of the vessel for injury. On the contrary, it is very difficult to consistently target the same vessel locations in the mouse model due to anatomic variations and the need for invasive exposure of the vessels. In zebrafish, venous thrombosis can be induced about 2 d postfertilization and is especially effective after hatching. However, arterial thrombosis cannot be induced effectively until 5–6 d postfertilization, when a sufficient amount of thrombocytes are in circulation. Following the laser-induced venous thrombosis of zebrafish larvae, red cells are the first components to adhere to vessel walls (unpublished), whereas in arterial thrombosis young thrombocytes adhere first, followed by mature

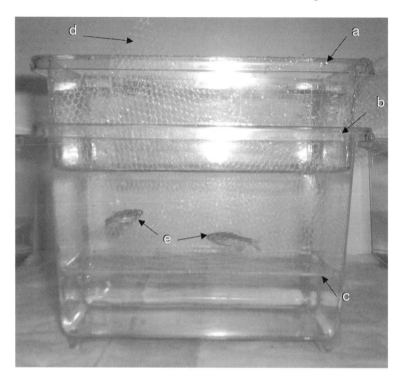

Fig. 1. The breeding tank is assembled with two 1-L tanks, with the bottom cut out from one tank. The bottomless tank is placed onto a mesh, and then placed into the tank with a bottom. The mesh is sterilized by autoclaving or ultraviolet treatment. (**a**) Top tank. (**b**) Bottom tank. (**c**) Top tank with bottom cut off. (**d**) Sterilized mesh. (**e**) Zebrafish breeding pair.

thrombocytes and young thrombocytes as independent clusters propagating the arterial thrombus.

3.1. Breeding Zebrafish

Zebrafish pairs are separated into individual 1-L tanks and fed three times daily with staple flakes, frozen brine shrimp, and fresh baby brine shrimp. The pair is then placed in a breeding tank at the end of a light cycle. The breeding tank is assembled with two 1-L tanks, with the bottom cut off from one tank (**Fig. 1**) (*see* **Note 1**). The bottomless tank is placed onto a mesh, and then inserted into the tank with a bottom such that fish cannot escape into the bottom tank where eggs would reside. The mesh is sterilized by either autoclaving or ultraviolet (UV) treatment. Within the first 2 h of the next light cycle, the fish begin to spawn, and dozens of eggs collect at the bottom of the tank under the protection of the mesh. After the fish are removed, the water is filtered through

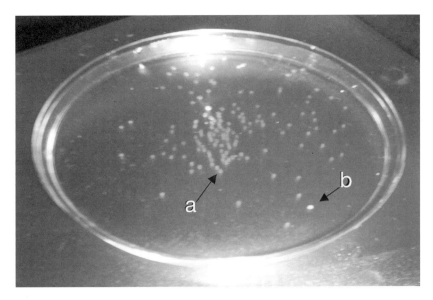

Fig. 2. Petri dish containing E3 media with freshly collected eggs. (**a**) Fertilized eggs. (**b**) Feces/junk material.

a brine shrimp net which retains the eggs. The net is immediately inverted over a Petri dish containing E3 media, which readily releases the eggs along with feces and other junk material (**Fig. 2**) (*see* **Note 2**). A plastic Pasteur pipet is used to gently separate the eggs from feces and junk material and placed in fresh E3 media, and this separation is repeated twice to increase their viability. Embryos and fish are maintained in the room maintained at 28.5°C. After hatching, the 3-d-old larvae are used for venous thrombosis assays, and others are saved for arterial thrombosis at 5–6 d postfertilization.

3.2. Mounting the Zebrafish Larvae in Agarose

Low-melt agarose is mixed with distilled water to make a 1% solution, boiled and refluxed in a microwave, and then is maintained at 35°C in a water bath (*see* **Note 3**). A glass microscopic slide is prepared by lightly coating one side of a rectangular gasket with petroleum jelly and pressing it onto the slide. For each assay, at least one dozen larvae are gently transferred from the Petri dish to a 2-mL Eppendorf tube along with excess media (*see* **Note 4**). The liquid level is slowly withdrawn with a pipet until it is reduced to 0.5 mL. Care is taken not to hurt the larvae in this process. Six microliters of a 10 mM Tricaine solution is added to the solution to anesthetize the larvae. The larvae stop moving within 30 s, and then 0.5 mL of the agarose solution is added and gently mixed by inversion and immediately but gently poured onto the prepared microscope slide. The larvae usually

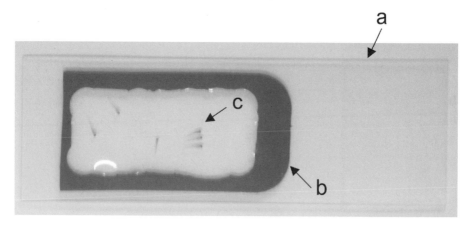

Fig. 3. A glass microscopic slide with rubber gasket with rubber gasket containing anesthetized larvae. (**a**) Glass slide (3 in. × 1 in. × 1 mm). (**b**) Rubber gasket. (**c**) Anesthetized larvae embedded in agarose.

position themselves flat on their side so the vessels are clearly visible, but some larvae require gentle reorientation under the dissection scope with a pipet tip as the agarose solidifies. At this time, the pattern of the larvae is roughly drawn on a paper and numbered so the larvae can be targeted according to a numbered scheme (**Fig. 3**).

3.3. Laser Ablations

The laser setup referred to previously is a nitrogen laser-pumped coumarin dye laser, configured according to the manufacturers' procedures (**Fig. 4**). The nitrogen laser repetition rate is set at 10 pulses per second and the pulse generator rate is set at 10 Hz. The coumarin laser attenuator plate is adjusted to power level 10 for the younger larvae and up to 14 for older larvae. Before each batch of larvae is placed on the scope, the accuracy of the laser is tested by placing a slide-shaped mirror on the stage and triggering the laser through the ×10 objective. The laser damages the mirror and allows a small beam of light through, which can be adjusted to be visible at the intersection of the cross-hairs embedded in the eyepiece. The prepared slide is placed under the microscope and viewed with a ×2 lens for orientation, and then individual larval vessels are located with the ×20 lens. The area for laser ablation is selected by counting five to six somites toward the caudal end from the anal pore (**Fig. 5**). Using a hand switch for the laser, the artery or vein is targeted and damaged for 5 s, with the subsequent thrombus formation clearly recorded onto videotape. At the start of an ablation, a hand is waived across the microscope's light source to mark the starting point of the laser pulse. Approximate TTA and TTO are recorded.

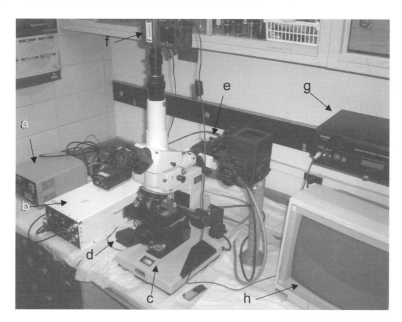

Fig. 4. Nitrogen laser-pumped coumarin dye laser set up, configured according to the manufacturer's procedures. (**a**) 100-W power supply unit for mercury lamp. (**b**) Thermo Laser Science nitrogen laser. (**c**) Nikon optiphot microscope. (**d**) Laser trigger. (**e**) Attenuator plate. (**f**) Nikon CoolPix 995 digital camera. (**g**) Hi-Fi VCR. (**h**) RGB monitor.

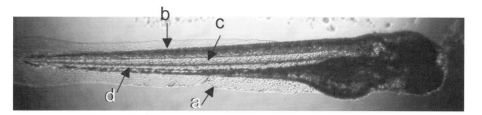

Fig. 5. A zebrafish larvae showing the sites of laser injury. (**a**) Anal pore. (**b**) Approximately the fifth or sixth somite from the anal pore. (**c**) Dorsal aorta. (**d**) Caudal vein.

The sequential images of thrombus formation in both artery and vein are shown in **Fig. 6**. After completion of ablations, the larvae continue to be monitored for the amount of time taken for thrombus dissolution and restoration of local circulation. The video is then reviewed to count the precise times taken for adherence and occlusion. The normal times for TTA, TTO, and TTD are approx 4 s, 21 s, and 90 min, respectively, for the vein; and 11 s, 75 s, and 5 min,

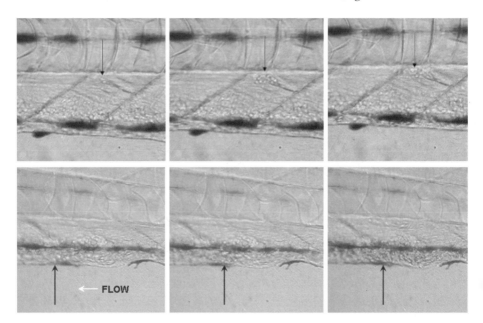

Fig. 6. Sequential still images taken from real-time videos of arterial (top panels) and venous (bottom panels) thrombus formation (shown by vertical arrows) in larvae at 120 hpf. Arterial images from left to right are at 10, 40, and 75 s postinjury. Venous images from left to right are preinjury and 10 and 20 s postinjury. Horizontal arrow shows the direction of blood flow marked as FLOW.

respectively, for the artery. Consistent departure from the normal times is considered to be caused by a mutation, which can be identified by linkage analysis using PCR-based microsatellite markers. The positional cloning approach is discussed in the other chapters of this volume.

4. Notes

1. There are many variations in the design of breeding tanks. Our design is a relatively simple, homemade design, as described in paragraph 2 of **Subheading 2.** This tank-in-tank design is inexpensive because it can even be constructed from two used plastic soda bottles or even empty milk cartons. Commercially available breeding tanks can range from $10 to $15.
2. In some laboratories, embryos are washed with 0.2% bleach, which usually prevents fungal infection, but this practice can sometimes be lethal to the embryos. We routinely use embryos that are gently washed two to three times with E3 media after removing feces and junk material and found this method yields viable embryos consistently.
3. We find that the temperature of the agarose is critical, as is the gentle mixing of the embryos.

4. In large-scale screenings, speed of mounting the larvae is essential. Previously we would mount one larva in each rubber gasket well, which turned out to be cumbersome. Our modification of placing all the larvae in a single rectangular well is more efficient. The numbering of the larvae is important as it becomes easier to keep track of the ablations, otherwise it may become difficult to detect which has been ablated by looking for a thrombus—in some cases, the thrombus may dissolve by the time one reaches the end of screening the slide. We have also noted that after identifying a mutant, we can recover it simply by releasing it from the agarose into clean water, thus resuscitating the larvae. This is important as such homozygous mutants can be grown, bred, and further evaluated.

Acknowledgments

This work was supported by National Institutes of Health grants HL63792 and HL77910.

References

1. Jagadeeswaran, P., Gregory, M., Day, K., Cykowski, M., and Thattaliyath B. (2005) Zebrafish: a genetic model for hemostasis and thrombosis. *J. Thromb. Haemost.* **3,** 46–53.
2. Sturtevant, A. H. (2001) Reminiscences of T. H. Morgan. *Genetics* **159,** 1–5.
3. Gregory, M., Hanumanthaiah, R., and Jagadeeswaran, P. (2002) Genetic analysis of hemostasis and thrombosis using vascular occlusion. *Blood Cells Mol. Dis.* **29,** 286–295.
4. Solnica-Krezel, L., Schier, A. F., and Driever, W. (1994) Efficient recovery of ENU-induced mutations from the zebrafish germline. *Genetics* **136,** 1401–1420.
5. Cheng, K. C. and Moore, J. L. (1997) Genetic dissection of vertebrate processes in the zebrafish: a comparison of uniparental and two-generation screens. *Biochem. Cell Biol.* **75,** 525–533.
6. Virchow, R. (1856) *Gesammelte Abhandlungen zur wissenschaftlichen Medicin.* Medinger Sohn and Co., Frankfurt.
7. Jagadeeswaran, P., Cykowski, M., and Thattaliyath, B. (2004) Vascular occlusion and thrombosis in zebrafish. *Methods Cell. Biol.* **76,** 489–500.
8. Thattaliyath, B., Cykowski, M., and Jagadeeswaran, P. (2005) Young thrombocytes initiate thrombus formation in zebrafish. *Blood* **106,** 118–124.
9. Jagadeeswaran, P. (2005) Zebrafish: a tool to study hemostasis and thrombosis. *Curr. Opin. Hematol.* **12,** 149–152.

13

Methods for Isolation of Endothelial and Smooth Muscle Cells and In Vitro Proliferation Assays

Ganapati H. Mahabeleshwar, Payaningal R. Somanath, and Tatiana V. Byzova

Summary

Angiogenesis, the formation of new blood vessel from pre-existing blood vessel, occurs in a variety of normal and pathological conditions. It is complex morphogenetic process involving the coordinate migration, invasion, and reorganization of several cell types including endothelial cells, pericytes, smooth muscle cells, and stromal fibroblasts. The angiogenic response begins with excess protease secretion to facilitate basement membrane remodeling, proliferation of endothelial cells, and endothelial cell migration to form capillary network and lumen closure. In this chapter, we describe the methods to isolate mouse and human endothelial cells, smooth muscle cells, which will provide abundant, convenient and useful tool for the investigation of many aspects of endothelial cell biology. The high degrees of functional diversity have been observed from endothelial cells derived from different organs, and within the different vascular beds of a given organ. Therefore, this apparent heterogeneity has highlighted the requirement for the endothelial cell isolation and culture from a variety of tissues of different species in order to establish more realistic in vitro angiogenic models.

Key Words: Endothelial cells; angiogenesis; aorta; matrigel; VEGF; smooth muscle cell; MTT; human umbilical vein endothelial cells; HUVEC.

1. Introduction

Over the past 20 yr, the study of angiogenesis has become a major hotspot in cardiovascular biology. It is an essential component of numerous inflammatory processes, and is particularly significant in cancer and cardiovascular research. Recently, several in vitro techniques have been developed to study angiogenesis more efficiently and more cost effectively than with in vivo models. In this chapter, we describe several in vitro techniques that are necessary for the study of angiogenesis.

From: *Methods in Molecular Medicine, vol. 129:*
Cardiovascular Disease: Methods and Protocols, Volume 2: Molecular Medicine
Edited by: Q. K. Wang © Humana Press Inc., Totowa, NJ

The aortic ring assay *(1)* is an interesting in vitro model in which a murine aortic ring is embedded in Matrigel, and is cultured in a controlled microenvironment. The rate of angiogenesis can, then, be assessed from the complex, branching network of microvessels that stem from the aortic ring. The isolation of murine endothelial cells from the aorta *(2)*, and the isolation of human endothelial cells from the umbilical vein *(3)*, can be a convenient and useful technique for the investigation of many aspects of endothelial cell biology. The most common experiments with endothelial cells compare the effects of pharmacological and physiological inhibitors or inducers. In order to assess microvascular angiogenesis, endothelial cells can be isolated from smaller blood vessels, such as those located in the mouse lung *(4)* and from Matrigel implants in mouse skin *(5)*. Vascular smooth muscle cells (SMCs) from the murine aorta *(6)* make good starting material for the study of growth factor regulated SMC activity. In this chapter, we describe the explant culture technique for the isolation of SMCs, which prevents most contamination from other cell types, particularly endothelial cells. Lastly, the cell proliferation assays using [3H]Thymidine *(7)* and MTT *(8)* are sound techniques that measure the proliferative response of vascular cells.

2. Materials

2.1. Aortic Ring Assay

1. 4- to 6-wk-old mice.
2. Anesthetic cocktail (ketamine 1 mL, xylasine 0.3 mL, saline 1.5 mL (*see* **Note 1**).
3. Microdissection scissors and forceps.
4. Sterile ice-cold 1X phosphate-buffered saline (PBS).
5. Syringe (1 mL) fitted with 23-G needle.
6. Scalpel blade.
7. Endothelial cell growth medium (Dulbecco's modified Eagle's medium [DMEM] with 25 mM HEPES [Invitrogen, Grand Island, NY], supplemented with 10% fetal bovine serum [FBS], 90 µg/mL heparin sulfate, 90 µg/mL endothelial cell growth factor, 10,000 U/mL penicillin, 10 mg/mL streptomycin).
8. Matrigel with/without growth factors (BD Biosciences, Bedford, MA) (*see* **Note 2**).
9. Six-well cell culture-treated plates (Corning Costar®, Corning, NY).
10. Inverted phase-contrast microscope, such as Leica.
11. Dispase (BD Biosciences).
12. Rat anti-mouse CD-31 antibody (BD Biosciences).

2.2. Isolation of Endothelial Cells From Murine Aorta

1. All the materials described under **Subheading 2.1.**
2. Orbital shaker (United Lab, St. Louis, MO).
3. Beckman Coulter Allegra™ 6 Centrifuge (Beckman Coulter).
4. Gelatin (Sigma, St. Louis, MO) (*see* **Note 3**).
5. Fibronectin (Roche, Indianapolis, IN).

2.3. Isolation of Microvascular Endothelial Cells From Murine Lung

1. 4- to 6-wk-old mice.
2. Anesthetic cocktail (ketamine 1 mL, sylasine 0.3 mL, saline 1.5 mL) (*see* **Note 1**).
3. Sterile ice-cold 1X PBS.
4. Micro-dissection scissors and forceps.
5. 60-mm sterile cell culture treated Petri plates (Becton Dickinson, Franklin Lakes, NJ).
6. Collagenase/dispase (Roche) (*see* **Note 4**).
7. Orbital shaker (United Lab).
8. Tissue strainer (Fisher).
9. Beckman Coulter Allegra 6 Centrifuge.
10. Endothelial cell growth medium (DMEM with 25 mM HEPES [Invitrogen], supplemented with 10% FBS, 90 µg/mL heparin sulfate, 90 µg/mL endothelial cell growth factor, 10,000 U/mL penicillin, 10 mg/mL streptomycin).
11. Rat anti-mouse CD-31 antibody (BD Biosciences).
12. Dynal MPC (Dynal ASA, Oslo, Norway).
13. Gelatin (Sigma), fibronectin (Roche), and trypsin/EDTA (Gibco).

2.4. Isolation of Endothelial Cells From Matrigel Implants in Skin

1. All the materials described in **Subheading 2.3.**
2. Matrigel with growth factors (BD Biosciences) (*see* **Note 2**).
3. Vascular endothelial growth factor (VEGF; R&D Systems, Minneapolis, MN) (*see* **Note 5**).
4. Heparin (Sigma).
5. 3-mL syringe fitted with 25-G needle.
6. Fur trimmer (WAHL clipper corporation, Sterling).
7. Dispase (BD Biosciences).

2.5. Isolation of Human Umbilical Vein Endothelial Cells

1. Fresh human umbilical cord (*see* **Note 6**).
2. 100-mm sterile cell culture-treated Petri plates (Becton Dickinson).
3. Surgical blades, clamps, and haemostatic forceps.
4. 50-mL syringe fitted with blunt-ended needle.
5. Collagenase (Sigma).
6. Falcon 50-mL sterile tubes.
7. Beckman Coulter Allegra 6 Centrifuge.
8. Endothelial cell growth medium (DMEM with 25 mM HEPES [Invitrogen], supplemented with 10% FBS, 90 µg/mL heparin sulfate, 90 µg/mL endothelial cell growth factor, 10,000 U/mL penicillin, 10 mg/mL streptomycin).
9. Gelatin (Sigma) (*see* **Note 3**).
10. 25-cm^2 cell culture flasks (Corning).

2.6. Isolation of Smooth Muscle Cells From Murine Aorta

1. 4- to 6-wk-old mice.
2. Micro-dissection scissors and forceps.

3. Ice-cold 1X PBS.
4. 60-mm sterile cell culture-treated Petri plates (Becton Dickinson).
5. 25-cm^2 cell culture flasks (Corning Incorporated, Corning, NY).
6. Trypsin/EDTA (Gibco).
7. DMEM (Invitrogen), supplemented with 10% FBS.

2.7. Cell Proliferation Assay Using ^3HThymidine

1. DMEM (Gibco).
2. Trypsin/EDTA (Cambrex).
3. Trypsin neutralizing solution (Cambrex).
4. Beckman Coulter Allegra 6 Centrifuge.
5. Hemocytometer (Fisher).
6. ^3HThymidine (ICN biochemicals and reagents).
7. Bovine serum albumin (BSA), trichloroacetic acid (TCA), sodium dodecyl sulfate (SDS), sodium hydroxide (Sigma).
8. Orbital shaker (United Lab).
9. Beckman β-scintillation counter.

2.8. MTT Cell Proliferation Assay

1. DMEM (Gibco).
2. RPMI-1640 without phenol red (Gibco).
3. MTT (Sigma).
4. 96-well cell culture plate (Corning).
5. Eppendorf 5415 R table-top centrifuge.
6. Isopropanol (Sigma).
7. Kinetic microplate reader (Molecular Devices).

3. Methods

3.1. Aortic Ring Assay

3.1.1. Isolation of Aorta From Mice

1. Mice 4–6 wk of age are injected with 50 µL anesthetic cocktail. Quickly remove the thoracic aorta using micro-dissection forceps and place it rapidly in ice-cold 1X sterile PBS. Gently flush the aorta with sterile ice-cold 1X PBS using 1-mL syringe fitted with 23-G needle to remove blood clots (**Fig. 1A–C**).
2. Using fine forceps, remove the fibro-adipose tissue and small lateral blood vessels. The aorta is cut into 1-mm rings using sterile scalpel blade under laminar airflow (**Fig. 1D–F**).
3. Wash the aortic rings further using sterile ice-cold 1X PBS (pH 7.4) and transfer them to endothelial growth medium.

3.1.2. Implantation and Maintenance of Aortic Rings In Vitro

1. Matrigel with/without growth factors is allowed to thaw at 4°C overnight. During the preparation of aortic rings, Matrigel is kept on ice to prevent any solidification.

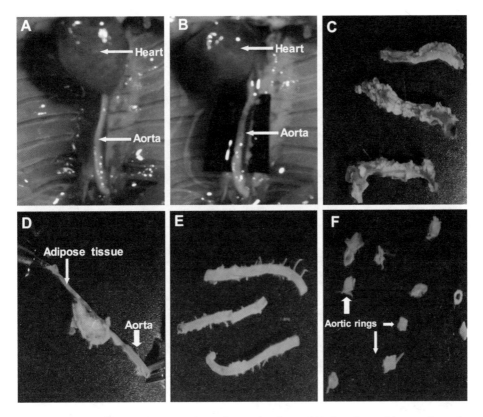

Fig. 1. Preparation of mouse thoracic aortic rings. (**A**) Loation of intact thoracic aorta and lateral blood vessels. (**B**) Thoracic aorta was surgically detached from lateral blood vessels and fibro-adipose tissue. (**C**) Mouse thoracic aorta was surgically removed and preserved on ice-cold culture medium. (**D–E**) Fibro-adipose tissues were carefully removed and aorta was cleaned and preserved on ice-cold 1X phosphate-buffered saline. (**F**) Cleaned aorta was cut into 1-mm rings and placed on ice-cold culture medium.

> All of the procedures should be performed under sterile laminar airflow for aseptic conditions.

2. Precool a six-well plate on ice and homogeneously coat the wells with 1 mL of Matrigel without introducing any air bubbles. These plates are placed at 37°C for 15 min to allow the Matrigel to solidify.
3. Insert four to six freshly prepared aortic rings in each well and pour a second layer of Matrigel above the aortic rings. Incubate the plates further for 15 min at 37°C to allow solidification of freshly added Matrigel. Slowly add the endothelial cell growth medium without disturbing the Matrigel. The endothelial cell sprouts will start to appear on the second day and grow rapidly between 5 and 12 d (**Figs. 2** and **3**).

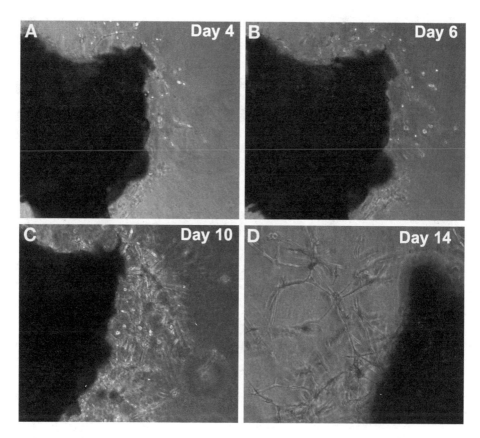

Fig. 2. Spontaneous angiogenic response of a mouse aortic ring embedded in growth factor-reduced matrigel. Mouse aortic rings were allowed to grow in growth factor-reduced matrigel without medium change for 2 wk. Photomicrographs were taken periodically.

4. Observe the aortic ring sprouts periodically under the phase-contrast microscope and take pictures when necessary.
5. In order to quantify the number of cells present in the sprouts, harvest the cells using dispase, wash in 1X PBS and subject the suspension for fluorescence-activated cell sorting (FACS) analysis using CD31 antibody.

3.2. Isolation of Endothelial Cells From Murine Aorta

1. To isolate the endothelial cells from the aorta, process aorta in a similar manner as described previously.
2. The aortic rings are implanted in Matrigel containing growth factors. The endothelial cell growth medium is added and maintained in a humidified incubator containing 5% CO_2 at 37°C.

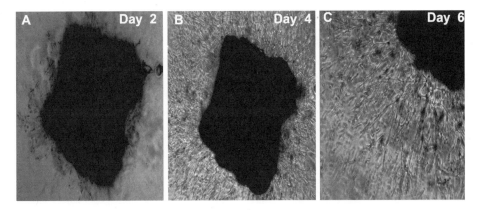

Fig. 3. Spontaneous angiogenic response of a mouse aortic ring embedded in growth factor-containing matrigel. Mouse aortic rings were allowed to grow in growth factor-containing matrigel without medium change for 7 d. Photomicrographs were taken periodically.

3. On the fourth day, decant the medium and remove aortic rings from the Matrigel carefully using sterile needle without disturbing the Matrigel. This process is essential to prevent the entry of contaminating fibroblasts and SMCs. The endothelial cells are allowed to proliferate in Matrigel until it reaches confluence.

4. To harvest the endothelial cells from Matrigel, wash the Matrigel plates carefully with sterile 1X PBS and further incubate with 0.5 mL of dispase for 30 min at room temperature on orbital platform with occasional shaking. Collect the supernatant carefully avoiding any undigested Matrigel. Dilute the supernatant with sterile, ice-cold 1X PBS (pH 7.4) and centrifuge at 320*g* for 5 min using Beckman Coulter centrifuge (Allegra 6 Centrifuge).

5. Wash the endothelial cell pellets twice with sterile, ice-cold 1X PBS and plate the cells on to tissue culture flasks precoated with 1% gelatin (w/v) or 0.01% (w/v) fibronectin. Culture and maintain the cells in endothelial growth medium.

3.3. Isolation of Microvascular Endothelial Cells From Murine Lung

1. Anesthetize 4- to 6-wk-old mice by injecting 50 μL of the anesthetic cocktail. Harvest the lungs and place them in sterile ice-cold 1X PBS. Chop the lungs and wash with a copious amount of sterile, ice-cold 1X PBS to remove a maximum amount of blood cells from the lung tissue.

2. Wash and mince lung tissues using a scalpel blade in 60-mm sterile Petri plates under filtered laminar airflow. Incubate the minced tissue with 3 mg/mL collagenase-dispase mixture for 4 h at room temperature with gentle shaking.

3. Remove the digest after 4 h and isolate cells from the tissue fragment using a tissue strainer (CELLECTOR® tissue sieve). Collect the supernatant and centrifuge at 320*g* for 5 min using Beckman Coulter centrifuge (Allegra 6 Centrifuge). Discard

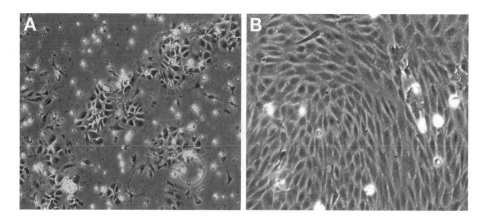

Fig. 4. Photomicrographs of mouse microvascular endothelial cells. (**A**) Phase-contrast photomicrographs of mouse microvascular endothelial cells after 2 d of plating. (**B**) Confluent monolayer of mouse microvascular endothelial cells after 7 d of plating.

    the supernatant and wash the cell pellets twice with sterile ice-cold 1X PBS. Resuspend the cells in endothelial cell growth medium.

4. Endothelial cells are isolated from the mixture of cell population using anti-CD31 antibody. Centrifuge and resuspend the cells in DMEM F12 medium and mix the suspension with 100 µL Dynabeads (Dynal MPC) and incubate further at 4°C for 15 min.

5. The endothelial cells bound to the magnetic beads are separated by trypsin digestion. After washing, these cells are plated on to tissue culture plates precoated with 1% (w/v) gelatin or 0.01% (w/v) fibronectin (**Fig. 4A,B**).

3.4. Isolation of Endothelial Cells From Matrigel Implants in Skin

1. Clean and remove the fur in the ventral region of the mice and subcutaneously inject with 0.5 mL Matrigel containing VEGF (60 ng/mL) and heparin (60 U/mL) at the ventral midline, using a 3-mL syringe fitted with a 25-G needle.

2. On day 5, sacrifice the mice, wipe the ventral region using alcoholic pads, and remove the Matrigels from skin with no contamination from skin tissue.

3. Wash the Matrigels in 1X PBS and digest using 2 mL dispase with constant shaking in an orbital shaker for 30 min at room temperature.

4. The rest of the procedure to obtain a pure culture of endothelial cells is essentially the same as discussed in **Subheading 3.3.**

3.5. Isolation of Human Umbilical Vein Endothelial Cells

1. Carefully clean the umbilical cord with clean gauze and place it on a tray. Placing one end in a Petri dish inside the culture hood, cut the end with a sterile surgical blade.

2. Screw the needle into the stopcock and look for the widest vessel. Place the needle into the vein. Open the clamp, place the free end of the cord inside the clamp and screw it tightly using surgical forceps.

3. Leave the clamped cord on a tray. Fill out 50-mL syringes with irrigation solution (1X PBS, pH 7.5). Fit the end of the syringe onto the top of the clamp and apply a gentle flow through the vein.

4. Squeeze the cord gently to remove remaining solution and lock the clamp. Fill out 50-mL syringes with 0.1% collagenase solution and clamp the free end with a hemostatic forceps and apply collagenase solution through the other end until the cord is moderately swollen. Lock the clamp. Place it onto a tray and leave them in the incubator for 20 min.

5. After this incubation time, remove the tray from the incubator. The cord must look softened because of the collagenase treatment. Again, fill 50-mL syringes with sterile irrigation solution, unlock the clamp, and place the end of the syringe into the cord. Hold the clamped end, flame the surgical scissor, and cut the cord carefully by holding the clamped end over a 50-mL falcon tube. Apply irrigation solution through the vein and collect the flow into the falcon tube. Squeeze it gently.

6. Collect the endothelial cells into the falcon tube (up to 50 mL per cord). Close the falcon tubes inside the tissue culture hood and place them into the centrifuge. Spin down samples at room temperature for 10 min at 320*g* using Beckman Coulter Allegra 6 Centrifuge. Pour off the supernatant.

7. Add endothelial growth media and resuspend cells. Place the cell suspension into a 25-cm^2 flask (typically three cords per flask). Place the flask into the incubator and observe the attached cells under phase contrast microscope.

3.6. Isolation of Smooth Muscle Cells From Murine Aorta

1. Aortic SMCs are isolated using a technique known as explant culture. Collect the mice aorta under aseptic condition as described previously.

2. Clean the aorta from fibro-adipose tissue and remove the blood clots by flushing with sterile, ice-cold 1X PBS. Endothelial cells are the major contaminant in SMC culture. Therefore, they must be removed before implantation into the matrigel. To remove endothelial cells, the intimal surface of the vessel is vigorously rubbed using a sterile cotton swab.

3. The cleaned aorta is transferred to a sterile 60-mm dish containing ice-cold 1X PBS (pH 7.4). Using sterile, sharp forceps, the entire intimal layer is removed from the adventitious layer and the aorta is minced into small pieces of 1–3 mm^2.

4. The minced pieces are spread evenly on the 60-mm dishes under the humidified conditions, which will allow adhesion of aortic pieces to Petri plates. Once these pieces adhere firmly to Petri plates, fresh, prewarmed media is added and the plate is placed in a humidified incubator containing 5% CO_2.

5. The cells usually start to sprout within 3–5 d. At the end of the second week, explants are carefully removed without disturbing the SMC outgrowths. The culture media is replaced and proliferative cells are allowed to grow for further 2–3 wk. Once SMCs form a monolayer, they are further subcultured using 25-cm^2 flasks.

3.7. Cell Proliferation Assay Using ^3H Thymidine

1. Deplete the cells in a serum-free medium 18–24 h before the experiment. Serum-starved cells are washed in 1X PBS and removed from the flask

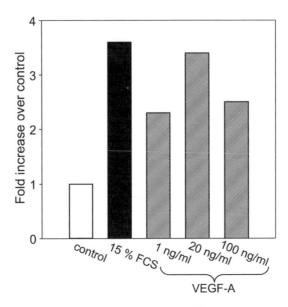

Fig. 5. Endothelial cell proliferation assay using [3H]Thymidine at a concentration of 1 μci/100 mL. These cells were allowed to proliferate for 24 h and [3H]Thymidine incorporation was measured by β-scintillation counter.

using trypsin-EDTA and thereby inactivating trypsin using trypsin neutralizing solution.

2. Transfer the cells after resuspension in Hank's balanced salt solution (HBSS) to a 50-mL sterile tube and centrifuge (Beckman Coulter Allegra 6 Centrifuge) at 320g for 10 min at room temperature. Discard supernatant and wash the cells using Iscove's modified Dulbecco's medium (IMDM) containing 5 μg/mL transferrin. After washing, resuspend the pellet in 1 mL IMDM containing 5 μg/mL transferrin.

3. Count the cells at this stage and make appropriate concentrations. Add [3H]Thymidine to the wells at a concentration of 1 μci/100 μL. Mix 200 μL of each sample with 200 μL of the one pretreated with [3H]Thymidine. Gently mix the sample and aliquot them in a sterile 96-well plate in quadruplicates of 100 μL each. Incubate the plate in a 37°C incubator at 5% CO_2 for 24 h.

4. After incubation, transfer the supernatant to a V-bottom plate. The cells are trypsinized, isolated, and mixed with respective supernatants in the V-bottom plates. Centrifuge (Beckman Coulter Allegra 6 Centrifuge) the V-bottom plates at 320g for 5 min. Discard the supernatant in a radioactive container. Wash the cells twice in 1X PBS and discard the washings also to the radioactive container.

5. Add 50 μL of 1X PBS containing 0.5% BSA to each well followed by 100 μL each of 20% TCA and incubate the plate overnight at 4°C. Discard the supernatant and wash the wells with PBS. Add 100 μL of 2% SDS with 0.2 M NaOH and incubate for 30 min with gentle shaking. Collect each sample and add to scintillation vials and subject to β-scintillation counting (**Fig. 5**).

3.8. MTT Cell Proliferation Assay

1. Plate cultured endothelial cells (10^3) in a 96-well plate and allow them to grow for overnight. Treat the cells with growth factors or inhibitors of your choice. Basic fibroblast growth factor (FGF)-2 is one of the strongest inducers of endothelial proliferation. VEGF also can be used; however, it is much less stable in culture media. If you are using any of endothelial growth factors, try to use several concentrations. It is important to remember that concentration response to the majority of growth factors is bell-shaped. Suggested concentrations of VEGF-A165 are 10, 20, 50, and 100 ng/mL.
2. Wash the endothelial cells with warm RPMI-1640 without phenol red medium.
3. Prepare the MTT working solution by diluting 1:10 of the 5-mg/mL stock.
4. Add 100 µL MTT working solution into each well being assayed. Incubate the 96-well plate at 37°C for 3 h.
5. At the end of the 3 h, aspirate the MTT solution from each well and wash the each well with 1X PBS carefully.
6. To each well, add 200 µL of acidic isopropanol (0.04 *M* HCl in absolute isopropanol) and incubate at room temperature for 15 min with gentle shaking.
7. At the end of 15 min, collect the supernatant from each well separately in a 0.5-mL Eppendorf tube and centrifuge at 9650*g* using Eppendorf table-top centrifuge for 5 min.
8. Transfer the supernatant into new tube. Absorbance of the dissolved dye is measured at wavelength of 570 nm with background substraction of 650 nm.

4. Notes

1. Anesthetic cocktail is stable at 4°C for 2 wk. Keep refrigerated or on ice while in use.
2. Thaw the Matrigel overnight at 4°C and always keep the Matrigel bottle on ice to prevent solidification.
3. Melt the gelatin in 1X PBS at 55°C for 30 min and filter-sterilize immediately. It can be stored at 4°C for 8–10 wk.
4. Collagenase-dispase stock solution can be stored as several aliquots at –20°C.
5. VEGF stock solution can be stored at a –80°C manual defrost freezer for 8 wk without detectable loss of activity.
6. Umbilical cord could be source of several human born pathogens, hence, handle and decontaminate the work area carefully.

Acknowledgments

The authors would like to thank Ilya Byzov and Joseph Potter for their help in preparation of the manuscript and Alla Gomer for technical assistance.

References

1. Reynolds, L. E., Wyder, L., Lively, J. C., et al. (2002) Enhanced pathological angiogenesis in mice lacking β_3 integrin or β_3 and β_5 integrins. *Nat. Med.* **8**, 27–34.
2. Magid, R., Martinson, D., Hwang, J., Jo, H., and Galis, Z. S. (2003) Optimization of isolation and functional characterization of primary murine aortic endothelial cells. *Endothelium* **10**, 103–109.

3. Xu, H. Q., Hao, H. P., Zhang, X., and Pan, Y. (2004) Morroniside protects cultured human umbilical vein endothelial cells from damage by high ambient glucose. *Acta Pharmacol. Sin.* **25,** 412–415.

4. Ewing, P., Wilke, A., Brockhoff, G., et al. (2003) Isolation and transplantation of allogeneic pulmonary endothelium derived from GFP transgenic mice. *J. Immunol. Methods* **283,** 307–315.

5. Dong, Q. G., Bernasconi, S., Lostaglio, S., et al. (1997) A general strategy for isolation of endothelial cells from murine tissues. Characterization of two endothelial cell lines from the murine lung and subcutaneous sponge implants. *Arterioscler. Thromb. Vasc. Biol.* **17,** 1599–1604.

6. Ray, J. L., Leach, R., Herbert, J. M., and Benson, M. (2001) Isolation of vascular smooth muscle cells from a single murine aorta. *Methods Cell Sci.* **23,** 185–188.

7. Byzova, T. V., Goldman, C. K., Pampori, N., et al. (2000) A mechanism for modulation of cellular responses to VEGF: activation of the integrins. *Mol. Cell.* **6,** 851–860.

8. Xiang, Y., Ma, B., Li, T., Gao, J. W., Yu, H. M., and Li, X. J. (2004) Acetazolamide inhibits aquaporin-1 protein expression and angiogenesis. *Acta Pharmacol. Sin.* **25,** 812–816.

14

Applications of Adenoviral Vector-Mediated Gene Transfer in Cardiovascular Research

Fang Xu, Delila Serra, and Andrea Amalfitano

Summary

Cardiovascular disease is a leading cause of morbidity and mortality worldwide. New studies are needed to explore novel therapeutic options for patients that are refractory to existing therapies. Gene transfer using adenoviral vectors has shown promising results in animal studies, and is now being tested in many clinical trials. In this chapter, the advantages of adenoviral vector-mediated gene transfer for cardiovascular disease applications, and the methods on how to construct, propagate, and evaluate adenoviral vectors, are discussed.

Key Words: Gene therapy; adenoviral vector; cardiovascular disease.

1. Introduction

Cardiovascular disease, a serious global health problem, is the leading cause of morbidity and mortality worldwide. Despite significant improvements in the diagnosis and treatment of cardiovascular disease, patients with severe forms of cardiovascular disease such as inoperable coronary artery disease (CAD), post-angioplasty and in-stent restenosis, and end-stage heart failure (HF) are still refractory to existing therapies. To improve the outcome of patients with severe cardiovascular diseases, ongoing efforts have been made to explore new forms of therapies as alternatives or adjuncts to the existing ones. Gene therapy studies in cardiovascular disease have drawn great attention because of the advantages of this form of therapy over the existing therapeutic modalities, advantages that include the possibility of long-term therapeutic effects after a single application and the targeted delivery of gene drugs, as well as a proven ability for easy to scale up for widespread use.

Clinical trials in cardiovascular gene therapy using nonvirally based (plasmid-based) and virally based vectors have been approved and are ongoing. In many

From: *Methods in Molecular Medicine, vol. 129:*
Cardiovascular Disease: Methods and Protocols, Volume 2: Molecular Medicine
Edited by: Q. K. Wang © Humana Press Inc., Totowa, NJ

instances, viral vector-based gene transfer systems outperform naked DNA/plasmid based systems as a result of a much higher gene transfer efficiency *(1)*. Of all virally based vectors, adenovirally based vectors are currently the most widely used of viral vectors, constituting 26% of all the vectors used in human gene therapy clinical trials worldwide (http://www.wiley.co.uk/genetherapy/clinical/). This usage has several major advantages, such as the fact that adenoviral vectors are nonintegrating vectors minimizing the risk of insertional mutagenesis; unlike integrating viral vectors such as those that are retrovirally or lentivirally based, adenoviral vectors infect both proliferating and quiescent cells, a point that is especially critical when considering cardiovascular applications, because adenoviral vectors are able to infect endothelial cells, fibroblasts, vascular smooth muscle cells (VSMCs), and also terminally differentiated cardiac myocytes. Adenoviral vectors are easy to scale up to high titers and can accommodate large gene inserts, allowing for the use of complex gene expression cassettes.

Before stepping into the discussion of adenovirally mediated gene therapy in cardiovascular disease, it is necessary to have a brief overview on adenoviral biology. Adenovirus, a "common cold"-causing reagent, was first isolated in 1953 when investigators were trying to establish cell-lines from adenoid tissue collected during tonsillectomy *(2)*. Subsequently, it has been determined that human adenoviruses, as members of the mastadenovirus family, are divided into five species, of which more than 50 serotypes have been identified. Among those identified, the genomes of serotypes 2, 5, 11, 12, 17, 21, 25, and 40 have been completely sequenced. Most of the adenoviral vectors used in gene therapy studies are based on serotype 2 or 5 of human adenovirus species group C.

In general, adenoviruses are nonenveloped viruses that are composed of a protein capsid and a double-stranded DNA/protein core *(3)*. As illustrated in **Fig. 1**, the viral capsid is of an icosahedronal structure with 20 equilateral triangle faces, 30 edges, and 12 vertices. There are three major capsid proteins, the hexon capsomer (a trimer of hexon polypeptide II), the penton base, and the fiber. The virus core is a protein–DNA complex that is composed of two basic core proteins (pV and pVII) and a linear double-strand DNA with a covalently bound terminal protein (TP) at each of the 5′ termini. The adenovirus genome is of about 36,000 bp in length.

Adenovirus serotype (Ad)5 virions primarily bind to the coxsackie and adenovirus receptor (CAR) on the target cell surface via the knob domain of the fiber proteins that protrudes out from the viral capsid *(4,5)*. Importantly, cardiac myocytes express low levels of the CAR receptor in the normal adult heart, but CAR expression levels increase dramatically in diseased hearts *(6,7)*. Endothelial cells express CAR constantly, whereas proliferating VSMCs, as well as injured VSMCs, express high level of CAR *(8)*. The interaction of penton base (containing an RGD motif) with $\alpha_v\beta_3/\alpha_v\beta_5$ integrins on the target cell surface

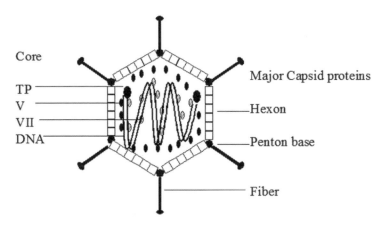

Fig. 1. Structure of an adenovirus. Step1: clone transgene expression cassette into a shuttle vector (also called a transfer vector).

facilitates and mediates the endocytosis of the adenovirus *(9)*. Recent reports demonstrated that heparin sulfate proteoglycans (HSPGs) on cell surfaces may also mediate Ad5 binding, via interaction with the fiber shaft *(10–12)*. Upon infection, the adenovirus life cycle is divided into early and late phases that are demarcated by viral DNA replication. The early phase includes the attachment and penetration of the virion to a target cell, the endosome escape of the dissembled virion, the passage of viral DNA into the nucleus, and the expression of multiple early genes including *E1*, *E2*, *E2*, and *E4*. *E1* provides the proper environment for transcription of other early genes, including the *E2* gene. *E2* encodes the viral DNA polymerase, the single-strand DNA binding protein and preterminal protein that are required for viral DNA replication. *E3* genes encode several immunomodulatory proteins, whereas the *E4* genes encode genes that further facilitate growth of the virus by interactions with the host protein synthesis machinery. After viral DNA replication, late viral gene expression dominates, and includes expression of all the virion structure proteins, facilitating the assembly of infectious progeny virus. The viral life cycle is complete when progeny viruses lyse the host cell at about 32–36 h after infection.

The great understanding of adenovirus biology directly led to the creation of adenoviral vectors. Several generations of adenoviral vectors have been constructed and tested in preclinical studies and clinical trials. These vectors are classified into two major groups.

One group of adenoviral vectors are *E1* and *E3* gene-deleted and are called the first-generation adenoviral vectors. The *E3* gene is not necessary for the viral life cycle in tissue culture systems, therefore the deletion of *E3* mainly provides cloning space to accommodate therapeutic gene carrying capacity.

A desired transgene is typically inserted into the viral genome in place of *E1*, although insertions into *E3* or *E4* regions have also been described. The deletion of *E1* also renders the vector nearly nonreplicable upon infection of target cells. The propagation of the *E1*-deleted first-generation adenoviral vectors in vitro thus requires a complementing cell line that provides *E1* functions *in trans*. The molecular construction and propagation of these "first-generation adenoviral vectors" will be described under **Subheadings 2.** and **3.** One of the limitations of the first-generation adenoviral vectors is that the transgene expression from them is many times found to be transient in vivo. This temporary transgene expression is desirable in some categories of cardiovascular gene therapy (such as therapeutic angiogenesis) in which only short-term expression of angiogenic cytokines is required to achieve beneficial biological effects *(13)*.

The other group of adenoviral vectors, also called second-generation adenoviral vectors, are further divided into helper virus-independent, multiply deleted vectors and helper virus-dependent, fully deleted adenovirus vectors *(14)*. The helper virus-independent, multiply deleted adenoviral vectors are derivatives of the first-generation viral vectors. In addition to the deletion of the *E1* and *E3* genes, other early viral genes such as viral *E2* genes (DNA polymerase, preterminal protein) or *E4* genes are deleted *(15)*. The additional deletions not only further increase the transgene-carrying capacities of the so-modified vectors, but also prolong the transgene expression duration and decrease toxicity associated with viral DNA replication and late viral gene expression *(16)*. To propagate these multiply deleted viral vectors, complementing cell lines that provide both *E1* and the corresponding deleted genes are required *(17)*.

The helper virus-dependent, fully deleted adenoviral vectors (or "gutted" adenoviral vectors) do not contain any adenoviral genome except the necessary *cis*-acting adenoviral genome sequences required for packaging of viral genomes, i.e., the inverted terminal repeats and the encapsidation signal sequence. The remaining vector contents are transgene expression cassettes of interest and stuffer sequence. As a result of the absence of expression of viral proteins, the helper-dependent adenoviral vectors also demonstrate a much-reduced toxicity and prolonged transgene expression relative to first-generation adenovirus-based vectors *(18)*. Propagation of the helper-dependent viruses, however, is more complicated than that of the first- or second-generation adenoviral vectors, requiring both a 293-cell line that coexpresses not only the *E1* genes but also the Cre recombinase *(19)*, as well as a co-infecting helper virus which provides *in trans* all of the viral proteins needed for completion of the viral life cycle. This system has been engineered to allow for preferential packaging of the fully deleted vector in lieu of the helper virus. The construction and propagation of both helper-independent and helper-dependent adenoviral vectors will be discussed in **Subheading 3.**

The different generations of adenoviral vectors described previously have been tested in various cardiovascular gene therapy applications, and each has demonstrated promising results. Some of these examples are discussed next.

Atherosclerosis features chronic inflammation as a prominent variable in its development. Oxidized low-density lipoproteins (LDLs) promote formation of foam cells, which secrete proinflammatory cytokine and exacerbate arterial wall inflammation *(20)*. To inhibit arterial wall inflammation in atherosclerosis, a first-generation *E1–, E3–* adenoviral vector expressing lipoprotein-associated phospholipase A2 (Lp-PLA2) was constructed and delivered into hypercholesterolaemic rabbits via intra-arterial infusion (1.15×10^{10} plaque-forming units [pfu]/animal). As a result, liver uptake of the vector resulted in hepatic secretion of the Lp-PLA2 protein directly into the circulation, facilitating formation of LDL particles with increased Lp-PLA2 activity. The LDL particles with increased Lp-PLA2 activity were subsequently isolated and tested in vitro. It was also found that the increased Lp-PLA2 activity (facilitated by adenoviral transduction in vivo) reduced LDL degradation and foam cell formation in vitro *(21)*. In another example, to protect against development of atherosclerosis, a second-generation helper-independent adenoviral vector expressing human apoE ([*E1–, E3–* polymerase-]AdapoE) was administrated intravenously (1×10^{10} or 6×10^{10} viral particles/animal) into apoE-deficient mice. After intravenous administration, the majority of the vectors were taken up by the mouse liver, which then secreted apoE into the circulation. Subsequently, elevated plasma levels of apoE were achieved, followed by reductions of plasma cholesterol and retarded progression of atherosclerosis *(22)*.

As described previously, systemic administration of adenoviral vectors typically results in liver sequestration of most of the adenovirus particles intravascularly infused into an animal. This normal function of the liver (and intrahepatic reticulo-endothelial systems) limits the level of transduction of other tissue targets, such as those found in the cardiovascular system. In many applications, however, cardiovascular targeting instead of liver targeting is desirable both to decrease systemic toxicity as well as to enhance gene transfer to cardiovascular tissues. Strategies have been devised to circumvent liver sequestration of adenoviruses while simultaneously increasing cardiovascular targeting. To help achieve targeted adenoviral vector delivery, localized vector delivery to vascular tissue using catheters has been extensively utilized. For example, the most common routes of adenoviral vector delivery into the heart are (1) catheter-mediated intracoronary delivery, which has been shown to result in 98% first-pass uptake of the adenoviral vectors by the heart *(23)*, and

(2) direct intramyocardial injection during coronary artery bypass grafting (CABG) or at thoracotomy (24–26).

Local delivery of adenoviral vectors has been used in many preclinical and clinical trials in cardiovascular gene therapy. The disease targets in cardiovascular gene therapy can be categorized into the following groups:

1. Arrhythmia (development of biological pacemaker).
2. HF.
3. Vascular disease (myocardial ischemia, peripheral vascular disease, lymphedema).

Studies of developing genetically engineered cardiac "pacemakers" are still in the early stages of development, but offer several exciting possibilities. These efforts are primarily attempting to overcome the shortcomings of the conventional electric pacemaker, such as limited battery life and the need for permanent catheter implantation into the heart, and/or to address lack of responsiveness to autonomic therapy. As one example, a first-generation adenoviral vector expressing the pacemaker gene *HCN2* (2–3×10^{10} fluorescent focus unit per dog) was delivered into the posterior division of the left bundle branch, with subsequent demonstration of the initiation of spontaneous rhythms in the so-treated canine heart (27,28).

Gene therapy using adenoviral vectors in treatment of HF is also a major thrust of preclinical efforts. To improve contractility of the myocardium, adenoviral vectors expressing β_2 adrenergic receptor (βAR) or the βAR kinase (βARK)1 inhibitor βARKct have been delivered in order to increase β-adrenergic responsiveness in failing hearts as well to facilitate increase myocardial contractility (29–31). A second strategy to increase heart contractility is to target calcium handling in cardiomyocytes. Furthermore, intracoronary delivery of a first-generation adenovirus overexpressing the calcium binding protein S100A can lead to increased myocardial contractile performance in vitro and in vivo (32–34).

Local delivery of adenoviral vectors for the potential treatment of vascular diseases is by far the most studied area in cardiovascular gene therapy. Adenoviral vectors expressing angiogenic cytokines have been tested to promote therapeutic angiogenesis, to alleviate symptoms of angina pectoris or intermittent claudication, to prevent postangioplasty and in-stent restenosis, or to prevent vein graft stenosis (13,35). Phase I clinical trials in which intramyocardial administration of a first-generation adenoviral vector expressing vascular endothelial growth factor (VEGF)121 (4×10^8 – 4×10^{10} particle units per patient) showed treadmill exercise assessment improvements in most individuals with severe CAD; this efficacy was accompanied by no evidence of systemic or cardiac-related adverse events related to vector administration (24,25). Phase I and II clinical trials with intracoronary delivery of first-generation adenoviral vectors expressing fibroblast growth factor (FGF)-4 (1×10^{10} viral particles per patient) showed encouraging trends toward evidence of improved myocardial perfusion *(23,36,37)*. In prevention of postangioplasty and in-stent restenosis, a phase II trial with percutaneous transluminal coronary angioplasty (PTCA) followed by gene transfer of a first-generation adenovirus expressing VEGF165 (2×10^{10} pfu/patient) showed significant myocardial perfusion in patients treated with the vector at the 6-mo follow-up visit *(1)*. For peripheral vascular diseases, such as intermittent claudication and lymphedema, multiple intramuscular injections, ex vivo transduction of vein grafts, intra-arterial delivery (with or without angioplasty), and periadventitial gene transfer of vascular growth factors by adenoviral vectors are all strategies tested in either animal models and/or afflicted patients *(38–41)*. In addition to gene transfer of angiogenic cytokines, adenoviral vectors expressing inducible nitric oxide synthase (iNOS) or Lp-PLA2 have also been shown to reduce neointima formation *(42,43)*.

Risks associated with adenovirally based gene transfer have been evaluated both in animal models and in human subjects. In animals, first-generation adenoviral vectors that have successfully transduced myocardium may also induce infiltration of leukocytes, but by using helper-dependent, fully deleted adenoviral vectors, this infiltration of leukocytes was diminished greatly *(44)*. In human subjects, aside from dose-dependent transient fevers and/or transient rises in some liver enzymes, local delivery of first-generation adenoviral vectors in patients revealed no major safety problems, i.e., there was no evidence of myocarditis *(37)*. As a side note, gene therapy approaches combined with adult stem cell therapy may further improve therapeutic outcomes *(45)*.

2. Materials

2.1. Preparation of Plasmid DNA and Homologous Recombination in Bacterial Cells

1. Standard plasmids for recombination-based assembly of adenovirus vectors (pAdEasy1 and transfer "shuttle" vectors) are available from Stratagene or from http://www.coloncancer.org/adeasy.htm.
2. Sterile Luria-Bertani (LB) broth. For 1 L, dissolve 10 g bacto-tryptone, 5 g bacto-yeast extract, and 10 g NaCl in 950 mL deionized water. Adjust the pH of the solution to 7.0 with NaOH and bring the volume up to 1 L. Autoclave on liquid cycle for 20 min at 15 lb/in.^{2}. Allow the solution to cool to 55°C and add antibiotic if needed. Store at 4°C.
3. LB-Agar plate with ampicillin or kanamycin. Prepare LB medium as in **step 1**, but add 15 g/L agar before autoclaving. Autoclave on liquid cycle for 20 min at 15 lb/in.^{2}. After autoclaving, cool to approx 55°C, add antibiotic (50 µg/mL of either ampicillin or kanamycin), and pour into plates. Let harden, then invert and store at 4°C.
4. 14-mL polystyrene round-bottom tubes, sterile.

5. Electrocompetent cells, *Escherichia coli* strains (XL1Blue, BJ5183), stored at –80°C.
6. T4 ligase, ligation buffer (1X): 50 mM Tris-HCl, 10 mM MgCl$_2$, 1 mM ATP, 10 mM dithiothreitol, 25 µg/mL bovine serum albumin, pH 7.5 at 25°C) stored at –20°C.
7. DNA Miniprep kits (Qiagen).
8. Buffer P1, 50 mM Tris-HCl, pH 8.0, 10 mM EDTA, 100 µg/mL RNase A. After RNase A addition, the buffer should be stored at 2–8°C. To make 1 L of solution, dissolve 6.06 g Tris base, 3.72 g Na2EDTA·2H$_2$O in 800 mL dH$_2$O. Adjust the pH to 8.0 with HCl. Adjust the volume to 1 L with dH$_2$O. Add 100 mg RNase A per liter of P1.
9. Buffer P2: 200 mM NaOH and 1% sodium dodecyl sulfate (SDS) (w/v). It should be stored at room temperature. To make Buffer P2, dissolve 8.0 g NaOH pellets in 950 mL dH$_2$O, 50 mL 20% SDS (w/v) solution. The final volume should be 1 L.
10. Buffer N3 (Qiagen) contains guanidine hydrochloride and acetic acid, and thus is harmful and an irritant.
11. Buffer EB: 10 mM Tris-HCl, pH 8.5, kept at room temperature.
12. 1% agarose gel: for 50 mL, 0.5 g of agarose, 50 mL of 1X TAE, 6 µL of ethidium bromide (10 mg/mL, store at room temperature, avoid light).
13. Gene Pulser electroporator; electroporation cuvet (1-mm gap, kept at –20°C).

2.2. Transfection of 293 Cells, Isolation of a Single Clone of Viral Vector, Propagation of Viral Vector

1. Dulbecco's modified Eagle's medium (DMEM) supplemented with 10% fetal bovine serum (FBS), 1X penicillin G/streptomycin/amphotericin B (Fungizone) (PSF; 100X, filtered through a 0.2-µm membrane; keep at –20°C); DMEM medium supplemented with 2% FBS only. Media kept at 4°C.
2. Humidified CO$_2$ incubator set at 37°C.
3. Calcium phosphate transfection kit: HEPES-buffered saline (HBS), 2 M CaCl, tissue culture sterile water; store kit at –20°C.
4. 60-mm cell culture plate.
5. 24-well cell culture plate.
6. 150-mm cell culture plate.
7. Pasteur pipet.
8. Inverted light microscope.
9. 10 mM Tris-HCl pH 8.0, kept at 4°C.

2.3. Purification of Viral Vector Via CsCl Banding

1. VWR Branson Sonifier 250.
2. 10% fresh sodium deoxycholic acid: 2.5 mL H$_2$O/0.25 g sodium deoxycholic acid.
3. RNase (10 mg/mL), DNase 1 (10 mg/mL), kept at –20°C; 2.0 M MgCl$_2$, kept at room temperature.
4. Freon trichlorotrifluoroethane.
5. 10 mM Tris pH 8.0, kept at 4°C.

6. Heavy CsCl, 1.45 g/mL CsCl in 10 mM Tris-HCl, pH 8.0; medium CsCl, 1.33 g/mL CsCl in 10 mM Tris-HCl, pH 8.0; light CsCl, 1.20 g/mL CsCl in 10 mM Tris-HCl pH 8.0; keep at room temperature.
7. Surespin 630 rotor (Sorvall, DuPont, maximum speed 30,000 rpm); ultracentrifuge tubes (25 × 89 mm, cat. no. 326823, Beckman); Sorvall Sure spin holder P/N79388; Sorvall ultracentrifuge, Ultra 80, Dupont.
8. 23_{G-1} needle.
9. Sorvall 11.5-mL clear-crimp centrifuge tubes, cat. no. 01087; Sorvall plugs/sleeves spare, cat. no. 03999; clamper (crimper, Sorvall SN 9603124, DuPont).
10. Sorvall T-1270 rotor, maximum 70,000 rev/min.
11. Ultra Pure Dialysis Tubing (Cellu Sep H1, cat. no. 1050-10, molecular weight cutoff [MWCO]: nominal 10,000; Membrane Filtration Products, Inc.), kept at 4°C.
13. Sterile 10% sucrose in 10X PBS, kept at 4°C.

2.4. Characterization of Adenoviral Vectors

1. OD_{260} assay: ultraviolet (UV)/Visible spectrophotometer, cuvet, 0.5% SDS.
2. CPE assay: DMEM medium supplemented with 10% FBS, 1X PSF, stored at 4°C; 293 cells; 24-well tissue culture plate; humidified CO_2 (5%) incubator; light microscope.
3. pfu assay: DMEM medium supplemented with 10% FBS, 1X PSF, stored at 4°C; 293 cells; 24-well tissue culture plate; humidified CO_2 (5%) incubator; 0.5% agarose in culture media; 0.5% neutral red in culture media; light microscope.
4. Blue-forming unit (bfu) assay: DMEM/10%FBS/1X PSF; 293 cells, six-well tissue culture plates, X-Gal staining kit, light microscope.
5. Fluorescent forming unit assay: DMEM/10%FBS/1X PSF; 293 cells; 24-well tissue culture plate; humidified CO_2 (5%) incubator; fluorescent microscope.
6. Replication-competent adenovirus (RCA) assay:

   a. Stock SDS solution 10%, room temperature.
   b. 1 M EDTA, room temperature.
   c. Proteinase K, 20 ng/µL, kept at –20°C.
   d. 3 M sodium acetate, keep at room temperature.
   e. tRNA 5 µg/µL, kept at –20°C.
   f. Phenol/chloroform (1:1), kept at 4°C.
   g. Countertop centrifuge.
   h. 100% ethanol, prechilled at –20°C.
   i. 10 mM Tris-HCl, pH 8.5, kept at room temperature.
   j. Wild-type adenovirus serotype 2 DNA (gibco-BRL), kept at –20°C.
   k. TE buffer.
   l. 10X PCR buffer, 25 nM dNTP, Taq DNA polymerase, kept at –20°C.
   m. Distilled, sterile water, kept at room temperature.
   n. Forward primer for detection of *E1* sequence, 5′GAC CCT GCG AGT GTG CGG 3′ reverse primer for detection of deleted *E1* sequence, 5′ GGT CAC AAG GGC GTC TCC AAG 3′.

o. Primers to adenovirus vector sequence to confirm presence of viral DNA: forward primer, 5′ CCA CAG CTC GCG GTT GAG 3′; reverse primer, 5′GAT CTA GCC CGC GCC C 3′.

p. 1% agarose gel: for 50 mL, 0.5 g of agarose, 50 mL of 1X TAE, 6 μL of ethidium bromide (10 mg/mL; store at room temperature, avoid light).

3. Methods

3.1. Construction, Propagation, Purification, and Characterization of First-Generation E1–, E3– Adenoviral Vectors

As aforementioned, adenoviral vectors are widely used tools both in the study of molecular biology and in the field of gene therapy because of several advantages of this viral vector, such as ease of scaling up, ability to transduce both proliferating and quiescent cells, and lack of risk of insertional mutagenicity and/or risk of associated malignancy, and so on. First-generation adenoviral vectors are *E1* and *E3* gene-deleted. These deletions render first generation adenoviral vectors replication defective and provide space for accommodating an up to 7.5-kb insert *(46)*. There are two traditional approaches to generating first-generation adenoviral vectors. The first involves the ligation of genomic subfragments of the adenoviral genome to a DNA fragment containing the desired transgene cassette. The scarcity of the unique restriction sites and the extremely low efficiency of large fragment ligation limits the use of this method, however *(47)*. The second and more widely utilized method involves cotransfection of two adenoviral DNA-containing fragments directly into 293 cells. Homologous recombination between the homologous portions of these two DNA fragments in 293 cells results in the generation of the full-length adenoviral vector genomes *(48)*. However, this method is also limited by low transfection efficiency into mammalian cells, as well as low homologous recombination rates in mammalian cells. These limitations also increase the possibility of generating revertant wild-type viruses and the need of plaque purification to generate pure viral vector clones.

A more recent system by which to generate recombinant adenoviral vectors, the "pAdEasy" system, is a more efficient and simplified system *(49)*. The gene of interest is cloned into a shuttle vector and then inserted into the adenovirus genome backbone (pAdEasy1) by homologous recombination, but in this instance, the recombination occurs in a highly recombinogenic strain of *E. coli.* The resultant recombinant plasmid containing the full-length adenovirus genome is then linearized (to release the viral ends into a native linear conformation) by restriction enzyme digestion and transfected into 293 cells.

This section focuses on the production of recombinant adenoviral vectors utilizing the pAdEasy-based system. **Figure 2** schematically illustrates an overview of the pAdEasy system. The adenoviral backbone vector, pAdEasy1, contains all

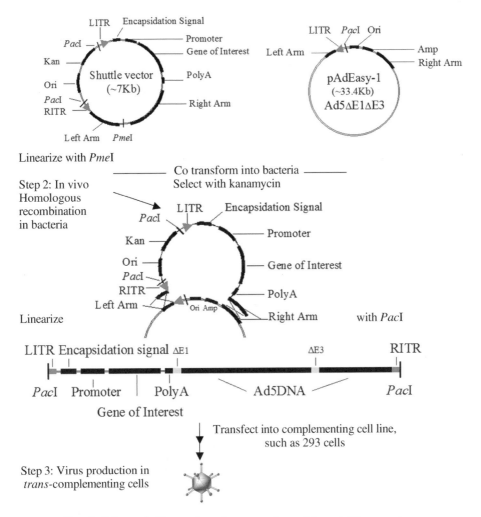

Fig. 2. Schematic illustration of an overview of the pAdEasy system.

of the Ad5 sequence except the *E1* and *E3* genes. The shuttle vector contains a polylinker for insertion of transgene; it also contains two arms, the left arm and the right arm, which mediate homologous recombination with the much larger viral backbone plasmid, pAdEasy1, after co-transformation into *E. coli* BJ5183. There are four types of transfer vectors that can allow for expression, or drive mammalian transcription of a given DNA sequence to meet different vector design requirements. These shuttle vectors are pShuttle, pshuttleCMV, pAdtrack, and pAdtrackCMV. After cloning in the transgene of interest in the polylinker of a desired shuttle plasmid, the shuttle plasmid is linearized with PmeI restriction enzyme and co-transformed into *E. coli* BJ5183 with circularized pAdEasy1.

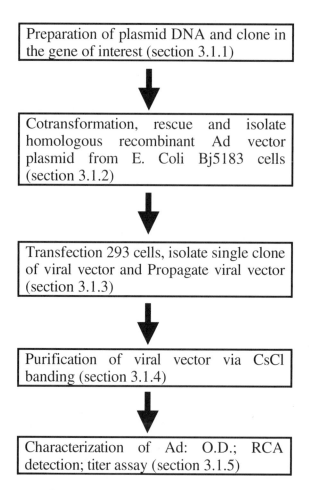

Fig. 3. Summary of the steps involved in the production of the first-generation adenoviral vectors.

Subsequent to homologous recombination in the BJ cells, and selection for kanamycin resistance, the recombinant adenoviral vector plasmid is then rescued and digested with *Pac*I restriction enzyme to facilitate transfection of the viral vector DNA into 293 cells. The recombinant viral vectors are then isolated, propagated and purified. **Figure 3** presents a summary of the steps involved in the production of the first-generation adenoviral vectors.

3.1.1. Preparation of Shuttle Plasmid DNA and Subcloning of a Gene of Interest

1. Inoculate 2×5 mL polypropylene tubes of LB supplemented with proper antibiotics (*see* **Note 1**) with either (1) a bacteria containing proper shuttle vector and

(2) *E. coli* containing the pAdEasy1 plasmid, respectively. Incubate culture at 37°C, and shake at 250–270 rpm for 14–16 h.

2. Pellet bacteria by centrifuging at 6000g for 10–15 min at 4°C. Aspirate supernatant.

3. Miniprep for typical plasmid DNA preparation following instruction along with the Qiagen® Miniprep kit. Briefly, resuspend bacterial pellet with 250 µL of buffer P1 with 100 µg/mL Rnase; transfer to a 1.5- to 2-mL Eppendorf tube and add 250 µL of buffer P2, invert the tube four to six times to mix; add 350 µL of buffer N3 and invert tube immediately by gently four to six times; centrifuge at about 17,900g in a table-top microcentrifuge; apply supernatant to spin column, centrifuge at the same force for 30–60 s; wash column by adding 0.75 mL buffer PE with ethanol added and spin for 30–60 s; discard flow through; and spin for additional 1 min at the same setting to remove residual wash buffer; place DNA binding column in a clean Eppendorf tube; elute plasmid DNA with 50–100 µL of Buffer EB. Note special precautions for isolation of the larger pAdEasy plasmid as outlined in manufacturer's instructions.

4. Clone gene of interest into shuttle vector: linearize purified shuttle vector DNA with suitable restriction enzyme present in the polylinker (*see* **Note 2**). The same restriction enzyme or enzyme bearing compatible ends is also used to excise the transgene expression cassette from its carrying plasmid (*see* **Note 3**). Alternatively, the transgene cassette may be generated from a PCR reaction utilizing primers "tailed" with the appropriate restriction site sequences. Ligate the two linearized DNA fragments (molar ratio of insert to vector ~3:1) in the presence of 1X ligation buffer and T4 ligase (*see* **Note 4**), and add water to constitute the proper total reaction volume. Let ligation reaction proceed for about 16 to 20 h in a 14°C water bath.

5. Transform electrocompetent bacteria cells such as XL-1 Blue (*see* **Note 5**) with ligated DNA from **step 4**: add 2 µL of ligation mix into 20 µL electrocompetent cells and mix gently, then transfer all of the cells to a chilled 1-mm electroporation cuvet. Electroporate the cells at 1.25 mV for 2–3 s, quickly add 1 mL of LB medium prewarmed at 37°C, and gently resuspend the cells. Transfer the solution to an Eppendorf tube and shake horizontally for 45 min to 1 h at 37°C. Spread 50–100 µL onto LB/kanamycin-inoculated selection plates. Invert plate and incubate overnight at 37°C.

6. The next day, pick colonies, grow in 5 mL LB/kanamycin medium for 14–16 h, miniprep, and purify putative shuttle/transgene-containing plasmid DNA as described in **step 3**. Cut about 1 µg plasmid DNA with a diagnostic restriction enzyme for 4 h. Run the digestion products on 1% agarose gel with ethidium bromide staining to confirm presence of transgene insert into the shuttle plasmid multiple cloning site; also confirm correct 5′–3′ orientation if cloning between the cytomegalovirus (CMV) promoter and polyadenylation sites present in pAdCMV shuttle, or pAdCMVGFP.

3.1.2. Cotransformation, Rescue, and Isolation of the Homologous Recombinant Adenoviral Vector Plasmid From E. coli BJ5183 Cells

1. Linearize shuttle vector containing the desired insert with *Pme*I restriction enzyme (*see* **Note 6**), let the reaction proceed for at lease 4 h, and check whether

the digestion is complete (*see* **Note 2**). Incomplete digestion will give increased background (i.e., shuttle plasmids rather than recombinant adenovirus genome-containing plasmids). **Note:** This may be unavoidable if the transgene contains a *Pme*I site, and thus partial digestion with *Pme*I is necessary; in this instance, more Kan^R colonies must be screened in **step 3**.

2. Homologous recombination in electrocompetent *E. coli* BJ5183 (*see* **Note 5**). The BJ5183 strain is recA proficient, and thus provides the recombinase that is required to efficiently perform the recombination event between the homologous portions of the insert bearing shuttle plasmid and the pAdEasy plasmid: mix 50–100 ng of linearized shuttle plasmid bearing the insert, a substantial amount (1 μg) of pAdEasy1 plasmid DNA purified from **step 3**, and 20 μL of electrocompetent *E. coli* BJ5183 and proceed with co-transformation by electroporation into electrocompetent BJ5183 cells as described in **Subheading 3.1.1., step 5**.

3. The next day, pick the *smallest* colonies on the plate and grow in miniculture for 12–16 h in LB/kanamycin, miniprep, and purify plasmid DNA as described in **Subheading 3.1.1., step 3**. Because successfully recombined plasmids will be much larger than nonrecombined shuttle plasmids (both are Kan^R), picking smaller colonies will select for those colonies harboring the larger (and desired) recombination product. As the yield of plasmid DNA grown in BJ5183 cells is very low, miniprep isolation of DNA from these cells will be at low concentrations, thus elute plasmid DNA from Qiagen columns with less volume of elution buffer (30 μL), digest half of the purified plasmid DNA volume with a diagnostic mapping restriction enzyme, and electrophoretically separate the digestion products in a 1% agarose gel. Once the clones harboring the correct homologous recombination plasmid are identified, we typically transfer the remaining adenovirus vector genome containing plasmid DNA into XL-1Blue cells to get higher yields of the recombinant Kan^R adenoviral plasmid.

3.1.3. Transfection of 293 Cells, Isolation of a Single Clone of Viral Vector, and Propagation of Viral Vector

1. Seed 2×10^5 293 cells (*E1*-transformed human embryonic kidney cells *[50,51]*) onto a 60-mm plastic cell culture plate approx 24 h prior to transfection. Incubate overnight at 37°C in a humidified CO_2 incubator. The confluency of the cells should be only about 50–70% at the time of transfection.

2. Digest 10 μg of recombinant adenoviral vector genome containing plasmid with *Pac*I (*see* **Note 7**) for more than 4 h, and run about 100 ng on gel to confirm that the digestion is complete as well as to confirm release of the bacterial sequences from the adenoviral vector genome sequences. The completely digested recombinant adenoviral plasmid will release a large fragment (near 36 kb), plus a smaller fragment of 3.0 or 4.5 kb (bacterial origin and Kan^R sequences).

3. When 293 cells on the 60-mm plate reach about 50–70% confluency, transfect the cells with *Pac*I-digested recombinant adenoviral plasmid using the calcium phosphate transfection method: label two Eppendorf tubes "A" and "B." To tube A, add 18 μL of 2 *M* CaCL (final CaCl concentration of 60 m*M*) and 10 μg of digested

DNA, and bring total volume to 150 µL with sterile water and gently mix. To tube B, add 150 µL of 2X HBS. Using a Pasteur pipet, slowly add solution A drop-wise to solution B while bubbling air through solution B with another pipet. Continue until solution A is depleted. This is a slow process that should be done over 1–2 min. A fine precipitate should form. Incubate at room temperature for 30 min. Add the precipitate drop-wise to the media of 293 cells on the 60-mm plate. Incubate overnight at 37°C in a humidified CO_2 incubator (*see* **Note 8**). Alternative transfection methods may be utilized as well.

4. The next day, harvest all cells and media on the plate (approx 5 mL), and increase volume to 36 mL by adding fresh medium. Mix the cells and split evenly into each well of three 24-well plates. Each well will now contain about 500 µL of the mixture; return the three plates into 37°C humidified CO_2 incubator.

5. Watch for cytopathic effect (CPE) (*see* **Note 9**) under an inverted light microscope and label the wells that shown signs of CPE. Typically, for the first-generation adenoviral vectors, CPE can be detected between 4 and 7 d posttransfection. When the cells in a well are totally detached and aggregated as a result of CPE (between 7 and 10 d posttransfection), harvest the cells and media into an Eppendorf tube and keep at –80°C until ready for propagation of virus. Theoretically, each well represents the growth of a single clone of the desired adenoviral vector, but if many wells show CPE, then the likelihood that a well contains more than a single clone of vector proportionally increases.

6. Propagate first-generation adenoviral vectors: freeze/thaw the cells collected from **step 5** in an Eppendorf tube three times (NEVER exceed 37°C during thawing) to lyse cells and liberate the virus. To expedite the procedure, freeze in dry ice/ethanol, and thaw in a 37°C water bath.

7. Infect 293 cells (typically in a 60-mm plate, seeded a day before the infection; the confluency of the cells at the time of infection should be around 80%) with a small portion (one-fifth) of the virus isolated in **step 5**. Briefly, aspirate media from the 60-mm plate containing 293 cells, add lysate from **step 6** to the cells (avoid adding cell debris into the culture plate) (*see* **Note 10**), supplement with just enough medium to cover the cells (~200–400 µL), and incubate at 37°C. Rock the plate every 15 min for 1 h to facilitate the binding of the viral vectors to the cells, while also keeping the cell monolayer moist. Rocking should be gentle to avoid detachment of the cells from the plate. After 1 h, add extra medium up to 5 mL and return the plate to the incubator (*see* **Note 11**). Because the adenoviral life cycle is about 36 h, if enough virus was added (insuring a multiplicity of infection >1), all of the cells infected will be detached from the plate over this time frame. Harvest all cells and media (5 mL in total) to a 15-mL conical tube. Keep at –80°C until ready for further propagation of virus.

8. Freeze/thaw the viral lysate as described in **step 6**, and use 1–5 mL of the lyaste to infect one 150-mm plate of nearly confluent 293 cells following the procedure, as described in **step 7**. Harvest all of the cells and media (20 mL in total) at 36 h postinfection into a 50-mL conical tube, and keep at –80°C until ready to use. Repeat this step until adequate amounts of cells have been infected to allow for

high-yield purification (20–90 150-mm plates of virus lysate, depending on the growth characteristics of a given vector) (*see* **Note 12**).

9. Scale up viral vector production by infecting up to 90- to 150-mm plates of 293 cells, each with 1 mL of lysate from **step 8**. At 36–72 h after infection (CPE maximally affecting all cells, depending on the respective vector), harvest all cells together with media and pellet cells at 2800 rpm for 15 min. Aspirate media (*see* **Note 13**).

10. Resuspend cell pellets in 10 m*M* Tris pH 8.0 to a final volume of approx 45 mL per four 50-mL conical tubes. Freeze (–80°C)/thaw (37°C) and resuspend the cell pellet three times. Store at –80°C until ready to proceed to viral vector purification by CsCl$_2$ banding.

3.1.4. Purification of Viral Vector Via CsCl Banding

1. Sonicate freeze/thawed virus in 10 m*M* Tris pH 8.0 from **Subheading 3.1.3.**, **step 10** for 5 min with a tapered microtip while keeping the virus on ice (use VWR Branson Sonifier 250, setting output control at 4–4.5, duty cycle percent at 40; use low energy levels, 70% microtip limits) (*see* **Note 14**).

2. Add sodium deoxycholic acid to 0.1% final concentration. Freshly make up 10% sodium deoxycholic acid each time in distilled H$_2$O. (2.5 mL H$_2$O/0.25 g). Sonicate for 5 min at same setting described in **step 1**. Incubate at 37°C for 30 min after adding RNase (10 mg/mL), 10 μL/mL virus; DNase 1 (10 mg/mL), 5 μL/mL virus; and 2.0 *M* MgCl$_2$, 10 μL/mL virus.

3. Add 50% volume of freon trichlorotrifluoroethane (T 180-4, Fisher or Sigma, cat. no. T5271, 500 mL, 1, 1, 2-TrichloroTrifluoroethane, F.W. 187.4, C2CL3, F3) prechilled to –20°C. On ice, place sonicator tip right at the interphase to form a complete viscous emulsion for 10–12 min. Spin at 2800 rpm for 15 min to separate the solution into two phases. Transfer the upper (aqueous) phase (~7.5 mL/tube) into a new 50-mL conical tube (keep lower Freon phase) and add 50% volume of chilled freon to the aqueous phase. Sonicate again till very viscous (for 5 min). Spin at 2800 rpm for 5 min. Save the top phase. Add 10 mL of 10 m*M* Tris pH 8.0 to saved Freon lower phase, and back extract by pipetting and sonicating for 5 min. Spin at 2800 rpm for 15 min. Transfer this top phase with those obtained from previous Freon extractions into a 50-mL conical tube (72 mL total).

4. Layer virus-containing suspensions onto the top of a CsCl step gradient. The centrifuge tube holds 38 mL. Subtract the total volume of virus supernatant (18–22 mL) and divide the number in half ([38 – 18]/2 = 10 mL). Layer 10 mL of sterile heavy CsCl (*density* = 1.45 g/mL, in Tris pH 8.0) into centrifuge tube and then layer sterile light CsCl (*density* = 1.2 g/mL) over this. Layer the virus supernatant (18 mL) carefully on top of this without disturbing each phase.

5. Balance each centrifuge tube pair (difference is no more than 0.001–0.002*g*).

6. Load centrifuge tubes into the Surespin 630 rotor (or equivalent) and spin at 20,000 rpm for 2 h.

7. After centrifugation, carefully remove the centrifuge tubes with forceps. Virus band should be a white turbid layer at interphase between heavy and light CsCl$_2$.

Use a 23_{G-1} needle, inserted just below the virus band level, and remove the virus in the smallest volume possible (~1–2 mL/tube).

8. Transfer isolated virus into an ultracentrifuge tube, and fill this with medium $CsCl_2$ (*density* = 1.33 g/mL, density of mature adenovirus virion) up to the tube neck, almost to the top, with no air bubbles or space left. Insert into the rotor and balance with another tube also filled with medium-density $CsCl_2$.

9. Load tubes in T120 rotor (or equivalent) and spin at 45,000 rpm at 4°C for at least 16 h.

10. After centrifugation, fix the centrifuge tube in holder. Place a 50-mL conical tube below the centrifuge tube to collect any drops from the centrifuge tube. Puncture a hole on the very top of the centrifuge tube with a 23_{G-1} needle. Remove the now obvious thick virus band with another 23_{G-1} needle inserted into the wall of the tube just below the viral band. Try to remove the virus into as small a volume as possible (~1–2 mL), save the virus in a 15-mL conical tube, and place on ice (*see* **Note 15**).

11. Add the adenovirus by glass Pasteur pipet to singly clamped dialysis tubing (rinsed very well with water before use). Clamp other end of dialysis tubing with a plastic clamp and leave air space inside the tubing. Dialyze the virus overnight against 10 m*M* Tris pH 8.0, with several changes of the dialysis buffer.

12. Remove the virus to a 15-mL conical tube and measure the virus volume. Add one-tenth volume of sterile 10% sucrose in 10X PBS to a final concentration of 1% sucrose in 1X PBS. Aliquot 100 μL of recombinant adenovirus to each prechilled 0.5-m tube. Store at –80°C and avoid repeated freeze/thawing of the virus.

3.1.5. Characterization of Adenoviral Vectors

The characterization of the purified adenoviral vector preparation includes determining the physical number of vector particles (VP) by optical absorbance at OD_{260}, and confirming lack of presence of revertant wild-type virus by use of an RCA assay.

There are several ways to determine the infectious titer of the viral vector preparation, including CPE assay, pfu assay, bfu assay, and/or a fluorescent focus-forming (ffu) assay. However, determining infectious unit concentrations of a given viral vector preparation is very prone to errors, as a result of numerous variables including the status of cells at the time of infection and lack of virus spread (which is typically limited to only several viral diameters in total distance). Thus, infectious titering methods will always underestimate the concentration of a given virus-containing solution. The method is also more labor-intensive. The inconsistency also makes it difficult to compare the results between reports/laboratories. Alternatively, measurement of the concentration of physical particles in vector preparation (by measuring absorbance of the virus solution at OD_{260}) is relatively easy and the nearly universally accepted standard for quantitaion of solutions containing purified adenoviruses. In fact, this method is made more useful by the production of a national adenovirus standard.

In order to establish a reference point for comparisons between studies using adenovirus-based vectors and to develop regulatory policy to guide more consistent, safer production of adenoviral vectors, the Adenovirus Reference Material (ARM) was developed under the guidance of the Adenovirus Reference Material Working Group (ARMWG) and the US Food and Drug Administration (FDA) through the donation of services and supplies by a large number of laboratories and organizations from the United States, Canada, France, the Netherlands, Germany, and the United Kingdom. All information regarding the development and characterization of the ARM can be found at the website http://www.wilbio.com, and the actual ARM is available from the American Type Culture Collection (ATCC) (http://www.atcc.org). The ARM consists of a purified wild-type Ad5. The particle concentration is 5.8×10^{11} particles/mL, and the infectious titer on HEK 293 cells is approx 7×10^{10} normalized adjusted standard infectious units (NIU)/mL (*see* **Note 16**). To evaluate the sensitivity of a lab's measurement of a respective adenoviral vector preparation, the ARM is measured using the procedure that routinely is used in a given laboratory, and the readout is compared and normalized to the ARM standard.

1. OD_{260} assay (*see* **Note 17**): take 5 µL of virus (postdialysis from **Subheading 3.1.4.**, **step 14**) and mix with 0.5% SDS, gently pipetting to avoid bubbles. Blank-spectrometer with 50 µL of 0.5% SDS at OD_{260}. Read the sample OD. OD_{260} in the range of 0.1 to 1.0 is appropriate; if the reading is lower or higher, adjust the dilution ratio by increasing or decreasing the amount of virus added. Additionally, the ratio of OD_{260} to OD_{280} should be around 1.3, reflective of a normal mature virion protein:DNA content. This ratio indicates the purity of the viral preparation. A ratio too high indicates possible unpackaged DNA contamination in the viral preparation, whereas a reading that is too low may indicate many empty capsids in the preparation. The following formula is used to calculate viral titer (optical particle unit [opu]): viral titer (opu/mL) = $OD_{260} \times$ viral dilution $\times 1.1 \times 10^{12}$. One absorbance unit at 260 nm is equivalent to 1.1×10^{12} adenoviral vector particles *(52)*.

2. Titering assay to assess the infectivity of the purified viral vectors: there are different ways to perform titering assay, which are dependent on the transgene that the viral vector encodes *(53,54)*. CPE assay and plaque assay are suitable for all viral vectors causing CPE. Infectious unit (IU)/mL or pfu/mL of the vector will be determined respectively in these two separate methods; for adenoviral vectors expressing the bacterial β-galactosidase gene *(lacZ)*, bfu/mL of virus is often performed; for adenoviral vectors carrying green fluorescent protein (GFP) or immunological detection of infected cells with fluorescent antibodies (such as against hexon), ffu/mL of virus can be performed. For first-generation adenoviral vectors, complementing 293 cell lines are also typically used in the titering assays. All titering assays are based on serial dilution of the viral vector preparations, counting the infectious events on the indicator cells after a given period of time after initial infection and incubation, and calculating the infectious events per milliliter of viral vector preparation.

Table 1
Loading of the First 24-Well Plate

1	2	3	4	5	6
a	20 µL dilute A	20 µL dilute A	20 µL dilute A	20 µL dilute A	20 µL dilute A
b	20 µL dilute A	20 µL dilute A	20 µL dilute A	20 µL dilute A	20 µL dilute A
c	20 µL dilute B	20 mL dilute B	20 µL dilute B	20 µL dilute B	20 µL dilute B
d	20 µL dilute B	20 µL dilute B	20 µL dilute B	20 µL dilute B	20 µL dilute B

The sensitivity of the titering assays is relatively lower and there is greater variability in the testing results. Successful infection of a cell by an adenovirus depends on the appropriate interaction of a given virion with a receptive cell. In the titering assay, the cells are attached to the bottom of the culture plates, but because the virion is very small (90 nm) in diameter, its diffusion rate in a solution is very low. Thus, perfectly viable and infectious virions present in the solution may not be detected, because they never interact with an indicator cell.

a. CPE assay:

i. Approximately 24 h before beginning the titration protocol, plate 293 cells into three 24-well plates. Carefully seed all wells at the same density ($\sim 10^5$ cells per well) in 500 µL of growth medium.

ii. Prepare serial dilutions of the virus as follows: make a 1:100 dilution by adding 10 µL virus stock to 990 µL sterile growth medium. First, starting with the 1:100 dilution, prepare serial 1:100 dilutions A, B, and C by transferring 10 µL diluted virus to 990 µL sterile growth medium. Next, starting with the C dilutions (1 to 10^8 of the original viral vector preparation), prepare serial 1:10 dilutions D, E, and F by transferring 100 µL diluted virus to 900 µL sterile growth medium.

iii. Remove three 24-well culture plates from the incubator and inspect the wells to ensure that the cells have attached to form an even monolayer. Add 20 µL diluted virus A to each well in columns 2–6, row a and b; add 20 µL diluted virus b to each well in columns 2–6, row c and d; and continue adding diluted virus following this modality until finishing loading viral dilution F to the bottom two rows of the third 24-well plate. Column 1 is used as negative control, i.e., no virus is added (**Table 1**).

iv. Cover the plate and incubate in a humidified CO_2 (5%) incubator for 10 d at 37°C.

v. Using a microscope, check each well for CPE 7–10 d after infection. For each row, count the number of wells having CPE. Wells are scored as CPE-positive even if only a few cells show cytopathic effects. If uncertain, compare the infected well with the noninfected control wells.

vi. Calculate viral titer, based upon where limiting dilution CPE occurs. **Table 2** shows an example of how one may want to calculate viral titer according to the number of CPE-positive wells.

Table 2
Calculating Viral Titer According to the Number of Cytopathic Effect (CPE)-Positive Wells

Dilution	CPE-positive wells
A	1×10^4 10 out of 10
B	1×10^6 10 out of 10
C	1×10^8 6 out of 10
D	1×10^9 4 out of 10
E	1×10^{10} 0 out of 10
F	1×10^{11} 0 out of 10

In this case, the infectious titer of this viral vector preparation is 4×5 (200 μL out of 1 mL of each dilution is added to 10 wells) $\times 1 \times 10 = 2 \times 10^{10}$ IU/mL of viral vector preparation.

The assay is useful for gross assessments of relative infectious units of a given preparation, and valid only if the following three conditions are met: the negative control wells show no visible signs of CPE nor growth inhibition; wells infected with the least dilute virus (10^4 in the example) are all CPE-positive; wells infected with the most dilute virus (10^{10-11} in the example) are all CPE-negative.

To increase the sensitivity of this method, much smaller and more wells (96-well plate) are used to perform the assay, and infectious unit calculations are based on the Spearman-Karber method (for detailed instructions, please refer to http://www.clontech.com/clontech/expression/adeno/adeno17.shtml).

For the completeness of the text, each of the following titer assays is summarized; detailed procedures can be found in **refs. *53*** and ***54***.

b. Plaque forming unit assay. This procedure is similar to the CPE assay, in terms of plating cells, making serial dilutions of viral vector preparations, incubating the diluted virus suspensions with the complementing 293 cells, counting plaques of adenovirus-killed cells in the monolayer, and calculating pfu per milliliter of viral vector preparation. The difference in this method over the CPE method detailed previously is that after incubation of the viral vector with the cells for 1 h, the viral inoculate is completely withdrawn and an overlay of 0.5% agarose in culture medium is added to the cell monolayer. The so-prepared plate is incubated for 7–10 d at 37°C, in a 5% CO_2 incubator. The agar overlay is used to keep the virus localized after cell lysis. At the end of incubation time (7–10 d), 0.5% neutral red in culture medium is added to the plates in a fresh agar overlay, and the dead cells centered at the point of initial infection are individually visualized and counted as a result of their inability to take up the dye. Multiplication of the number of plaques by the dilution factor gives the pfu per milliliter of a given viral preparation. This method is cumbersome, less sensitive, and subject to even greater variability.

   c. bfu assay. This assay is suitable for first-generation adenoviral vectors express-
      ing a *LacZ* transgene. The outline of the procedure is as follows: plate cells,
      make serial dilutions of viral vector preparations, incubate the virus-containing
      suspensions with the complementing 293 cells for 12–24 h, withdraw media,
      and proceed to a standard procedure of staining mammalian cells utilizing the
      chromogenic substrate of *LacZ*, X-gal. One then simply counts the number of
      blue-staining cells and calculates bfu per milliliter of viral vector preparation
      based on the dilution factor.
   d. ffu assay. This assay is mostly suitable for first-generation adenoviral vectors
      expressing GFP. The outline of the procedure is as follows: plate the cells,
      make serial dilutions of viral vector preparations, incubate the viral containing
      solutions with the complementing 293 cells, and count the green fluorescence
      cells present in each well at 12–24 h after infection of the cells. This number
      is then multiplied by the dilution factor to yield GFP-forming units per milli-
      liter of the original virus preparation. For immunological detection of infected
      cells with fluorescent antibodies, please refer to **ref. 54**.
3. RCA detection assay. Because 293 cells were originally created by transfection of
   sheared human Ad5 DNA into fetal kidney cells, and are immortalized as a result
   of the presence of the adenoviral *E1* genes, they are utilized to transcomplement
   the growth of *E1*-deleted adenovirus vectors. The limited overlap homology
   between the integrated adenovirus *E1* sequences and the adenovirus DNA sequences
   present in the recombinant adenoviral vectors can potentially allow for a very low
   frequency of homologous recombination to occur, resulting in the production of
   RCA. The likelihood that a given adenovirus vector preparation contains an RCA
   increases with each amplification of that preparation *(55)*. Thus, it is strongly recommended that all amplifications be initiated with virus stock at the lowest possible passage number. The use of bacterial plasmids to facilitate generation of
   infectious virus clones offers the greatest protection against this problem. For
   safety considerations in preclinical and clinical studies, it is necessary to detect
   and limit RCA to less than one RCA for every 3×10^{10} viral particles. Several
   methods to detect RCA in a given adenovirus vector preparation have been
   described, with several groups having developed quantitative RCA detection
   methods based on sensitive PCR-based techniques, utilizing DNA primers that
   hybridize to the areas either within or flanking the native adenovirus *E1* sequences
   (56,57). A detailed procedure is described next.
   a. Step 1: extraction of virion DNA from purified stock. To 100 μL of CsCl$_2$-
      purified virus, add SDS and EDTA to final concentrations of 0.5% and 5 m*M*,
      respectively, to both disrupt viral capsids, and to inhibit endogenous DNases.
      Incubate this mixture at room temperature for 10 min and add 1 μL proteinase
      K (20 ng/μL) and incubate at 55°C for 2 h to overnight. Add one-tenth volume
      of 3 *M* sodium acetate, mix, and add 1 μL tRNA (5 μg/μL), mix, add equal vol-
      ume of phenol/chloroform (1:1), and spin for 5 min at maximum speed in
      counter-top centrifuge to separate the phases. Save the supernatant, add 2.5 vol
      of cold 100% ethanol, mix, and precipitate virion DNA overnight at –20°C.

Centrifuge at 4°C for 15 min after precipitation, save the DNA pellet, and allow to air-dry for 5–10 min. Resuspend the DNA in 30–50 µL 10 m*M* Tris-Cl, pH 8.5.

b. Step 2: make wild-type Ad2 DNA (Gibco-BRL) standards (*see* **Note 18**). Purified Ad2 DNA at a concentration of 0.3 µg/µL is diluted as follows:

i. Dilution A: 1 µL of 0.3 µg/µL of Ad2 DNA in 990 µL of TE (7.8 × 10^6 genome/µL).
ii. Dilution B: 10 µL of Dilution A in 990 µL of TE (7.8 × 10^4 genome/µL).
iii. Dilution C: 10 µL of Dilution B in 990 µL of TE (7.8 × 10^2 genome/µL).
iv. Dilution D: 100 µL of Dilution C in 900 µL of TE (7.8 × 10^1 genome/µL).
v. Dilution E: 100 µL of Dilution D in 900 µL of TE (7.8 genome/µL).
vi. Dilution F: 100 µL of Dilution E in 900 µL of TE (0.78 genome/µL, <1 genome/µL).

c. Step 3: vector reversion PCR assay. The total reaction of the PCR is 100 µL. For each standard, add 90 µL of PCR mix and 1 µL of each wild-type adenoviral DNA dilution standard (A–F), respectively; for each testing tube, add 90 µL of PCR mix and 10, 1, and 0.1 µL of purified virion DNA, respectively; add water to constitute a volume of 100 µL in each tube. Set a negative tube by adding 10 µL of water to 90 µL of PCR reaction mix. Set two sets of tubes for the reactions, one set for primer detection of the *E1* deletion (detection of 2.2 kb PCR fragment) and the other for using primers capable of hybridizing to a nondeleted portion of adenovirus vector genome to confirm the presence of viral DNA in each reaction (detection of 1.2 kb PCR fragment).
PCR reaction in 100 µL total volume:

i. 10 µL of reaction buffer.
ii. 1 µL of forward primer (100 ng/µL) (either *E1*-specific or adenoviral genome-specific; *see* **Subheading 2.**).
iii. 1 µL of reverse primer (100 ng/µL) (either *E1*-specific or adenoviralH genome-specific; *see* **Subheading 2.**).
iv. 1 µL of dNTPs at 25 m*M*.
v. 0.5–1 µL of Taq (Roche) DNA polymerase (1–3 U/uL) distilled, sterile water to a volume of 90 µL.
vi. DNA template and water in final volume of 10 µL.
Thermocycler conditions: 94°C for 3 min; 94°C denaturing for 30 s, 55°C annealing for 20 s, 72°C extension for 1 min, repeat for 35 cycles; 72°C extension for 10 min; 4°C pause.
Run PCR reaction products out on a 1% agarose gel and stain with ethidium bromide to visualize reaction products and confirm absence of *E1* sequences in the preparation.
Interpretation of the results: the detection of the 2.2-kb *E1* fragment in the Ad2 wild-type genome will confirm that the assay was correctly carried out, and also validates the sensitivity of the assay; the detection of the 1.2-kb PCR fragment in viral DNA extracted from the purified viral vectors confirm the

presence of amplifiable adenovirus DNA in the extracts. If a sample tests positive with the *E1*-specific primers, then this sample is positive for RCA; we recommend discarding the entire stock after autoclaving, and reisolating the virus from bacterial plasmid stage.

To avoid RCA, a cell line designated as PER.C6 was developed. This cell line incorporates the Ad5 *E1*-encoding sequence (Ad5 nucleotides 459–3510) under the control of the human phosphoglycerate kinase (PGK) promoter. Because there is no sequence overlap between this adenovirus *E1* DNA sequence and that of most first-generation adenovirus vectors (typically *E1* deleted for Ad5 nucleotides 459–3510) there is a decreased (but not obviated) propensity to generate RCA during the propagation of first-generation adenoviral vectors in PER.C6 cells *(58)*.

3.2. Second-Generation, Helper-Independent Adenoviral Vectors

First-generation adenoviral vectors have demonstrated many advantages; however, when used at higher multiplicity of infection (MOI; the average number of adenvoiral particles that infect a single target cell in a specific experiment), low levels of viral DNA replication can occur despite the deletion of the *E1* genes. This is likely owing to the presence of "*E1*-like" factors in target cells *(59,60)*. This low level of viral replication leads to expression of viral early and late genes and can result in associated cytotoxicities as well as in the elimination of the transduced target cells by CD8+ cytotoxic T-lymphocytes (CTL) in vivo *(61)*. To further reduce the possibility of adenoviral vector replication in vivo, multiple deleted adenoviral vectors were developed. These vectors comprise additional specific viral genome deletions in addition to the *E1* and *E3* deletions. These multiple deletions also reduce the possibility of producing RCA when propagating the viral vectors in vitro, as multiple recombination events would be required to recapitulate a wild-type virus genome in the multiply transcomplementing cell lines used to propagate these vectors. These deletions have been introduced into the pAdEasy1 plasmid system, which can also be homologously recombined with typical shuttle plasmids to yield the multiply deleted second-generation adenoviral vector. A complementing cell line is required to transcomplement the multiple genes deleted in these vectors, in lieu of the typical 293 cells. For example, an adenoviral vector with *E1*, DNA polymerase, and preterminal protein-coding genes deleted was constructed, and propagated to very high titers on a transcomplementing cell line co-expressing *E1*, viral DNA polymerase, and preterminal proteins. Thus, the generation of first-generation adenoviral vectors and that of second-generation, helper-independent adenoviral vectors differ only in the initial cloning steps and the need for use of a different cell line. The transfection, propagation, purification, and characterization of the resultant vectors are identical to those procedures detailed for isolation of first-generation adenoviral vectors (please refer to **Subheading 3.1.**). When tested in vivo, it was shown that this class of adenovirally based vectors persists in vivo and has reduced toxicity, relative to first-generation adenovirus vectors *(15–17)*.

3.3. Second-Generation, Helper-Dependent Adenoviral Vectors

As aforementioned, further adenoviral modifications have been introduced to eliminate the low level of viral DNA replication of the first-generation viral vector and decrease the cytotoxicity associated with this replication. Another approach to achieve this is to generate helper-dependent adenoviral vectors. This vector is devoid of all viral coding sequences and only contains the *cis*-acting elements that are necessary for viral DNA replication, i.e., the inverted terminal repeats (ITR) on both ends and the packaging signal that is close to the left ITR. The helper-dependent vector can accommodate transgene cassettes up to the size of 37 kb. In most cases, the trangene inserts are much smaller than 37 kb, and a stuffer DNA fragment (noncoding eukaryotic DNA) is also inserted into the vector to facilitate efficient viral packaging into the capsids *(62)*. The helper-dependent adenoviral vector is so named because there is no cell line that can transcomplement the entire adenoviral protein encoding genome (>60 proteins), thus the growth of the helper-dependent adenoviral vectors is solely dependent on co-infection of cells with a helper virus that provides all viral proteins *in trans* during viral propagation.

Attempts have been made to decrease contamination of the helper virus present in the final helper-dependent viral stock. A *Cre/Lox*P method was developed to further reduce helper virus contamination *(19)*. *Lox*P sites were introduced into the *E1–*, *E3–* helper virus genome which flank the packaging signal in the helper viral genome. A 293-cell line expressing the p1 bacterial phage-derived *Cre* recombinase was also isolated. In this manner, shortly after the helper virus infects the *Cre*-producing 293 cells, the packaging signal sequence in the helper viral genome is excised by *Cre/Lox*P recombination, rendering the helper viral genome unpackageable into the viral capsid. In contrast, the helper-dependent vector genome contains an intact packaging signal, and thus its genome can be packaged into the capsids produced from the helper virus. Propagation of the helper-dependent vector starts with transfection of a linearized helper-dependent vector plasmid followed by co-infection with the helper virus into 293/*Cre*-positive cells. About 48 h postinfection, when there are about 90% CPE appearing in the plates, the cells are harvested and repeatedly freeze/thawed to release infectious viruses. This lysate now primarily containing helper-dependent viruses are used to infect more *Cre*-positive 293 cells, again with co-infection of the helper virus. After several rounds of harvesting and co-infection, the helper-dependent viruses are purified by $CsCl_2$ banding. PCR is performed after the purification to detect helper virus contamination in the purified helper-dependent vector. With this *Cre/LoxP* method, the contamination of the helper virus is reduced to 0.1–1%. For detailed procedures on optimized propagation of helper-dependent viral vectors, please refer to **refs. *63*** and ***64***.

4. Notes

1. pAdEasy-1 plasmid is a 33.4-kb plasmid containing the Ad5 genome with *E1* (Ad5 nucleotides 1–3533) and *E3* (Ad5 nucleotides 28,130–30,820) regions deleted. This plasmid contains a copy of the ampicillin resistance gene; thus, to select bacteria containing this plasmid, the LB media is supplemented with 75 µg/mL of ampicillin. All shuttle plasmids are kanamycin-resistant; thus, to grow bacteria bearing this plasmid, 50 µg/mL of kanamycin is added to LB media.
2. One unit of restriction enzyme digests 1 µg of plasmid DNA per hour, or 1 U of restriction enzyme digests 10 µg plasmid DNA overnight. Assure complete digestion of the shuttle vector to avoid high background in the ligation reaction. Treatment of linearized plasmid DNA with alkaline phosphatase 1 U/10 µg DNA at 37°C for 1–2 h may reduce religation and further reduce the background. After digestion is complete, heat inactivate enzyme if possible.
3. Expression cassette is less than 7–8 kb, and the transgene product should be nontoxic.
4. Do not add more than 1% by volume of T4 ligase; glycerol content in the enzyme storage solution inhibits ligase activity.
5. Reuse of thawed cells is not recommended, because it may reduce future transformation efficiency; rather, freeze cells in small aliquots to avoid repetitive freeze/thaws.
6. Avoid presence of *Pme*I sites in transgenes to be subcloned into shuttle plasmids. If a *Pme*I site is present, partial digestion of the insert containing shuttle plasmid is recommended before proceeding to homologous recombination.
7. Avoid presence of *Pac*I sites in transgenes. If a *Pac*I site cannot be avoided, partial digestion of the recombinant adenoviral plasmid DNA is recommended before proceeding to transfection.
8. Starting from this step, several general considerations must be kept in mind. The National Institutes of Health and Center for Disease Control have designated adenoviruses as Level 2 biological agents. This distinction requires the maintenance of a Biosafety Level 2 facility for work involving this virus and others like it. (http://www.clontech.com/clontech/expression/adeno/adeno22.shtml). The virus packaged by transfecting HEK 293 cells with the adenovirally based vectors are capable of infecting human cells. These viral supernatants could, depending on the gene insert, contain a potentially hazardous recombinant virus. A Biosafety Cabinet must be used for all manipulations, including (but not limited to) pipetting, harvesting infected cells, loading, and opening containers. Minimize aerosols. Use sterile, cotton-plugged pipet tips for all pipetting. No work with adenovirus is permitted on the open bench. Perform work in a limited-access area. Centrifugation must be done in closed containers and using sealed rotors.

Decontaminate potentially infectious wastes before disposal, as UV lighting and bleach solution (10%) will kill the virus. Personal protection should include a double layer of gloves, lab coats, and protective eye-goggles.

9. Adenoviruses produce a characteristic CPE in cell culture, which consists of the rounding and clustering of cells with development of refractile intranuclear inclusion bodies. The CPE may start at the periphery of the culture before spreading throughout the plate. Infected cells eventually become rounded and the cell sheet disintegrates.

10. Cell debris is toxic to cells. Always spin down and remove cell debris after freeze/thawing virus lysates and before infection.

11. When passing 293 cells, DMEM with 10% FBS is used. When infecting the cells, DMEM with only 2% FBS is used. Serum factors in FBS may decrease the infectivity of the virus.

12. It is important to have enough media to cover the cells during the rocking steps to prevent cell detaching from the plate. For example, the minimum amount of media allowed for a 60-mm plate is 1 mL; for one 100-mm plate, 2 mL; and for one 150-mm plate, 4 mL. If the viral lysate used in the infection is less than the minimal volume, supplement with DMEM with 2% FBS. For example, if 1 mL of viral lysate is used to infect one 150-mm plate of cells, add of 3 mL DMEM with 2% FBS.

13. Although there are viruses in the media, the majority of the viruses are still attached to or included in the cells before the freeze/thaw procedure. It is important to remember to isolate all the infected cells *prior* to freeze/thawing.

14. The virus is not stable at room temperature. Always put virus-containing solutions or cell cultures on ice when collecting viruses. Thaw the virus on ice as well when ready for the experiment. Always use aerosol tips when pipetting.

15. As the density of the mature adenoviral particle is around 1.33 g/L and is different from those of other intermediates or empty viral capsid, the purified viral preparation should contain minimal contamination by empty viral capsids or other intermediate viral particles.

16. Normalized adjusted standard is a mathematical model developed to calculate the minimum required infectious virion concentration for an observed number of infectious events and to estimate the maximum number of expected hits if all of the virions in a preparation were infectious (*53*).

17. OD_{260} assay is for determining the titer of concentrated stocks of purified adenovirus. It should not be used for measuring virus in crude cell lysates or in culture supernatant, because serum and other factors in growth media interfere with the absorbance at 260 nm.

18. One microgram of Ad2 DNA equals 2.6×10^{10} molecule of Ad2 genome.

References

1. Hedman, M., Hartikainen, J., Syvanne, M., et al. (2003) Safety and feasibility of catheter-based local intracoronary vascular endothelial growth factor gene transfer in the prevention of postangioplasty and in-stent restenosis and in the treatment of

chronic myocardial ischemia: phase II results of the Kuopio Angiogenesis Trial (KAT). *Circulation* **107,** 2677–2683.

2. Rowe, W. P., Huebner, R. J., Gilmore, L. K., Parrott, R. H., and Ward, T. G. (1953) Isolation of a cytopathogenic agent from human adenoids undergoing spontaneous degeneration in tissue culture. *Proc. Soc. Exp. Biol. Med.* **84,** 570–573.

3. Volpers, C. and Kochanek, S. (2004) Adenoviral vectors for gene transfer and therapy. *J. Gene Med.* **6(Suppl 1),** S164–S171.

4. Bergelson, J. M., Cunningham, J. A., Droguett, G., et al. (1997) Isolation of a common receptor for Coxsackie B viruses and adenoviruses 2 and 5. *Science* **275,** 1320–1323.

5. Tomko, R. P., Xu, R., and Philipson, L. (1997) HCAR and MCAR: the human and mouse cellular receptors for subgroup C adenoviruses and group B coxsackieviruses. *Proc. Natl. Acad. Sci. USA* **94,** 3352–3356.

6. Noutsias, M., Fechner, H., de Jonge, H., et al. (2001) Human coxsackie-adenovirus receptor is colocalized with integrins alpha(v)beta(3) and alpha(v)beta(5) on the cardiomyocyte sarcolemma and upregulated in dilated cardiomyopathy: implications for cardiotropic viral infections. *Circulation* **104,** 275–280.

7. Fechner, H., Noutsias, M., Tschoepe, C., et al. (2003) Induction of coxsackievirus-adenovirus-receptor expression during myocardial tissue formation and remodeling: identification of a cell-to-cell contact-dependent regulatory mechanism. *Circulation* **107,** 876–882.

8. Nasuno, A., Toba, K., Ozawa, T., et al. (2004) Expression of coxsackievirus and adenovirus receptor in neointima of the rat carotid artery. *Cardiovasc. Pathol.* **13,** 79–84.

9. Wickham, T. J., Mathias, P., Cheresh, D. A., and Nemerow, G. R. (1993) Integrins alpha v beta 3 and alpha v beta 5 promote adenovirus internalization but not virus attachment. *Cell* **73,** 309–319.

10. Dechecchi, M. C., Tamanini, A., Bonizzato, A., and Cabrini, G. (2000) Heparan sulfate glycosaminoglycans are involved in adenovirus type 5 and 2-host cell interactions. *Virology* **268,** 382–390.

11. Smith, T. A., Idamakanti, N., Rollence, M. L., et al. (2003) Adenovirus serotype 5 fiber shaft influences in vivo gene transfer in mice. *Hum. Gene Ther.* **14,** 777–787.

12. Dechecchi, M. C., Melotti, P., Bonizzato, A., Santacatterina, M., Chilosi, M., and Cabrini, G. (2001) Heparan sulfate glycosaminoglycans are receptors sufficient to mediate the initial binding of adenovirus types 2 and 5. *J. Virol.* **75,** 8772–8780.

13. Yla-Herttuala, S. and Martin, J. F. (2000) Cardiovascular gene therapy. *Lancet* **355,** 213–222.

14. Amalfitano, A. (1999) Next-generation adenoviral vectors: new and improved. *Gene Ther.* **6,** 1643–1645.

15. Hodges, B. L., Serra, D., Hu, H., Begy, C. A., Chamberlain, J. S., and Amalfitano, A. (2000) Multiply deleted [E1, polymerase-, and pTP-] adenovirus vector persists despite deletion of the preterminal protein. *J. Gene Med.* **2,** 250–259.

16. Everett, R. S., Hodges, B. L., Ding, E. Y., Xu, F., Serra, D., and Amalfitano, A. (2003) Liver toxicities typically induced by first-generation adenoviral vectors can be reduced by use of E1, E2b-deleted adenoviral vectors. *Hum. Gene Ther.* **14,** 1715–1726.

17. Amalfitano, A. and Chamberlain, J. S. (1997) Isolation and characterization of packaging cell lines that coexpress the adenovirus E1, DNA polymerase, and preterminal proteins: implications for gene therapy. *Gene Ther.* **4,** 258–263.
18. Amalfitano, A. and Parks, R. J. (2002) Separating fact from fiction: assessing the potential of modified adenovirus vectors for use in human gene therapy. *Curr. Gene Ther.* **2,** 111–133.
19. Parks, R. J., Chen, L., Anton, M., Sankar, U., Rudnicki, M. A., and Graham, F. L. (1996) A helper-dependent adenovirus vector system: removal of helper virus by Cre-mediated excision of the viral packaging signal. *Proc. Natl. Acad. Sci. USA* **93,** 13,565–13,570.
20. Ross, R. (1999) Atherosclerosis: an inflammatory disease. *N. Engl. J. Med.* **340,** 115–126.
21. Turunen, P., Jalkanen, J., Heikura, T., et al. (2004) Adenovirus-mediated gene transfer of Lp-PLA2 reduces LDL degradation and foam cell formation in vitro. *J. Lipid Res.* **45,** 1633–1639.
22. Harris, J. D., Graham, I. R., Schepelmann, S., et al. (2002) Acute regression of advanced and retardation of early aortic atheroma in immunocompetent apolipoprotein-E (apoE) deficient mice by administration of a second generation [E1(-), E3(-), polymerase(-)] adenovirus vector expressing human apoE. *Hum. Mol. Genet.* **11,** 43–58.
23. Grines, C. L., Watkins, M. W., Mahmarian, J. J., et al. (2003) A randomized, double-blind, placebo-controlled trial of Ad5FGF-4 gene therapy and its effect on myocardial perfusion in patients with stable angina. *J. Am. Coll. Cardiol.* **42,** 1339–1347.
24. Rosengart, T. K., Lee, L. Y., Patel, S. R., et al. (1999) Six-month assessment of a phase I trial of angiogenic gene therapy for the treatment of coronary artery disease using direct intramyocardial administration of an adenovirus vector expressing the VEGF121 cDNA. *Ann. Surg.* **230,** 466–470.
25. Rosengart, T. K., Lee, L. Y., Patel, S. R., et al. (1999) Angiogenesis gene therapy: phase I assessment of direct intramyocardial administration of an adenovirus vector expressing VEGF121 cDNA to individuals with clinically significant severe coronary artery disease. *Circulation* **100,** 468–474.
26. Patel, S. R., Lee, L. Y., Mack, C. A., et al. (1999) Safety of direct myocardial administration of an adenovirus vector encoding vascular endothelial growth factor 121. *Hum. Gene Ther.* **10,** 1331–1348.
27. Rosen, M. R., Robinson, R. B., Brink, P., and Cohen, I. S. (2004) Recreating the biological pacemaker. *Anat. Rec. A. Discov. Mol. Cell Evol. Biol.* **280,** 1046–1052.
28. Plotnikov, A. N., Sosunov, E. A., Qu, J., et al. (2004) Biological pacemaker implanted in canine left bundle branch provides ventricular escape rhythms that have physiologically acceptable rates. *Circulation* **109,** 506–512.
29. Tevaearai, H. T. and Koch, W. J. (2004) Molecular restoration of beta-adrenergic receptor signaling improves contractile function of failing hearts. *Trends Cardiovasc. Med.* **14,** 252–256.
30. Most, P., Eicher, C., Volkers, M., Pleger, S. T., and Katus, H. A. (2004) Hope for a broken heart? *Trends Biotechnol.* **22,** 487–489.

31. Shah, A. S., White, D. C., Emani, S., et al. (2001) In vivo ventricular gene delivery of a beta-adrenergic receptor kinase inhibitor to the failing heart reverses cardiac dysfunction. *Circulation* **103,** 1311–1316.

32. Most, P., Pleger, S. T., Volkers, M., et al. (2004) Cardiac adenoviral S100A1 gene delivery rescues failing myocardium. *J. Clin. Invest.* **114,** 1550–1563.

33. Hajjar, R. J. (2005) Cardiac gene therapy: kick-starting calcium cycling in rats. *Gene Ther.*

34. Hoshijima, M. (2005) Gene therapy targeted at calcium handling as an approach to the treatment of heart failure. *Pharmacol. Ther.* **105,** 211–228.

35. Yla-Herttuala, S., Markkanen, J. E., and Rissanen, T. T. (2004) Gene therapy for ischemic cardiovascular diseases: some lessons learned from the first clinical trials. *Trends Cardiovasc. Med.* **14,** 295–300.

36. Grines, C. L., Watkins, M. W., Helmer, G., et al. (2002) Angiogenic Gene Therapy (AGENT) trial in patients with stable angina pectoris. *Circulation* **105,** 1291–1297.

37. Grines, C., Rubanyi, G. M., Kleiman, N. S., Marrott, P., and Watkins, M. W. (2003) Angiogenic gene therapy with adenovirus 5 fibroblast growth factor-4 (Ad5FGF-4): a new option for the treatment of coronary artery disease. *Am. J. Cardiol.* **92,** 24N–31N.

38. Laitinen, M., Pakkanen, T., Donetti, E., et al. (1997) Gene transfer into the carotid artery using an adventitial collar: comparison of the effectiveness of the plasmid-liposome complexes, retroviruses, pseudotyped retroviruses, and adenoviruses. *Hum. Gene Ther.* **8,** 1645–1650.

39. Fuster, V., Charlton, P., and Boyd, A. (2001) Clinical protocol. A phase IIb, randomized, multicenter, double-blind study of the efficacy and safety of Trinam (EG004) in stenosis prevention at the graft-vein anastomosis site in dialysis patients. *Hum. Gene Ther.* **12,** 2025–2027.

40. Bhardwaj, S., Roy, H., Karpanen, T., et al. (2005) Periadventitial angiopoietin-1 gene transfer induces angiogenesis in rabbit carotid arteries. *Gene Ther.* **12,** 388–394.

41. Yla-Herttuala, S. and Alitalo, K. (2003) Gene transfer as a tool to induce therapeutic vascular growth. *Nat. Med.* **9,** 694–701.

42. Barbato, J. E. and Tzeng, E. (2004) iNOS gene transfer for graft disease. *Trends Cardiovasc. Med.* **14,** 267–272.

43. Turunen, P., Puhakka, H., Rutanen, J., et al. (2005) Intravascular adenovirus-mediated lipoprotein-associated phospholipase A2 gene transfer reduces neointima formation in balloon-denuded rabbit aorta. *Atherosclerosis* **179,** 27–33.

44. Fleury, S., Driscoll, R., Simeoni, E., et al. (2004) Helper-dependent adenovirus vectors devoid of all viral genes cause less myocardial inflammation compared with first-generation adenovirus vectors. *Basic Res. Cardiol.* **99,** 247–256.

45. Askari, A., Unzek, S., Goldman, C. K., et al. (2004) Cellular, but not direct, adenoviral delivery of vascular endothelial growth factor results in improved left ventricular function and neovascularization in dilated ischemic cardiomyopathy. *J. Am. Coll. Cardiol.* **43,** 1908–1914.

46. Benihoud, K., Yeh, P., and Perricaudet, M. (1999) Adenovirus vectors for gene delivery. *Curr. Opin. Biotechnol.* **10,** 440–447.

47. Rosenfeld, M. A., Siegfried, W., Yoshimura, K., et al. (1991) Adenovirus-mediated transfer of a recombinant alpha 1-antitrypsin gene to the lung epithelium in vivo. *Science* **252**, 431–434.
48. Bett, A. J., Haddara, W., Prevec, L., and Graham, F. L. (1994) An efficient and flexible system for construction of adenovirus vectors with insertions or deletions in early regions 1 and 3. *Proc. Natl. Acad. Sci .USA* **91**, 8802–8806.
49. He, T. C., Zhou, S., da Costa, L. T., Yu, J., Kinzler, K. W., and Vogelstein, B. (1998) A simplified system for generating recombinant adenoviruses. *Proc. Natl. Acad. Sci. USA* **95**, 2509–2514.
50. Graham, F. L., Smiley, J., Russell, W. C., and Nairn, R. (1977) Characteristics of a human cell line transformed by DNA from human adenovirus type 5. *J. Gen. Virol.* **36**, 59–74.
51. Graham, F. L. and van der Eb, A. J. (1973) Transformation of rat cells by DNA of human adenovirus 5. *Virology* **54**, 536–539.
52. Maizel, J. V., Jr., White, D. O., and Scharff, M. D. (1968) The polypeptides of adenovirus. I. Evidence for multiple protein components in the virion and a comparison of Types 2, 7A and 12. *Virology* **36**, 115–125.
53. Nyberg-Hoffman, C., Shabram, P., Li, W., Giroux, D., and Aguilar-Cordova, E. (1997) Sensitivity and reproducibility in adenoviral infectious titer determination. *Nat. Med.* **3**, 808–811.
54. Weaver, L. S. and Kadan, M. J. (2000) Evaluation of adenoviral vectors by flow cytometry. *Methods* **21**, 297–312.
55. Lochmuller, H., Jani, A., Huard, J., et al. (1994) Emergence of early region 1-containing replication-competent adenovirus in stocks of replication-defective adenovirus recombinants (delta E1 + delta E3) during multiple passages in 293 cells. *Hum. Gene Ther.* **5**, 1485–1491.
56. Ishii-Watabe, A., Uchida, E., Iwata, A., et al. (2003) Detection of replication-competent adenoviruses spiked into recombinant adenovirus vector products by infectivity PCR. *Mol. Ther.* **8**, 1009–1016.
57. Suzuki, E., Murata, T., Watanabe, S., et al. (2004) A simple method for the simultaneous detection of E1A and E1B in adenovirus stocks. *Oncol. Rep.* **11**, 173–178.
58. Fallaux, F. J., Bout, A., van der Velde, I., et al. (1998) New helper cells and matched early region 1-deleted adenovirus vectors prevent generation of replication-competent adenoviruses. *Hum. Gene Ther.* **9**, 1909–1917.
59. Imperiale, M. J., Kao, H. T., Feldman, L. T., Nevins, J. R., and Strickland, S. (1984) Common control of the heat shock gene and early adenovirus genes: evidence for a cellular E1A-like activity. *Mol. Cell. Biol.* **4**, 867–874.
60. Nevins, J. R., Imperiale, M. J., Kao, H. T., Strickland, S., and Feldman, L. T. (1984) Detection of an adenovirus E1A-like activity in mammalian cells. *Curr. Top. Microbiol. Immunol.* **113**, 15–19.
61. Yang, Y., Nunes, F. A., Berencsi, K., Furth, E. E., Gonczol, E., and Wilson, J. M. (1994) Cellular immunity to viral antigens limits E1-deleted adenoviruses for gene therapy. *Proc. Natl. Acad. Sci. USA* **91**, 4407–4411.

62. Bett, A. J., Prevec, L., and Graham, F. L. (1993) Packaging capacity and stability of human adenovirus type 5 vectors. *J. Virol.* **67,** 5911–5921.
63. Ng, P., Parks, R. J., and Graham, F. L. (2002) Preparation of helper-dependent adenovirus vectors. *Methods Mol. Med.* **69,** 371–388.
64. Palmer, D. and Ng, P. (2003) Improved system for helper-dependent adenoviral vector production. *Mol Ther.* **8,** 846–852.

15

Murine and HIV-Based Retroviral Vectors for In Vitro and In Vivo Gene Transfer

Ronald W. Alfa and Armin Blesch

Summary

The success of experimental gene therapy is dependent on the ability to safely and efficiently introduce transgenes into the target cell or tissue. Retroviral-based vectors, notably those derived from Moloney murine leukemia virus (MLV) and lentiviral vectors derived from HIV, have proven to be valuable gene transfer vehicles as a result of their ease of production and their ability to mediate long-term transgene expression. One of the most widely used methods for viral vector production is based on the transient transfection of viral vector plasmid DNA into a producer cell line. Here, we describe protocols to produce and standardize high quality MLV-based retroviral and HIV-based lentiviral vectors for ex vivo and in vivo gene delivery.

Key Words: Gene therapy; lentivirus; retrovirus; HIV; virus producer cells.

1. Introduction

Gene therapy offers a promising means for the treatment of acquired and genetic disease. Although a variety of viral (and nonviral) gene delivery methods have been described, the ability of retroviruses to stably integrate into the host genome and to mediate long-term transgene expression have made retroviral vectors an attractive tool for the delivery of transgenes in vitro and in vivo. Murine retroviral vectors with a wide array of host ranges and lentiviral vectors with high infectious titers can be relatively easily produced. The capacity of lentiviral vectors to transduce both dividing and nondividing cells and improvements in the safety and production of retroviral vectors have further increased their utility as transfer vehicles for gene therapy applications.

Before addressing specific methods, we will briefly review some fundamental retroviral biology valuable to the understanding of the principles underlying safe and effective vector production.

From: *Methods in Molecular Medicine, vol. 129:*
Cardiovascular Disease: Methods and Protocols, Volume 2: Molecular Medicine
Edited by: Q. K. Wang © Humana Press Inc., Totowa, NJ

1.1. Retroviral Biology

All retroviruses exhibit the same basic structural elements. The viral particle is a lipid-enveloped capsid enclosing the viral 7–12 kb long RNA genome (in complex with nucleocapsid proteins) and essential viral enzymes. The retroviral genome is organized into three or four genes: *gag, pol,* and *env* and often *pro.* The *gag* open reading frame (ORF) encodes a single precursor poly-protein from which the structural proteins are derived. In addition, the *gag* ORF also encodes several proteins involved in particle budding *(1)*. *Pro* encodes a protease responsible for processing of *gag* proteins and maturation of the viral particle. Two additional enzymes, reverse transcriptase and integrase, are encoded by *pol*. These key enzymes allow the viral RNA to be reverse-transcribed to DNA and mediate its integration into the host genome *(2)*. The envelope gene, *env,* encodes the TM and SU subunits of the envelope glycoproteins.

In concert with viral proteins, several *cis*-acting sequences within the genome serve essential roles in gene expression, reverse transcription, and integration of the provirus. The viral RNA contains long terminal repeats (LTRs) at the 5′ and 3′ ends, composed of sequences designated U3, R, and U5. During reverse transcription of viral RNA, the 5′ U5 region and the 3′ U3 region are duplicated resulting in identical LTR sequences at each end of the proviral DNA. Transcription is driven by promoter and enhancer elements within the U3 region. The repeat sequences, designated R, allow reverse transcriptase to "jump" between strands during reverse transcription. A GU-rich region within the U5 sequence facilitates the recognition of a poly-adenylation signal within the R region by the cellular machinery. Two additional elements, primer binding sequence (PBS) and psi (ψ), are necessary for efficient reverse transcription and packaging of the viral RNA into virions.

Complex retroviruses such as lentivirus exhibit several additional regulatory and accessory genes. The tat and rev proteins are important in viral replication and enhance transcription and transport of unspliced viral RNA out of the nucleus, respectively *(3)*. The accessory proteins vpr, vpu, vif, and nef comprise a group of HIV virulence factors but are not essential for lentivirus replication *(4)*.

Following entry into the cell, the viral RNA genome is released into the cytoplasm and reverse-transcribed to DNA. During reverse transcription, the 5′ U5 and 3′ U3 are replicated, resulting in identical flanking LTRs. As a result, heterologous sequences placed in either region will also be replicated. Once reverse-transcribed, proviral DNA then associates with viral and cellular proteins forming a preintegration complex (PIC) *(5,6)*. Finally, nuclear localization of the PIC culminates in the integration of the virus into the host genome. Although lentiviral PICs are actively transported into the nucleus, PICs of simple retroviruses, such as Moloney murine leukemia virus (MLV), cannot penetrate the nuclear membrane; as a result, MLV-based vectors can only transduce actively dividing cells *(7–11)*.

1.2. MLV Vector Systems

The fundamental aim in producing a clinically efficacious retroviral vector system is the packaging of a viral RNA containing an expression cassette for the gene of interest but lacking any viral genes necessary for replication and pathogenesis. To create such a system, the viral structural genes (*gag, pol, env*) are supplied on one or more separate transcription units with heterologous promoters and polyadenylation signals. The separation of components onto multiple transcription units minimizes the risks of producing replication competent virus through recombination events. The transfer vector or transgene construct contains the necessary *cis*-acting sequences for packaging of its RNA including the packaging signal (ψ), a fragment of the *gag* coding region ($\psi+$) for improved titer *(12)*, the PBS, and the LTRs.

Two approaches have been characterized for the production of recombinant retroviral vectors. By generating a stable cell line expressing some or all viral structural genes, large quantities of viral stocks can be produced over extended passages *(13)*. Stable introduction of the transfer plasmid/transgene construct into these cells, followed by expansion and characterization of single cell clones, results in stable retroviral producer cells for a specific gene. Protocols for the generation of stable retroviral producer cell lines have been described elsewhere *(14–16)*. Alternatively, transient transfection methods can generate viral stocks of high titers in limited quantities, though more quickly, for short-term usage *(17,18)*.

In recent years, several additional modifications have increased the efficacy and safety of retroviral vectors. Although sufficiently high titers for in vitro transduction could be achieved, titers for in vivo transduction were inadequate *(19)*. To increase viral RNA production, and thereby viral titers, the viral U3 promoter/enhancer in the transfer vector was replaced with a more robust cytomegalovirus (CMV) enhancer leading to a notable increase in viral titers **(Fig. 1)** *(20)*. Further improvements in the safety of retroviral vectors were achieved by introducing deletions into the 3′ LTR. The presence of a promoter/enhancer in the wild-type 3′ LTR can potentially lead to the insertional activation of cellular genes located at the integration site. Deletion of promoter/enhancer sequences in the U3 region of the 3′ LTR results in self-inactivating (sin) vectors **(Fig. 1)** *(21,22)*. Sin vectors require an internal promoter for transgene expression, as the promoter/enhancer activity in the 5′ LTR is lost upon duplication of the 3′ LTR during reverse transcription. Sin vectors can also not be reactivated when transduced cells are infected by wild-type virus.

Retroviral tropism, or the range of cells that can be transduced, is largely dependent on the interaction of the viral envelope glycoprotein with the specific proteins on the host cell membrane *(23)*. To modify vector tropism, a wide array of heterologous envelope glycoproteins can be incorporated into

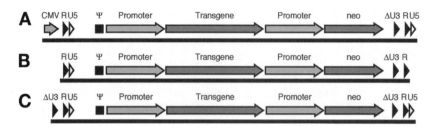

Fig. 1. Schematic outline of a prototypical self-inactivating (SIN) retroviral vector. **(A)** In the retroviral transfer plasmid viral RNA production is driven by cytomegalovirus (CMV) promoter in the 5′ long terminal repeats (LTR) replacing the 5′ U3 region. The 3′ LTR contains a deletion in the U3 region (ΔU3) and transgene expression is driven by an internal promoter. **(B)** Retroviral RNA transcribed from the transfer plasmid is packaged into virus particles in the producer cell line. **(C)** Upon transduction of the target cell, reverse transcription and integration into the genome, the partially deleted U3 region (ΔU3) from the 3′ LTR, is duplicated into the 5′ LTR and thereby inactivates the promoter activity of the 5′ LTR.

retroviral particles (pseudotyping) resulting in ecotropic, amphotropic, or pantropic viral vectors *(24)*. Pseudotyping can also result in higher stability of vectors, e.g., pseudotyping with the vesicular stomatitis virus (VSV)-G envelope glycoprotein allows the concentration of viral vectors by ultracentrifugation *(25–27)*.

1.3. Lentiviral Systems

The production of lentiviral vectors involves the same principles as MLV production. One of the best-characterized systems is based on HIV-1, and therefore the contamination with wild-type virus represents a big safety concern.

The first recombinant lentiviral vector system was based on the co-transfection of three recombinant plasmids into 293T cells. The packaging construct (helper plasmid) contained all HIV sequences, except for the envelope coding region and the 5′ and 3′ LTRs, which were replaced by a heterologous promoter and a poly-adenylation signal, respectively. The transfer/transducing plasmid carried the transgene and all wild-type HIV cis-acting sequences. The third plasmid, a VSV-G envelope gene with heterologous transcriptional signals, was used for pseudotyping *(28)*. This system produced mostly recombinant virus but the presence of most wild-type genomic elements and sequence overlaps between the transfer plasmid and the helper plasmid resulted in a small amount of pseudotyped replication-competent HIV-1 virus due to recombination events.

To further increase the safety of lentiviral systems, several modifications were introduced in subsequent applications. The first substantial safeguard involved the elimination of all viral accessory genes (*vif, vpr, vpu,* and *nef*) *(4,29)*. The tat

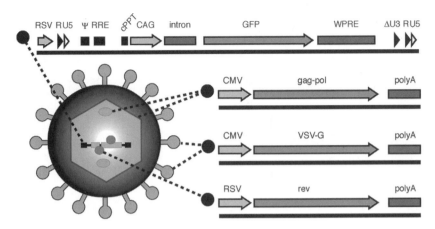

Fig. 2. Plasmids for the production of pseudotyped lentiviral vectors. The 5′ U3 region in the transfer vector (top) is replaced by an RSV promoter to drive viral RNA production. A mutation in the 3′ U3 region disrupts enhancer activity following reverse transcription and integration of the provirus. The rev response element (RRE) serves as a binding site for the rev protein, permitting the transport of unspliced RNA out of the nucleus for packaging. The transgene green fluorescent protein (GFP) is placed under the control of a cytomegalovirus (CMV)/β-actin promoter (CAG), which becomes the only active enhancer/promoter in the provirus following transduction of target cells. In addition, a woodchuck post-transcriptional response element (WPRE) is often included to stabilize the mRNA. For virus production, *gag-pol, env* (VSV-G), and *rev* are provided in trans on three distinct plasmids to avoid the risk of replication competent virus production. The schematic to the left outlines the regions of the viral particle provided by different plasmids. (RSV, Rous sarcoma virus promoter/enhancer; cPPT, central poly-purine tract; VSV-G, vesicular stomatitis virus G protein coding region; poly A, polyadenylation signal).

and rev proteins, although not crucial for basal HIV gene expression, play important roles in regulating gene expression. The tat protein is necessary for efficient transcription from the 5′ LTR and rev facilitates the export of viral RNA from the nucleus. To circumvent the need for the tat protein, the U3 region of the 5′ LTR in the transfer plasmid was replaced by a heterologous promoter. In addition, the genome was further dissected by moving the *rev* gene onto an additional expression plasmid *(30)*. Last, to construct a sin lentiviral vector, a deletion has been introduced into the U3 element of the 3′ LTR *(22,31)*. The current lentivirus vector production methods involve co-transfection of 293T cells with four distinct plasmids encoding the *gag–pol* genes, the *rev* gene, the VSV-G envelope, and a sin transfer vector plasmid with internal promoter for transgene expression **(Fig. 2)**.

2. Materials

2.1. Cell Culture and Transfection

1. Dulbecco's modified Eagle's medium (DMEM) (Gibco/BRL, Bethesda, MD) supplemented with 10% fetal calf serum, 1% penicillin-streptomycin-glutamine (100X stock) (Invitrogen, Carlsbad, CA).
2. 2.0 M $CaCl_2$: 29.4 g $CaCl_2$-$2H_2O$ (MW 147) per 100 mL distilled H_2O (*see* **Note 2**).
3. 2X HEPES-buffered saline (HBS), pH 7.0: 280 mM NaCl (MW 58.44), 100 mM HEPES SigmaUltra H7523 (MW 238.3) (Sigma-Aldrich, St. Louis, MO), 1.5 mM Na_2HPO_4, distilled H_2O (*see* **Note 3**).
4. Endotoxin-free plasmid DNA (*see* **Note 4**).
5. HEK 293T cell line for lentiviral vector production (American Type Culture Collection [ATCC], Manassas, VA), Phoenix 293T for retroviral producer cells (Nolan Group, http://www.stanford.edu/group/nolan) or other 293 cell-based murine retroviral producer cell lines (*see* **Note 5**).
6. Hank's balanced salt solution (HBSS) without phenol red with calcium and magnesium (Gibco/BRL).
7. HV Durapore 250-mL, 0.45-μm filter units (Millipore Corporation, Bedford, MA).

2.2. Titer Determination—MLV Vectors

1. NIH/3T3 Cell line (ATCC, Manassas, VA).
2. DMEM (Gibco/BRL) supplemented with 10% fetal calf serum, 1% penicillin-streptomycin-glutamine (100X stock) (Invitrogen).
3. 10 mg/mL Polybrene in H_2O (Sigma, St. Louis, MO). Store at 4°C.
4. Brilliant Blue G Solution (MW: 854.02): 1 g Brilliant Blue per liter 75% ethanol/5% acetic acid. Can be stored at room temperature.
5. Dulbecco's phosphate-buffered saline (DPBS) (Gibco/BRL).
6. G418 50 mg/mL active concentration. Store at –20°C.

3. Methods

3.1. MLV Retroviral Vector Production

1. Day 1: plate 5×10^6 retroviral producer cells such as Phoenix ampho per 100-mm plate (*see* **Notes 5** and **6**) and briefly swirl the plates to equally distribute the cells.
2. Day 2: transfection (per 100-mm plate).

   a. Three hours prior to transfection, replace the culture medium with 10 mL of fresh medium.
   b. Dilute 10 μg retroviral plasmid DNA (transfer vector) in 175 μL H_2O.
   c. Add 25 μL 2 M $CaCl_2$ to the DNA in H_2O.
   d. Aliquot 200 μL 2X HBS into a second tube and drop-wise add the $CaCl_2$-DNA solution to the 2X HBS while mixing well (*see* **Note 7**).
   e. Incubate the transfection mixture for 20–30 min at room temperature (*see* **Note 8**).
   f. Briefly vortex and add the transfection mixture drop-wise to the cells.

g. Gently shake the plate to properly distribute precipitate and incubate the cells overnight at 37°C and 5% CO_2.

3. Day 3: examine the cells and replace the medium with 6 mL of fresh medium (*see* **Note 9**). Incubate the cells overnight at 37°C in 10% CO_2.

4. Day 4: harvest the virus containing supernatants and filter through a 0.45-μm filter. Store the aliquots at –70°C (*see* **Note 10**).

3.2. Titer Determination: MLV Vectors

This protocol assumes that the vector contains a G418 resistance gene. G418 is utilized to select for transduced cells following addition of diluted virus. Over the 7- to 10-d selection, transduced cells form G418-resistant colonies that can be visualized using a protein stain. This protocol can be modified if other selection markers are incorporated in the retroviral vector such as hygromycin or zeocin resistance by using the appropriate selection drug.

1. Plate three 60-mm tissue culture dishes per viral supernatant to be tested at a density of 5×10^5 NIH/3T3 cells per dish in 4 mL cell culture medium, two plates for the virus to be tested and one plate as negative control.

2. After 24 h, replace medium with fresh medium containing 4 μg/mL polybrene and add 0.1 or 10 μL of viral supernatant filtered through a 0.45-μm filter (*see* **Note 11**).

3. After 24 h, split one-tenth of the cells from each plate into a 60-mm dish and five-tenths into a 100-mm dish. Discard the remaining cells. Include G418 in the culture medium (500 μg/mL).

4. Change medium twice per week and monitor over the subsequent 7–10 d for cell survival and colony formation.

5. After visible colonies have formed, and all cells in the negative control have died, rinse the cells with ice-cold DPBS, fix and stain for 5 min with Brilliant Blue G solution.

6. To determine virus titer, wash the cells twice with DPBS and quantify the number of colonies. Based on the volume of virus added, calculate the titer in colony-forming units (cfu) per milliliter (*see* **Note 12**).

3.3. Lentiviral Vector Production

1. Seed 10 plates of 293T cells at a density of 1×10^6 cells per 150-mm tissue culture dish in 15 mL of medium. Incubate the cells for 72 h (over the weekend) at 37°C in 10% CO_2 (*see* **Note 13**).

2. Day 1: reseed the 10 plates of 293T cells into 12 plates at a density of 1×10^7 cells per 150-mm tissue culture dish in 15 mL of medium. Incubate the cells overnight at 37°C in 10% CO_2 (*see* **Note 6**).
    Day 2: transfection (per 150-mm plate).

    a. Dilute viral packaging and transfer vector plasmid DNA to a final volume of 12.6 mL in H_2O (*see* **Note 14**).

    b. Add 1.8 mL of 2 *M* $CaCl_2$ to the DNA/H_2O mixture ($CaCl_2$ final concentration 250 m*M*).

    c. Aliquot 14.4 mL 2X HBS to a second tube and drop-wise add $CaCl_2$–DNA solution to HBS while mixing well (*see* **Note 7**).

    d. Incubate the transfection mixture for 20–30 min at room temperature (*see* **Note 8**).

    e. Briefly vortex and add the transfection mixture drop-wise to the cells.

    f. Gently shake the plate to properly distribute the precipitate and incubate the cells overnight at 37°C and 10% CO_2.

4. Day 3: examine the cells and replace the medium with 15 mL of fresh medium (*see* **Note 15**). Incubate the cells overnight at 37°C in 10% CO_2.

5. Day 4: collection of supernatants.

    a. Harvest the supernatant from all plates and filter immediately through a 250-mL, 0.45-μm filter unit. Store the supernatant at 4°C overnight or proceed immediately to concentration of virus.

    b. Add fresh medium (15 mL) to the plates and incubate the cells overnight at 37°C in 10% CO_2 (*see* **Note 15**).

6. Day 5: collection of supernatants and concentration of virus *(see* **Note 16***)*. Harvest the supernatant from all plates and pass through a 0.45-μm filter unit. Store the supernatant at 4°C until centrifugation.

    a. Centrifuge the filtered supernatants in 30-mL polyallomer conical tubes at 69,000*g* for 2 h at 4°C.

    b. Carefully remove the supernatants (*see* **Note 17**), resuspend the pellets in 200 μL of HBSS each, and pool in 3-mL polyallomer centrifuge tube (*see* **Note 18**). Store the pellets at 4°C until all pellets have been collected.

    c. After the last pellets have been collected, wash each tube with an additional 100 μL of HBSS to retrieve any remaining virus and pool this wash volume with the collected pellets in a single 3-mL conical centrifuge tube.

    d. Centrifuge the pooled resuspended pellets at 69,000*g* for 2 h at 4°C.

    e. Very carefully remove the supernatant and resuspend the pellet in 100–200 μL of HBSS (*see* **Note 19**).

    f. Shake the suspended virus at room temperature for 1 h, briefly spin down the undissolved pellet (10-s microfuge spin) and aliquot the viral supernatant. The virus aliquots should be stored at –80°C.

3.4. Titer Determination: Lentivirus Vectors

The titer of lentivirus stocks can be determined using one of two methods: analysis of p24 capsid antigen levels or by measuring the infectivity of the virus stock assuming your construct expresses a reporter gene such as green fluorescent protein (GFP). Levels of p24 antigen generally correlate to the number of infectious particles per stock if similar methods and viral plasmids are used. If the transfer vector does not contain a reporter gene, p24 levels can be compared with a GFP-expressing virus stock to estimate the number of infectious units (IU) per milliliter (*see* **Note 20**).

1. Seed 5×10^4 293T cells per well in a 24-well plate in 1 mL of cell culture medium.
2. Make serial dilutions of the concentrated virus stock from 10^{-3} to 10^{-7} in cell culture medium (*see* **Note 21**).
3. Add 10 µL of each dilution per well in triplicates and incubate the cells for 2 d at 10% CO_2 at 37°C.
4. To determine infectivity of the virus (IU/mL), count the number of reporter GFP-positive colonies under a fluorescent microscope after 48 h. Based on the dilution factor of virus added, the virus titer can be determined (*see* **Note 22**).

3.5. Transduction of Target Cells

Following determination of titer, the recombinant virus can be used to transduce target cells in vitro or in vivo. Transduction with MLV-based vectors is restricted to actively dividing cells and thus, these systems show the most efficacy in vitro. In contrast, the ability of lentiviral vectors to transduce nondividing cells makes these systems a useful tool for in vivo gene transfer. Methods for in vivo transduction are largely dependent on the target tissue and, thus, a generalized protocol cannot be given. Instead, the reader should refer to relevant literature in the area of interest. A brief protocol for in vitro transduction with MLV-based retroviral vectors is described next:

1. One day prior to transduction, cells should be split to an appropriate density such that they are in an exponential growth phase at the time of transduction.
2. To transduce the cells, mix an appropriate volume of cell culture medium with polybrene to yield a final concentration of 4 µg/mL (*see* **Note 11**).
3. Add an appropriate amount of virus to achieve the desired multiplicity of infection (MOI; *see* **Note 23**) to the polybrene-medium solution and use this to feed the cells. Cell exposure to virus can be repeated on consecutive days to reach the desired MOI.
4. If the vector contains a selection marker, such as neomycin resistance, change the cell culture medium to medium containing an appropriate concentration of G418 following cell transduction (*see* **Note 24**) to select against nontransduced cells. Alternatively, if the vector contains a fluorescent reporter gene, transduced cells may be sorted by fluorescence-activated cell sorting (FACS) as early as 2 d following transduction.

4. Notes

1. The viral supernatants produced by these methods might contain hazardous virus depending on the gene expressed. Appropriate caution should be taken especially with amphotropic or VSV-G pseudotyped viruses and institutional and governmental guidelines should be followed.
2. 2 *M* $CaCl_2$ should be sterile filtered and stored at –20°C in 50-mL aliquots. The solution may be stored for several months without loss of transfection efficiency.
3. Adjust the pH to 7.0 with NaOH solution. Appropriate pH is absolutely critical for precipitate formation and good transfection efficiency; be sure to correctly calibrate

your pH meter. For frequent vector production it is useful to make several stocks, ranging in pH from 6.9 to 7.05, and assay the transfection efficiency of each stock to ensure optimal transfection. Store in aliquots at –20°C.

4. We generally use endotoxin-free Qiagen kits for the preparation of plasmid DNA. However, kits from other manufacturers might work as well. Many MLV-based retroviral transfer plasmids and lentiviral plasmids are commercially available.

5. The HEK 293T cell-line is the cell line of choice for viral vector production because it can be easily transfected using calcium phosphate or lipid-based methods. Transfection efficiencies can be as high as 90%, yielding supernatants with high viral titers. The Phoenix cell line has been developed by Nolan and colleagues for retroviral production and is a 293T-based cell line stably expressing viral packaging genes *(13)*. Several variants of the cell line are available expressing amphotropic or ecotropic envelope proteins or expressing only the *gag-pol* genes and lacking an envelope protein. Several cell lines are also commercially available such as the EcoPack™ 2-293 AmphoPack™ 293 and GP2-293 cell lines from Clontech or the Retro-X system from Stratagene.

6. Cells should be 70–80% confluent at the time of transfection. It might be necessary to adjust the precise cell number, as passage number, different batches of FBS, and culture conditions can alter the doubling time of the cells and, therefore, the cell density at the time of transfection. In addition, for routine maintenance of cells, never let cells reach 100% and split cells every 2–3 d. This will ensure optimal cell conditions for transfection.

7. The slow, drop-wise addition of DNA to 2X HBS solution is very important for proper precipitate formation; DNA-CaCl$_2$ should be added at a rate of about one drop every other second. Continuously mix the transfection mixture by bubbling with an autopipetor while adding DNA-CaCl$_2$ drop-wise with a 1-mL pipet.

8. The incubation time is essential for precipitate formation. Short incubation times will result in little precipitate and subsequently, poor transfection efficiencies. Also, the mixture should not be incubated too long; long incubation times may result in a course precipitate, which will also adversely affect transfection efficiency.

9. Upon inspection, you should notice a very fine/sandy precipitate all over the plate at high magnification under the microscope. If your transfer vector includes a fluorescent reporter gene, examine fluorescence to determine transfection efficiency. For sufficient viral production, at least 50% of cells should be transfected at this point. Gently swirl the plate before removing the medium to ensure resuspension and removal of precipitate. Be sure to prewarm fresh medium to 37°C before addition; 293T cells are sensitive to thermal shock and will shrink and detach if medium is not prewarmed or if the cells are left outside the incubator for long times. Last, gently and slowly add the fresh medium to the side of the dish to avoiding disrupting the cell monolayer.

10. MLV-based vectors can be concentrated as described later for lentiviral vectors. However, only retroviral vectors pseudotyped with VSV-G envelope are sufficiently stable to be efficiently concentrated. In this case, a retroviral producer cell

line expressing only the *gag-pol* genes is used and 10 μg retroviral vector (transfer plasmid) is co-transfected with 3 μg VSV-G coding plasmid.

11. Polybrene is a cationic polymer and increases the transfection efficiency in vitro about 10- to 100-fold.

12. Good viral titers in supernatants of retroviral producer cells are usually around 10^6 cfu/mL, but can be as high as 10^8 cfu/mL depending on transfection efficiency, retroviral producer cells, and retroviral plasmid used.

13. It is convenient to begin the lentivirus production protocol on a Friday. The cells are then incubated over the weekend to be reseeded on Monday (day 1), continuing over the remainder of the week.

14. Viral packaging plasmids and transfer vector plasmid should be added in the following quantities (for 12 × 150 mm plates): 176 μg pMDLg/pRRE (coding for *gag-pol*), 68 μg pRSV-Rev (*rev* coding plasmid), 95 μg pCMV-VSV-G (VSV-G envelope), and 270 μg HIV transfer vector.

15. Again, whenever replacing the medium, be sure it is prewarmed to 37°C to avoid thermal shock of the cells. At a high cell density, cells are especially susceptible to stress. Add fresh medium slowly and very gently to the side of the dish being careful not to dislodge the cells.

16. Viral supernatants can also be partially concentrated by filtration using a molecular weight cut off filter of 100 kD followed by ultracentrifugation. Storage of viral supernatants at 4°C should be limited to 48 h, otherwise viral titers will significantly drop.

17. When aspirating the supernatants, be careful not to dislodge the small viral pellet. Slowly aspirate the media with a glass pipet attached to a vacuum source to the halfway point on the conical tube. Next, place the pipet against the (halfway point) wall of the tube and gently tip the tube to allow the remaining supernatant to flow toward the pipet. This technique allows one to remove the supernatant while minimizing the risk of aspirating the viral pellet. If additional virus containing supernatant must be centrifuged, the virus pellet can remain in the tubes and new virus containing supernatant can be added on top followed by another round of centrifugation.

18. To collect the pellets, first transfer a small volume of HBSS (about 4 mL) to an appropriately sized disposable vessel. Use a 1000-μL pipetman and a single tip to add 200 μL of HBSS to each conical tube. With the same tip, collect and transfer all the pellets to the 3-mL polyallomer conical centrifuge tube—use of the same tip will minimize loss of virus. To collect the pellets from each tube, gently break them up with the 1000-μL pipetor. Avoid creating bubbles in the solution.

19. To resuspend the pellet, use a 100-μL pipetor and a single tip to break up the pellet, being careful not to introduce bubbles. As the pellet is resuspended, the solution should become milky white and opaque.

20. p24 ELISAs are available from a number of commercial suppliers with detailed manufacturer's instructions. Each viral particle contains approx 2000 molecules of p24 (MW: 24 kDa), and one picogram p24 equals therefore approx 10^4 viral particles. Although the number of infectious particles present in a given sample can

vary, a well-packaged virus will exhibit an infectivity range from 1 infectious unit (IU) per 200–2000 particles. As such, the infectivity of a particular stock can be approximated to be 5–50 IU/pg p24 or 5×10^6 to 5×10^7 IU/µg p24. A good concentrated virus stock typically contains a p24 concentration of about 100–250 µg/mL.

21. Add 1 µL of virus stock to 1000 µL media to yield a 10^{-3} dilution. Next, add 100 µL of this (and subsequent) dilutions to 900 µL of medium to produce serial dilutions up to 10^{-7}.

22. For example, if the 10^{-3} dilution corresponding to 0.01 µL virus contains 10 reporter positive cell foci (i.e., transduced cells), the viral titer is 10 IU per 0.01 µL, or 10^6 IU/mL. Good virus stocks generally range from 5×10^8 to 10^{10} IU/mL. This can vary depending on how strong a reporter gene is expressed in the cell line used to determine the infectious titer and on the susceptibility of the cells to lentiviral transduction. It is, therefore, sometimes difficult to compare viral titers from laboratory to laboratory unless the same protocol is used. As an alternative to the counting of green colonies, serial dilutions of GFP expressing virus can be used to transduce a known number of 293T cells, and the percentage of GFP positive cells can be determined by FACS analysis 2–3 d later to calculate viral titers. Parameters should be determined such that only 1–5% of cells are GFP-positive to avoid multiple infections of the same cells, which will result in an underestimation of viral titers.

23. To calculate the amount of virus to add *(x)*, the following formula is used: for an MOI of Y: *x* mL *virus = number of cells in the flask* $\times$ *Y / virus titer* (in cfu/mL). The MOI is an important consideration to achieve the appropriate copy number per cell. If it is essential that cells contain no more than one copy, an MOI of 0.1 should be used. The amount of virus to be added also depends on the percentage of dividing cells. Very high MOI will not only result in multiple copies of the transgene per cell but can lead to cell fusion.

24. The exact amount of G418 to be used will depend on the cell type and should be determined experimentally prior to selection. Incubate cells with a dilution series of G418 (100–1000 µg/mL active concentration) to determine the minimum amount of G418 sufficient to kill nontransduced cells.

Acknowledgments

This work was supported by grants from the Paralyzed Veterans of America/Spinal Cord Research Foundation, International Spinal Research Trust, Christopher Reeve Paralysis Foundation, Spinal Cord Injury Research Fund of California, and the National Institute of Neurological Disorders and Stroke (NS46466).

References

1. Pages, J. C. and Bru, T. (2004) Toolbox for retrovectorologists. *J. Gene Med.* **6(Suppl 1),** S67–S82.

2. Weiss, R. (1998) Viral RNA-dependent DNA polymerase RNA-dependent DNA polymerase in virions of Rous sarcoma virus. *Rev. Med. Virol.* **8**, 3–11.
3. Southgate, C., Zapp, M. L., and Green, M. R. (1990) Activation of transcription by HIV-1 Tat protein tethered to nascent RNA through another protein. *Nature* **345**, 640–642.
4. Kim, V. N., Mitrophanous, K., Kingsman, S. M., and Kingsman, A. J. (1998) Minimal requirement for a lentivirus vector based on human immunodeficiency virus type 1. *J. Virol.* **72**, 811–816.
5. Farnet, C. M. and Bushman, F. D. (1997) HIV-1 cDNA integration: requirement of HMG I(Y) protein for function of preintegration complexes in vitro. *Cell* **88**, 483–492.
6. Bushman, F. D. (1999) Host proteins in retroviral cDNA integration. *Adv. Virus Res.* **52**, 301–317.
7. Bukrinsky, M. I., Haggerty, S., Dempsey, M. P., et al. (1993) A nuclear localization signal within HIV-1 matrix protein that governs infection of non-dividing cells. *Nature* **365**, 666–669.
8. Gallay, P., Swingler, S., Aiken, C., and Trono D. (1995) HIV-1 infection of nondividing cells: C-terminal tyrosine phosphorylation of the viral matrix protein is a key regulator. *Cell* **80**, 379–388.
9. Gallay, P., Swingler, S., Song, J., Bushman, F., and Trono, D. (1995) HIV nuclear import is governed by the phosphotyrosine-mediated binding of matrix to the core domain of integrase. *Cell* **83**, 569–576.
10. Roe, T., Reynolds, T. C., Yu, G., and Brown, P. O. (1993) Integration of murine leukemia virus DNA depends on mitosis. *EMBO J.* **12**, 2099–2108.
11. Miller, D. G., Adam, M. A., and Miller, A.D. (1990) Gene transfer by retrovirus vectors occurs only in cells that are actively replicating at the time of infection. *Mol. Cell Biol.* **10**, 4239–4242.
12. Linial, M. L. and Miller, A. D. (1990) Retroviral RNA packaging: sequence requirements and implications. *Curr. Top Microbiol. Immunol.* **157**, 125–152.
13. Pear, W. S., Nolan, G. P., Scott, M. L., and Baltimore, D. (1993) Production of high-titer helper-free retroviruses by transient transfection. *Proc. Natl. Acad. Sci. USA* **90**, 8392–8396.
14. Blesch, A. (2004) Lentiviral and MLV based retroviral vectors for ex vivo and in vivo gene transfer. *Methods* **33**, 164–172.
15. Palmer, T. D. and Gage, F. H. (1996) Delivery of gene products to the central nervous system by grafting retrovirally engineered neuronal and nonneuronal cells, in *Protocols for Gene Transfer in Neuroscience: Towards Gene Therapy of Neurological Disorders,* (Lowenstein, P. R. and Enquist, L.W., eds.). John Wiley and Sons Ltd, New York pp. 235–262.
16. Miller, A. D., Trauber, D. R., and Buttimore, C. (1986) Factors involved in production of helper virus-free retrovirus vectors. *Somat. Cell Mol. Genet.* **12**, 175–183.
17. Miller, A. D., Miller, D. G., Garcia, J. V., and Lynch, C. M. (1993) Use of retroviral vectors for gene transfer and expression. *Methods Enzymol.* **217**, 581–599.
18. Soneoka, Y., Cannon, P. M., Ramsdale, E. E., et al. (1995) A transient three-plasmid expression system for the production of high titer retroviral vectors. *Nucleic Acids Res.* **23**, 628–633.

19. Palu, G., Parolin, C., Takeuchi, Y., and Pizzato, M. (2000) Progress with retroviral gene vectors. *Rev. Med. Virol.* **10**, 185–202.
20. Naviaux, R. K., Costanzi, E., Haas, M., and Verma, I. M. (1996) The pCL vector system: rapid production of helper-free, high-titer, recombinant retroviruses. *J. Virol.* **70**, 5701–5705.
21. Yee, J. K., Moores, J. C., Jolly, D. J., et al. (1987) Gene expression from transcriptionally disabled retroviral vectors. *Proc. Natl. Acad. Sci. USA* **84**, 5197–5201.
22. Miyoshi, H., Blomer, U., Takahashi, M., Gage, F. H., and Verma, I. M. (1998) Development of a self-inactivating lentivirus vector. *J. Virol.* **72**, 8150–8157.
23. Varmus, H. (1988) Retroviruses. *Science* **240**, 1427–1435.
24. Miller, A. D. (1996) Cell-surface receptors for retroviruses and implications for gene transfer. *Proc. Natl. Acad. Sci. USA* **93**, 11,407–11,413.
25. Chen, S. T., Iida, A., Guo, L., Friedmann, T., and Yee, J. K. (1996) Generation of packaging cell lines for pseudotyped retroviral vectors of the G protein of vesicular stomatitis virus by using a modified tetracycline inducible system. *Proc. Natl. Acad. Sci. USA* **93**, 10,057–10,062.
26. Burns, J. C., Friedmann, T., Driever, W., Burrascano, M., and Yee, J. K. (1993) Vesicular stomatitis virus G glycoprotein pseudotyped retroviral vectors: concentration to very high titer and efficient gene transfer into mammalian and nonmammalian cells. *Proc. Natl. Acad. Sci. USA* **90**, 8033–8037.
27. Yee, J. K., Miyanohara, A., LaPorte, P., Bouic, K., Burns, J. C., and Friedmann, T. (1994) A general method for the generation of high-titer, pantropic retroviral vectors: highly efficient infection of primary hepatocytes. *Proc. Natl. Acad. Sci. USA* **91**, 9564–9568.
28. Naldini, L., Blomer, U., Gage, F. H., Trono, D., and Verma, I. M. (1996) Efficient transfer, integration, and sustained long-term expression of the transgene in adult rat brains injected with a lentiviral vector. *Proc. Natl. Acad. Sci. USA* **93**, 11,382–11,388.
29. Zufferey, R., Nagy, D., Mandel, R. J., Naldini, L., and Trono, D. (1997) Multiply attenuated lentiviral vector achieves efficient gene delivery in vivo. *Nat. Biotechnol.* **15**, 871–875.
30. Dull, T., Zufferey, R., Kelly, M., et al. (1998) A third-generation lentivirus vector with a conditional packaging system. *J. Virol.* **72**, 8463–8471.
31. Zufferey, R., Dull, T., Mandel, R. J., et al. (1998) Self-inactivating lentivirus vector for safe and efficient in vivo gene delivery. *J. Virol.* **72**, 9873–9880.

16

Efficient Transfection of Primary Cells Relevant for Cardiovascular Research by nucleofection®

Corinna Thiel and Michael Nix

Summary

Cell types that are important for cardiovascular research, e.g., cardiomyocytes, endothelial cells, or adult stem cells, are often hard to isolate, culture, and transfect. Low-transfection efficiencies are a major limitation because, in many cases, results achieved with surrogate model cell lines, if any at all are available for the primary cell type of interest, do not reflect the situation in the primary cell. We have demonstrated that unprecedented transfection results are achieved with primary cells when novel electroporation conditions are combined with a treatment of the cells in specific solutions that help stabilize the cells in the electrical field. This led to the development of the new proprietary transfection technology nucleofection®. Nucleofection has proved to be successfully applicable to a variety of primary cells and other hard-to-transfect cell lines, and, thus, opens unique perspectives for novel experimental setups as therapeutic strategies. Herein we present protocols for the efficient nucleofection of human umbilical vein endothelial cells, human coronary artery endothelial cells, smooth muscle cells (e.g., pig vascular smooth muscle cells), neonatal rat cardiomyocytes, and human mesenchymal stem cells and depict some results obtained with such transfected cells.

Key Words: Transfection; nucleofection®; cardiovascular research; primary cells; endothelial cells; cardiomyocytes; smooth muscle cells; stem cells.

1. Introduction

The transfer of genes, either unmodified or engineered, into cells is an invaluable technology to study a gene's function or gene products. In vitro applications of a transfection technology include promoter analysis or studies of intracellular signaling pathways, as well as the development of therapeutic strategies such as tissue engineering (*1–4*) or gene therapy (*2,3,5,6*). In the past, mainly cell lines have been used for transfection studies because they are more readily available and usually more amenable to transfection. However, cell lines

From: *Methods in Molecular Medicine, vol. 129:*
Cardiovascular Disease: Methods and Protocols, Volume 2: Molecular Medicine
Edited by: Q. K. Wang © Humana Press Inc., Totowa, NJ

are artificial model systems that do not necessarily reflect the biochemical status of a given primary cell *(7–9)*. In some cases model cell lines may not even be available (e.g., for cardiomyocytes) *(5,6)*. Transfection of primary cells still is cumbersome when applying common methods such as calcium phosphate, DEAE-dextran, or liposome-mediated transfer, which lead to low transfection efficiencies *(6,10,11)*. Viral methods generally are more efficient but often associated with time-consuming vector generation as well as high biological safety levels *(12)*.

We describe here a novel electroporation-based method called nucleofection, and ready-to-use transfection protocols for primary cells *(3,4,13–15)* that are relevant for cardiovascular research. Nucleofection offers advantages over traditional transfection methods and allows for new experiments and strategies toward a clinical use of modified primary cells.

2. Materials

2.1. Nucleofector®

1. Nucleofector device.
2. Nucleofector kits containing specific Nucleofector solutions, supplements, certified cuvets, and certified plastic pipets.

2.2. Human Umbilical Vein Endothelial Cells

1. Human umbilical vein endothelial cells (HUVECs) (e.g., Cambrex, cat. no. CC-2519).
2. Endothelial growth medium (EGM)-2 BulletKit (Cambrex, cat. no. CC-3162).
3. ReagentPack™ Subculture Reagent Kit containing trypsin/EDTA, HEPES-buffered saline (HBS), and trypsin neutralizing solution (TNS) (Cambrex, cat. no. CC-5034).
4. 75- and 162-cm^2 flasks.
5. Six-well plates.
6. 50-mL tubes.
7. HUVEC Nucleofector Kit (amaxa GmbH, cat. no. VPB-1002).

2.3. Human Coronary Artery Endothelial Cells

1. Human coronary artery endothelial cells (HCAECs) (e.g., Cambrex, cat. no. CC-2585).
2. Culture medium: EGM-2-MV BulletKit (Cambrex, cat. no. CC-3202).
3. 0.5% trypsin/0.2% EDTA (Invitrogen/Gibco, cat. no. 15400-054).
4. ReagentPack Subculture Reagent Kit containing trypsin/EDTA, HBS, and TNS (Cambrex, cat. no. CC-5034).
5. 75- and 162-cm^2 flasks.
6. Six-well plates.
7. 50-mL tubes.
8. HCAEC Nucleofector Kit (amaxa GmbH, cat. no. VPB-1001).

2.4. Human Mesenchymal Stem Cells

1. Human mesenchymal stem cells (HMSCs), adult (Cambrex, cat. no. PT-2501).
2. Mesenchymal stem cell growth medium (MSCGM) BulletKit (Cambrex, cat. no. PT-3001).
3. ReagentPack Subculture Reagent Kit containing trypsin/EDTA, HBS, and TNS (Cambrex, cat. no. CC-5034).
4. 0.5% trypsin/0.2% EDTA (Invitrogen/Gibco, cat. no. 15400-054).
5. Human MSC Nucleofector Kit (amaxa GmbH, cat. no. VPE-1001).

2.5. Smooth Muscle Cells (Various Species)

1. Culture medium: smooth muscle growth medium (SmGM)-2 BulletKit (Cambrex, cat. no. CC-3182) or Dulbecco's modified Eagle's medium (DMEM) supplemented with 10% fetal calf serum (FCS), 2 mM glutamine, 100 U/mL penicillin, and 100 µg/mL streptomycin.
2. ReagentPack Subculture Reagent Kit containing trypsin/EDTA, HBS, and TNS (Cambrex, cat. no. CC-5034).
3. 0.5% trypsin/0.2% EDTA (Invitrogen/Gibco, cat. no. 15400-054).
4. Basic Nucleofector Kit for Primary Smooth Muscle Cells (amaxa GmbH, cat. no. VPI-1004).

2.6. Rat Cardiomyocytes/Neonatal

1. Culture medium: DMEM/F12 medium (American Type Culture Collection [ATCC], cat. no. 30-2006) supplemented with 5% horse serum (PAA Laboratories, cat. no. B15-021), 0.2% bovine serum albumin (BSA) (Sigma, cat. no. A-4161), 2 mM L-glutamine (Invitrogen/Gibco, cat. no. 250300-164), 3 mM sodium pyruvate (Sigma, cat. no. S-8636), 0.1 mM ascorbate (Sigma, cat. no. A-4034), 1 µg/mL insulin, 1 µg/mL transferrin, 10 µg/mL sodium selenite (ITS Tri-Mix Invitrogen/Gibco, cat. no. 513000044), 0.02 mM cytosine β-D-arabinofuranoside (Sigma, cat. no. C-1768), 0.1 U/mL penicillin, 100 mg/mL streptomycin.
2. Adhesion medium: DMEM/F12 medium (e.g., ATCC, cat. no. 30-2006) supplemented with 10% FCS (ATCC, cat. no. 30-2020), 2 mM glutamine, 0.1 U/mL penicillin, 100 mg/mL streptomycin.
3. HEPES buffer (20 mM HEPES-NaOH, pH 7.6, 130 mM NaCl, 3 mM KCl, 1 mM NaH$_2$PO$_4$, 4 mM glucose [Sigma, cat. no. G-7021]). Use sterile-filtered or autoclaved salt stock solutions. Store glucose stock solution (sterile-filtered) at –20°C.
4. Enzyme buffer (for digestion): add 16.8 mg collagenase type II (Invitrogen, cat. no. 17101015), 48 mg pancreatin (Sigma, cat. no. P-3292), and 1.8 mg DNAse I (Roche, cat. no. 104159) freshly to 120 mL HEPES buffer (sufficient for ~50 neonatal hearts). Sterile filter the solution under a laminar flow.
5. Prepare a 1% gelatin (Sigma, cat. no. G-1890) solution in bidest water by autoclaving. Incubate dishes or cover slips with sufficient amount of gelatin solution for at least 2 h at 37°C. Remove solution and let dry, ideally under germicidal ultraviolet light.

Table 1
Culture Parameter of Primary Cells

Cell type	Medium	Seeding concentration (per cm²)	No. of cells per T75 flask[a]	Confluency before splitting	Maximal passage number
HUVECs	EGM-2	2×10^3	$2\text{–}3 \times 10^6$	90%	10
HCAECs	EGM-2-MV	5×10^3	$5\text{–}7 \times 10^5$	70%	10
HMSCs	MSCGM	$2\text{–}3 \times 10^3$	$1\text{–}2 \times 10^6$	85%	9
pVSMCs	SmGM-2	5×10^3	$8\text{–}10^6$	80%	15
SMCs	DMEM, 10% FCS	5×10^3	$8\text{–}10 \times 10^6$	80%	15
Rat cardiomyocytes	DMEM/F12	Freshly isolated	$(0.8\text{–}1 \times 10^6$ per heart)	–	–

[a]Dependent on confluency.

DMEM, Dulbecco's modified Eagle's medium; EGM, endothelial growth medium; FCS, fetal calf serum; HCAECs, human coronary artery endothelial cells; HMSCs, human mesenchymal stem cells; HUVECs, human umbilical vein endothelial cells; MSCGM, mesenchymal stem cell growth medium; pVSMC, pig vascular smooth muscle cells; SMGM, smooth muscle growth medium; SMCs, smooth muscle cells.

6. D-PBS, calcium and magnesium-free (Invitrogen/Gibco, cat. no. 14190-094).
7. 6-cm plastic Petri dishes.
8. 10-cm plastic dishes.
9. Ficoll, Percoll.
10. Rat Cardiomyocyte-Neonatal Nucleofector Kit (amaxa GmbH, cat. no. VPE-1002).

3. Methods

3.1. Preparation of Primary Cells for nucleofection

3.1.1. Cultivation of HUVECs, HCAECs, or HMSCs (see **Table 1**)

1. Thaw cells and seed them with a density of $2\text{–}4 \times 10^3$ cells per cm².
2. Replace medium two to three times per week (5–6 mL medium per 75-cm² flask).
3. Passage cells if they are 70–90% confluent.

3.1.2. Preparation of HUVECs, HCAECs, or HMSCs for nucleofection

3.1.2.1. PREPARATION OF HUVECS FOR NUCLEOFECTION

1. Split HUVECs 2 d before nucleofection.
2. Use 90% confluent cells for nucleofection experiments.
3. A 75-cm² flask (90% confluency) contains about $2\text{–}3 \times 10^6$ cells.

3.1.2.2. PREPARATION OF HCAECs FOR NUCLEOFECTION

1. Passage HCAECs 3–4 d before nucleofection.
2. Use 70% confluent cells for nucleofection experiments.
3. A 75-cm² flask (70% confluency) contains about 5–7×10^5 cells.

3.1.2.3. PREPARATION OF HMSCs FOR NUCLEOFECTION

1. Passage HMSCs 6–7 d before nucleofection.
2. Use 85% confluent cells for nucleofection experiments.
3. A 75-cm² flask (85% confluency) contains about 1–1.5×10^6 cells.

3.1.3. Isolation and Cultivation of Smooth Muscle Cells (e.g., Vascular Smooth Muscle Cells) From Various Species for nucleofection (see **Table 1**)

1. Prepare the cells out of the thoracic aorta by enzymatic digestion *(16)*.
2. Plate the cells with a density of 2×10^6 cells per 75-cm² flask.
3. Replace medium twice per week (5–6 mL medium per 75-cm² flask).
4. Use 80% confluent cells for nucleofection experiments.
5. A 75-cm² flask (80% confluency) contains about 8–10×10^6 cells.

3.1.4. Isolation of Neonatal Rat Cardiomyocytes for nucleofection (**17,18**) (see **Note 1**)

1. Every medium, HEPES buffer, and D-PBS should be prewarmed to 37°C (*see* **Notes 2** and **3**). Another aliquot of D-PBS must be ice-cold.
2. Depending on the experimental setup, 10–20 hearts of 2- to 3-d-old rats are required.
3. You may expect a yield of 0.8–1×10^6 cardiomyocytes per heart.
4. Sacrifice 2- to 3-d-old rats and excise hearts from all pups.
5. Store the excised hearts in D-PBS (calcium and magnesium-free) on ice.
6. Squeeze hearts gently with forceps to expel blood from the lumen.
7. Transfer hearts into fresh ice-cold D-PBS.
8. Move ventricles to a dry 6-cm dish and mince tissue as fine as possible with a scalpel blade.
9. Transfer minced neonatal heart tissue into 20 mL of warm digestion buffer (HEPES buffer and enzymes) in a 50-mL tube and incubate for 5 min in a 37°C water bath. Mix with a microstirrer or by gentle shaking (*see* **Notes 4** and **5**).
10. Let the cells settle for 5 min, remove supernatant, add new prewarmed digestion buffer and repeat enzyme treatment six to seven times.
11. Let cells settle down and wash once with prewarmed HEPES buffer (without enzymes) containing 5% horse serum.
12. Spin down for 1 min at 340*g*.
13. Resuspend in adhesion medium (20 mL per 10 hearts) and plate cell suspension on uncoated 10-cm dishes.
14. Incubate for 1–1.5 h at 37°C/5% CO_2. Repeat this step. Fibroblasts will stick and spread on the plate while cardiomyocytes remain in suspension.

15. As an alternative to **steps 11** and **12**, cardiomyocytes can be purified by Ficoll-Paque™ Plus or Percoll® gradient centrifugation (not recommended; *see* **Note 6**).
16. Collect and count the cells.
17. Continue directly with nucleofection. If it is necessary, store cells in warm medium or buffer (*see* **Note 7**).

3.2. Nucleofection of Primary Cells

1. Cultivate the required number of cells (*see* **Notes 8–10**) (**Table 1**).
2. Prepare 1–5 µg plasmid DNA per sample (*see* **Notes 11–13**).
3. Prewarm the cell-specific supplemented Nucleofector solution to room temperature.
4. Prepare the six-well plates by filling the appropriate number of wells with 2 mL of the cell-specific culture medium containing serum and supplements and preincubate plates in a humidified 37°C/5% CO_2 atmosphere (*see* **Notes 14–16**).
5. Remove the medium from the primary cell culture.
6. Wash cells once with approx 10 mL HBS or D-PBS.
7. Aspirate HBS or D-PBS.
8. Harvest the cells by trypsinization (HUVECs, HCAECs, HMSCs) or take freshly isolated cells (neonatal rat cardiomyocytes).
9. Add trypsin/ EDTA solution to cover the cell layer.
10. Incubate the cells for 3–5 min at 37°C until they start to detach.
11. If the majority of the cells have dislodged, add TNS to stop trypsinization.
12. Remove the cell suspension from the flask by pipetting.
13. Take an aliquot of the trypsinized cell suspension and count the cells to determine the cell density.
14. Centrifuge the required number of cells at 90–200*g* for 10 min at room temperature.
15. Discard the supernatant completely so that no residual medium covers the cell pellet.
16. Resuspend the cell pellet in the specific supplemented and prewarmed Nucleofector solution to a final concentration of 0.5– 1×10^6 cells per 100 µL (*see* **Notes 17–21**).
17. Add 1–5 µg DNA per 100 µL of the cell/Nucleofector solution mixture (*see* **Notes 11–13**).
18. Transfer 100 µL nucleofection sample into an amaxa-certified cuvet and close the cuvet with the blue cap.
19. Insert the cuvet into the Nucleofector cuvet holder.
20. Select the cell specific Nucleofector program (*see* **Note 18**).
21. Press the button "start" (Nucleofector device II) or rotate the carousel clockwise to the final position and press the "X" key to start the program (nucleofector device I).
22. Take the cuvet out of the holder.
23. Add approx 500 µL of the preincubated medium of the six-well plates with the certified plastic pipet to the sample (*see* **Notes 14** and **22**).
24. Transfer the complete cell suspension into the prepared six-well plates.
25. Press any key to reset the Nucleofector device.
26. Repeat **steps 18–25** for every single sample.
27. Incubate Nucleofected cells in a humidified 37°C/5% CO_2 incubator.

Figure 1 shows the transfection efficiency of HUVECs, which is as high as 90%.

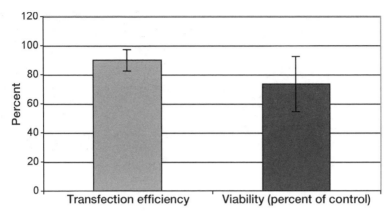

Fig. 1. Transfection efficiency of human umbilical vein endothelial cells 24 h post-nucleofection®. Cells were nucleofected with program A-034 and a plasmid encoding maxGFP™.

3.3. Cultivation of nucleofected Primary Cells

1. Depending of the gene of interest, expression might be detectable after 4–6 h (*see* **Note 23**).
2. Normally cells are analyzed after a 24–48 h incubation period.

3.4. Analysis of nucleofected Primary Cells

3.4.1. Nucleofected Cells Can be Analyzed by Fluorescence Microscopy (e.g., Cardiomyocytes, Vascular Smooth Muscle Cells) (see *Figs. 2 and 3*)

1. Aspirate and discard medium from each well.
2. Wash nucleofected cells with culture medium or D-PBS.
3. Cover the nucleofected cells with fresh culture medium.
4. Depending on the reporter plasmid, expression can be directly observed by fluorescence microscopy (e.g., green fluorescent proteins [GFP]).
5. It is also possible to fix the nucleofected cells before observation in the fluorescence microscope (e.g., with 4% paraformaldehyde in D-PBS).

3.4.2. Nucleofected Cells Can be Analyzed by Flow Cytometry (HUVECs, HCAECs, HMSCs, Smooth Muscle Cells) (see *Fig. 1*)

1. Aspirate and discard medium.
2. Wash cells with 1 mL D-PBS.
3. Add 300 μL trypsin/EDTA and incubate at 37°C until the cells detach.
4. Add 400 μL D-PBS/0.5% BSA per well to stop trypsinization.
5. Rinse the cells from the well and transfer into a 1.5-mL reaction tube.
6. Centrifuge for 10 min at 200*g* at 4°C and discard supernatant.
7. Resuspend the pellet in 400 μL D-PBS/BSA.

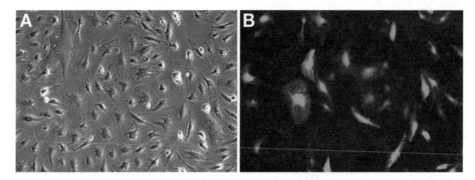

Fig. 2. Human coronary artery endothelial cells (HCAECs) were nucleofected using the HCAEC Nucleofector Kit and a plasmid encoding the fluorescent protein eGFP. Twenty-five hours post-nucleofection, cells were analyzed by light (**A**) and fluorescence microscopy (**B**).

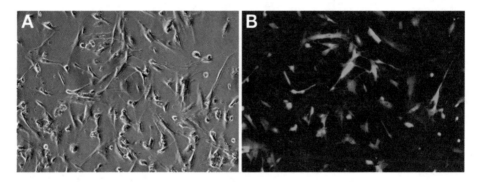

Fig. 3. Human mesenchymal stem cells (HMSCs) were nucleofected using the HMSC Nucleofector Kit and a plasmid encoding the fluorescent protein eGFP. Twenty-four hours post-nucleofection, cells were analyzed by light (**A**) and fluorescence microscopy (**B**).

8. Add 1 μL propidium iodide (10 μg/mL) to stain dead cells and mix well.
9. Analyze each sample by flow cytometry.

3.4.3. Nucleofected Cells Can be Analyzed by Antibody Staining and Flow Cytometry

1. Aspirate and discard medium.
2. Wash adherent cells with 1 mL D-PBS.
3. Add 300 μL trypsin/EDTA and incubate at 37°C until the cells detach.
4. Add 400 μL D-PBS/0.5% BSA per well to stop trypsinization.
5. Rinse the cells from each well and transfer the cell suspension to a 1.5-mL tube.
6. Centrifuge the cell suspension for 10 min at 200*g* at 4°C and discard supernatant.

7. Resuspend the pellet in 100 µL of a fluorescent dye-conjugated antibody against the respective surface marker appropriately diluted in D-PBS/0.5% BSA.
8. Incubate for 10 min on ice in the dark.
9. Wash each sample with 1 mL D-PBS/0.5% BSA.
10. Centrifuge cells for 10 min at 200g at 4°C and discard supernatant.
11. Resuspend the cell pellet in 400 µL D-PBS/0.5% BSA per sample.
12. Add 1 µL propidium iodide (10 µg/mL) to stain dead cells and mix well.
13. Analyze each sample by flow cytometry.

4. Notes

1. The isolation and culture of cardiomyocytes requires experience. Make sure that these processes are established in your hands before setting out to transfect cardiomyocytes.
2. It is essential for good cell viability to complete the isolation and transfection procedures as fast as possible. Make sure that required reagents (medium, solutions, etc.) and material (cuvets, dishes, etc.) are ready before sacrificing the animals and starting the preparation.
3. During the whole isolation process, cardiomyocytes should be handled in 37°C warm buffers (D-PBS, HEPES buffer, and so on). Cold solutions will impair cardiomyocyte functionality.
4. Do not resuspend the cardiomyocytes by pipetting. Tap the tube to resuspend the cell pellet.
5. Use 1000 µL or larger pipet tips to transfer the cells, even for the 100 µL volume. Otherwise the cells will be damaged by shear forces.
6. It is recommended to purify cardiomyocytes by the adhesion step. Percoll or Ficoll-Paque Plus may alter the characteristics of the cellular membrane.
7. Nucleofect only freshly isolated cardiomyocytes.
8. It is possible to use self-isolated HUVECs, HCAECs, and HMSCs for nucleofection.
9. Do not use HUVECs or HCAECs after passage number 10, or HMSCs after passage number 9, for nucleofection (**Table 2**). Trypsin treatment of HUVECs and HCAECs after passage 10 and HMSCs after passage 9 might be more difficult and may severely damage cells and decrease viability in combination with nucleofection. Nucleofection of HUVECs and HCAECs after passage 10 and HMSCs after passage 9 may also result in substantially lower gene transfer efficiency.
10. Use the Basic Nucleofector Kit for smooth muscle cells from species other than human.
11. We recommend using 2 µg pmaxGFP (supplied as positive control in each Nucleofector Kit), 1–5 µg specific plasmid DNA, or 0.5–3 µg specific siRNA per nucleofection sample.
12. The quality and the concentration of DNA used for nucleofection plays a critical role for the efficiency of gene transfer. Plasmid purification should be performed with QIAGEN EndoFree® Plasmid Kits. The purified DNA should be resuspended in deionized water or TE buffer (10 mM Tris-HCl, 1 mM EDTA, pH 8.0) with a

Table 2
Nucleofection Parameter of Primary Cells

Cell type	Confluency before nucleofection	Maximal passage number for nucleofection	No. of cells per sample	Nucleofector program[a]
HUVECs	90%	10	$0.5–1 \times 10^6$	A-034
HCAECs	70%	10	5×10^5	S-005
HMSCs	85%	9	$4–5 \times 10^5$	U-023
pVSMCs	80%	15	$0.5–1 \times 10^6$	A-033
SMCs	80%	15	$0.5–1 \times 10^6$	A-033, D-033, P-013, P-024, U-025
Rat cardiomyocytes	–	–	2×10^6	G-009

[a]Nucleofector® II; for Nucleofector® I, *see* detailed protocol.
For abbreviations, *see* **Table 1**.

concentration between 1 and 5 µg/µL. The A260:A280 ratio for the purity of the plasmid DNA for nucleofection should be at least 1.8.

13. We recommend performing two control samples to assess the initial quality of cell culture and the potential influences of nucleofection or amount/purity of DNA on cell viability. Control 1: Cells + Solution + DNA – Nucleofector program; and control 2: Cells + Solution – DNA + Nucleofector program.

14. It could be advantageous to purge the cardiomyocytes off the cuvet with warm RPMI supplemented with 10% horse serum. After a short incubation in Eppendorf cups at 37°C, cardiomyocytes were plated into six-well plates containing the recommended culture medium.

15. Supplemented medium stored for more than 2 d at 4°C should not be used for nucleofection. This will decrease cell viability and reduce transfection efficiency.

16. Supplemented EGM-2, EGM-2-MV, and MSCGM media should be stored in 40-mL aliquots at –20°C.

17. Optimal cell number for one nucleofection sample is 2×10^6 (recommended minimal cell number for one nucleofection sample 8×10^5 cells; recommended maximal cell number for one nucleofection sample 4×10^6 cells).

18. Optimal Nucleofector programs: for HUVECs, A-034 (Nucleofector II), A-34 (Nucleofector I); for HCAECs, S-005 (Nucleofector II) and S-05 (Nucleofector I), and for HMSCs, U-023 (for high transfection efficiency) or C-017 (for high cell survival) (Nucleofector II), U-23 or C-17 (Nucleofector I) (**Table 2**).

Optimal Nucleofector program for pig vascular smooth muscle cells: A-033 (Nucleofector II), A-33 (Nucleofector I) (**Table 2**). For cells from other mammalian species, test all Nucleofector programs (A-033, D-033, P-033, P-024, U-025) indicated in the Basic Kit protocol included in the kit. Optimal

Nucleofector program for rat cardiomyocytes, G-009 (Nucleofector II), G-09 (Nucleofector I) (**Table 2**).

19. Optimal cell number per nucleofection sample for HUVECs is $0.5-1 \times 10^6$ (recommended minimum cell number per nucleofection sample 2×10^5 cells; recommended maximum cell number per nucleofection sample 5×10^6 cells). For HCAECs, it is 5×10^5 (recommended minimum cell number per nucleofection sample 2×10^5 cells; recommended maximum cell number per nucleofection sample 5×10^5 cells). For HMSCs, it is $4-5 \times 10^5$ (recommended minimum cell number per nucleofection sample 2×10^5 cells; recommended maximum cell number per nucleofection sample 6×10^5 cells. Optimal cell number per nucleofection sample for rat cardiomyocytes is 2×10^6 (recommended minimal cell number per nucleofection sample is 8×10^5 cells; recommended maximum cell number per nucelofection sample is 4×10^5) (**Table 2**).

20. For optimal expression levels, HUVECs should be stored in Nucleofector Solution as shortly as possible. Therefore, it is beneficial to centrifuge each sample separately and resuspend in Nucleofector Solution immediately before nucleofection.

21. The minimal recommended cell number per nucleofection sample is 2×10^5 cells. A lower cell number may lead to a major increase in cell mortality.

22. Avoid storing the cell suspension longer than 15 min in specific Nucleofector Solution, as this reduces cell viability and transfection efficiency.

23. It is possible to check transfection efficiency and viability 2 h after Nucleofection by evaluating the proportion of cells attached in the cultured wells with the microscope.

References

1. Jiang, Y., Jahagirdar, B. N., Reinhardt, R. L., et al. (2002) Pluripotency of mesenchymal stem cells derived from adult marrow. *Nature* **418,** 41–49.
2. Huttmann, A., Li, C. L., and Duhrsen, U. (2003) Bone marrow-derived stem cells and "plasticity". *Ann. Hematol.* **82,** 599–604.
3. Haleem-Smith, H., Derfoul, A., Okafor, C., et al. (2005) Optimization of high-efficiency transfection of adult human mesenchymal stem cells in vitro. *Mol. Biotechnology* **30,** 9–20.
4. Tuli, R., Tuli, S., Nandi, S., et al. (2003) TGF-beta-mediated chondrogenesis of human mesenchymal progenitor cells involves N-cadherin and MAP kinase and wnt signalling crosstalk. *J. Biol. Chem.* **278,** 41,227–41,236.
5. Baksh, D., Song, L., and Tuan, R. S. (2004) Adult mesenchymal stem cells: characterization, differentiation, and application in cell and gene therapy. *J. Cell. Mol. Med.* **8,** 301–316.
6. Hamm, A., Krott, N., Breibach, I., Blindt, R., and Bosserhoff, A. K. (2002) Efficient transfection method for primary cells. *Tissue Eng.* **8,** 235–245.
7. Barlic, J., McDermott, D. H., Merrell, M. N., Gonzales, J., Via, L. E., and Murphy, P. M. (2004) Interleukin (IL)-15 and IL-2 reciprocally regulate expression of the chemokine receptor CX3CR1 through selective NFAT1- and NFAT2-dependent mechanisms. *J. Biol. Chem.* **279,** 48,520–48,534.
8. Lin, B., Kolluri, S. K., Lin, F., et al. (2004) Conversion of Bcl-2 from protector to killer by interaction with nuclear orphan receptor Nur77/TR3. *Cell* **116,** 527–540.

9. Harriague, J. and Bismuth, G. (2002) Imaging antigen-induced P13K activation in T cells. *Nat. Immunol.* **3**, 1090–1096.
10. Lakshmipathy, U., Pelacho, B., Sudo, K., et al. (2004) Efficient transfection of embryonic and adult stem cells. *Stem Cells* **22**, 531–543.
11. Nagahata, T., Sato, T., Tomura, A., Onda, M., Nishikawa, K., and Emi, M. (2005) Identification of RAI3 as a therapeutic target for breast cancer. *Endocr. Relat. Cancer* **12**, 65–73.
12. Lehrman, S. (1999) Virus treatment questioned after gene therapy death. *Nature* **401**, 517, 518.
13. Hannah, M. J., Hume, A. N., Arribas, M., et al. (2003) Weibel-Palade bodies recruit Rab27 by a content-driven, maturation dependent mechanism that is independent of cell type. *J. Cell. Sci.* **116**, 3939–3948.
14. Peister, A., Mellad, J. A., Wang, M., Tucker, H. A., and Prockop, D. J. (2004) Stable transfection of MSCs by electroporation. *Gene Therapy* **11**, 224–228.
15. Potapova, I., Plotnikov, A., Lu, Z., et al. (2004) Human mesenchymal stem cells as a gene delivery system to create cardiac pacemakers. *Circ. Res.* **94**, 952–959.
16. Chamley-Campell, J., Campell, G., and Ross, R. (1979) The smooth muscle cell in culture. *Physiol. Rev.* **59**, 1–61.
17. Bergmann, M. W., Loser, P., Dietz, R., and von Harsdorf, R. (2001) Effect of NF-κB Inhibition on TNFα-induced apoptosis and downstream pathways in cardiomyocytes. *J. Mol. Cell Cardiol.* **33**, 1223–1232.
18. von Harsdorf, R., Li, P. F., and Dietz, R. (1999) Signaling pathways in reactive oxygen species-induced cardiomyocyte apoptosis. *Circulation* **99**, 2934–2941.

17

Cell Adhesion and Migration Assays

Dmitry A. Soloviev, Elzbieta Pluskota, and Edward F. Plow

Summary

Adhesion and migration are basic responses of living cells to environmental stimuli. Such responses are central to a broad range of physiological processes, such as the immune response, repair of injured tissues, and prevention of excessive bleeding. Cell adhesion and migration also contributes to pathologies, including vascular and inflammatory diseases, as well as tumor growth and metastasis. These cellular responses depend on engagement of adhesion receptors by components of the extracellular matrix or molecules present on the surface of other cells. Hence, cell adhesion and migration assays are crucial methods in cell biology. In this chapter, several detailed protocols describing cell adhesion and migration assays are presented, and advantages and disadvantages of each method are discussed.

Key Words: Methods; cell migration; cell adhesion; integrins; Mac-1; iC3b.

1. Introduction

The adhesive state of a cell is one of its fundamental and defining characteristics, and the capacity of a cell to change its adhesive properties and migrate is essential for its response to environmental stimuli. Cell adhesion and migration depend on interactions of adhesion receptors on the cell surface with immobile constituents of the extracellular matrix or on the surface of other cells. Migration, as opposed to firm adhesion, requires the variable regulation of the interactions mediated by these adhesion receptors. The adhesion receptors include a variety of membrane proteins (e.g., members of the cadherin, selectins, integrin, and immunoglobulin [Ig] families) and nonproteins (e.g., glycosaminoglycans) that directly contact the extracellular constituents as well as numerous modulators that can either stimulate or suppress adhesive responses. Linkage of these adhesion receptors, directly or indirectly, to the

From: *Methods in Molecular Medicine, vol. 129:*
Cardiovascular Disease: Methods and Protocols, Volume 2: Molecular Medicine
Edited by: Q. K. Wang © Humana Press Inc., Totowa, NJ

cytoskeleton of the cell is essential to allow development of firm adhesion and to achieve the regulation needed to mediate cell migration.

In describing methods used to measure cell adhesion and migration, we will use cells expressing a particular integrin family member and recognizing a specific ligand. Altogether, there are more than 20 integrins (reviewed in **ref. *1***). Each integrin is a noncovalent heterodimer composed of an α- and a β-subunit. Each subunit consists of a short intracellular cytoplasmic tail, a single transmembrane domain, and a large extracellular domain. The ligand binding site is formed at the interface between the extracellular domains of each subunit *(2)*. The integrin of focus is $\alpha_M\beta_2$, which is also known as Mac-1, CD11b/18, or complement receptor (CR)3. It is a member of the β_2-subfamily of integrins, which are also known as the leukocyte integrins, reflecting their cellular distribution *(3)*. $\alpha_M\beta_2$ is notorious for its capacity to bind many different and structurally unrelated ligands; it has the most extensive ligand repertoire of all the integrins, with more than 30 ligands having been identified *(4)*. Among its many ligands is the complement degradation product, iC3b, which will be used for illustrative purposes in describing $\alpha_M\beta_2$-mediated adhesion and migration *(5,6)*. iC3b is formed following activating and then inactivating cleavages of the third component of the complement system *(7)*. The generation of iC3b provides one of the best examples in which a novel function is ascribed to a proteolytic degradation product of a parent molecule. The biological importance of iC3b resides in its function as the major, naturally occurring opsonin. It was the recognition of iC3b by leukocytes that led to the original identification and designation of $\alpha_M\beta_2$ as CR3. Activation of complement on foreign pathogens leads to formation of iC3b on their surface, which then serves as an attractant and an adhesive substrate for $\alpha_M\beta_2$-bearing inflammatory cells, ultimately leading to the destruction of the microorganisms *(4)*. Supporting the functional importance of this ligand–adhesion receptor interaction, individuals lacking the β_2 integrins, leukocyte adhesion deficiency (LAD) *(8)*, and mice lacking $\alpha_M\beta_2$ show increased susceptibility to infections *(9)*. iC3b recognition by $\alpha_M\beta_2$-bearing macrophages also has been implicated in recognition and destruction of tumor cells *(10)*.

In the description that follows, the human embryonic kidney (HEK)293 cell line transfected to express $\alpha_M\beta_2$ is used as the integrin-bearing cell for adhesion and migration assays. However, the assays described are applicable to many cell types, including blood cells naturally expressing $\alpha_M\beta_2$, and to cells expressing other integrins. Integrins, including $\alpha_M\beta_2$, can exist in low affinity or high affinity states, and *activation* of the integrins maximizes the adhesive and migratory responses they mediate. Such activation is achieved through stimulation of the cells. The agonists that induce integrin activation are cell-type specific, and physiological agonists usually induce activation by engaging

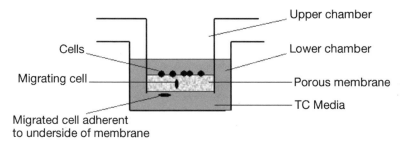

Fig. 1. The Boyden chamber. The lower and upper chambers are separated by a porous membrane through which cells can migrate. Chemotactic gradients are formed by placing different concentrations of the test ligand in the upper and lower chambers. The cells respond by moving toward the ligand and squeezing through the pore of the membrane. Usually, migrated cells remain attached to the underside of the membrane.

G protein-coupled receptors. In the model system described next, PMA is used as a model agonist to activate $\alpha_M\beta_2$. Ligand binding to integrins is divalention-dependent. Manganese not only supports ligand binding but also can activate integrins; magnesium supports ligand binding; and calcium can either support or suppress (as it does in the case of $\alpha_M\beta_2$) ligand binding. In the described assays, a buffer containing both Mg^{2+} and Ca^{2+} is used as the divalent ion condition to approach physiological conditions, but in investigating a novel ligand–integrin interaction, divalent ion conditions should be varied to maximize the chances for detection.

2. Materials

1. HEK293 cells that express $\alpha_M\beta_2$ on their surface. Such cells are developed by cotransfecting the HEK293 cells with the cDNAs for the α_M- and β_2-subunits in mammalian expression vectors *(11,12)*.
2. Tissue culture-treated 48-well plates (e.g., Costar 3548, Corning Inc. Corning, NY).
3. 6.5-mm-diameter (24-well format) Boyden chambers, such as TC-treated Costar Transwell plates and inserts 3421, with 5-μm pore size (*see* **Fig. 1**).
4. Purified iC3b (R&D Systems, Minneapolis, MN).
5. Phosphate-buffered saline (PBS): 0.15 M NaCl, 10 mM Na-phosphate buffer, pH 7.4.
6. 0.5% (w/v) polyvinylpyrrolidone (PVP), MW 360,000 in PBS.
7. Enzyme-free cell dissociation buffer (CDB) (Invitrogen, Carlsbad, CA).
8. Hanks' balanced salt solution (HBSS).
9. 1% (w/v) bovine serum albumin (BSA) in HBSS, containing 2 mM $CaCl_2$ and 2 mM $MgCl_2$ (HBSS, Ca^{2+}/Mg^{2+}).
10. Trypan Blue solution.
11. Dulbeco's modified Eagle's medium (DMEM)/F12 media (without fetal bovine serum [FBS]), containing $CaCl_2$ and $MgSO_4$.
12. CyQuant Cell Proliferation Kit (Molecular Probes, Eugene, OR).

13. Optical microscope and hemacytometer.
14. −70°C freezer.
15. Fluorescence multiwell plate reader with filters at 485 nm for excitation and 530 nm for emission, (e.g., Cytofluor II by Applied Biosystems, Perkin Elmer).
16. CO_2 incubator.

3. Methods

3.1. Adhesion Assays

1. Coat tissue culture-treated, 48-well plates overnight at 4°C with 200 µL/well of various concentrations of purified iC3b in triplicate at each concentration. At least three wells should be left uncoated as controls (*see* **Note 1**).
2. Remove the protein solution and *postcoat* all wells, including control wells, with 0.5 mL 0.5% PVP for 1 h room temperature (RT) (*see* **Note 2**).
3. Wash the plate free of nonbound material twice with 0.5 mL PBS.
4. Detach and harvest HEK293/ $\alpha_M\beta_2$ cells from culture dish(es) with CDB treatment for 5 min at RT and wash the recovered cells twice by centrifugation in HBSS.
5. Resuspend the cell pellet in 1 mL HBSS containing 1% BSA and Ca^{2+}/Mg^{2+}, and count viable cells using a hemacytometer and Trypan Blue solution.
6. Dilute the cells suspension with HBSS containing 1% BSA, Ca^{2+}/Mg^{2+} to 5×10^5 viable cells per milliliter and add 200 µL per well to the iC3b-coated plates as well as to the uncoated control wells.
7. Incubate the plates with cells for 30 min in the CO_2 incubator to allow the cells attach to the immobilized iC3b (*see* **Note 3**).
8. Rinse the plate three times with 1 mL PBS and freeze them immediately at −70°C until ready to proceed to the further steps. The plates may be stored for several months but should be frozen for at least 3 h (*see* **Note 4**).
9. Remove plates from the freezer and allow them to thaw to RT for 30 min.
10. During this time, the CyQuant reagent may be prepared by diluting 20-fold with lysis buffer and 400-fold with the fluorescent dye as specified in the CyQuant kit.
11. Dispense the CyQuant reagent into the wells, 500 µL/well, and let the plate stand 30 min in the dark or covered completely with aluminum foil.
12. Read the fluorescence in microplate fluorescence reader using a 485-nm filter for excitation and a 530-nm filter for emission.
13. Calculate mean fluorescence from each set of triplicates at the same protein coating concentration, and subtract the mean fluorescence of the triplicates from the noncoated control wells (*see* **Note 5**).
14. Inhibit cell adhesion (*see* **Note 6**).
15. *See* **Note 7a–c** for alternative methods.

3.2. Migration Assays (13)

1. Prepare serial dilutions of iC3b with DMEM/F12 and dispense them in 600-µL aliquots into wells of a 24-wells TC plate, in duplicate or more every concentration and adding only DMEM/F-12 to control wells (*see* **Note 8**).

2. Detach and harvest HEK293/$\alpha_M\beta_2$ cells at confluence from culture dish(es) by CDB treatment for 5 min at RT and wash the cells twice in DMEM/F12 (*see* **Note 9**).

3. Resuspend the cell pellet in 1 mL DMEM/F-12 and count viable cells, using hemacytometer and Trypan Blue solution.

4. Insert transwells (upper chambers) into wells and add 150 µL DMEM/F12 into each upper chamber (*see* **Note 10**).

5. Dilute the cell suspension with DMEM/F12 to 10^7 viable cells/mL and distribute it in 50-µL aliquots to each upper chamber.

6. Cover the plate with a lid and incubate it in humidifying CO_2 incubator overnight (16–20 h).

7. After incubation, aspirate media from all upper and lower chambers and carefully wipe the membranes INSIDE of upper chambers with cotton-tipped applicators.

8. Put all upper chambers back into wells and freeze the plate immediately to –70°C until ready for further steps (up to several months), but not less than 3 h.

9. Remove plates from the freezer and allow them to thaw to RT for 30 min.

10. During this time, prepare CyQuant reagent by diluting cell lysis buffer 20-fold and fluorescent dye 400-fold with dH_2O.

11. Dispense CyQuant reagent into the lower chambers (plate wells), 600 mL/well and let the plate stand for 30 min in the dark or cover completely with aluminum foil.

12. Read the fluorescence in a microplate fluorescence reader.

13. Calculate mean fluorescence from each duplicate point with the same protein concentration, and subtract from the mean fluorescence of control wells (*see* **Note 11**).

14. Inhibit the migration (*see* **Note 12**).

15. Modifiy the methods (*see* **Note 13a–d**).

16. Discrimination between chemotactic/chemokinetic effects: "checkerboard assay" (*see* **Note 7a**) and migration under agarose (*see* **Note 14b**).

4. Notes

1. The 48-well plates are more practical for cell adhesion assays than 96-well plates because cells tend to cling to the sidewalls of the plates nonspecifically and it is more difficult to effectively wash the smaller 96-well configuration. It is necessary to use a range of coating concentrations. Adhesion is dose-dependent and often reaches a plateau as the cells saturate the available ligand (*see* **Fig. 2**). However, with some ligands, maximal adhesion is followed by a decline at higher ligand concentrations. Hence, dose titrations of ligand, typically coating concentrations in the range of 0.1–10 µg/mL, should be performed.

2. PVP is used as a preferred postcoat. BSA, which is often used for this purpose, can serve as a ligand for $\alpha_M\beta_2$ when it denatures *(14)*. In most adhesion assays involving other ligand–receptor pairs, 1% BSA in PBS is suitable.

3. $\alpha_M\beta_2$–ligand interactions are temperature- and divalent cation-dependent *(15)*. For other cell types and receptors, the incubation time and temperature may vary. Typically, an incubation time of 20–60 min is appropriate, and temperatures of

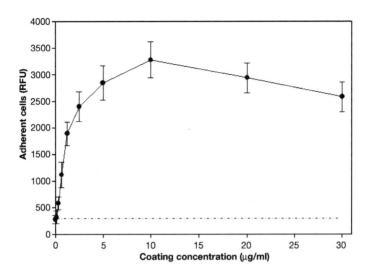

Fig. 2. Adhesion of human embryonic kidney (HEK)293/$\alpha_M\beta_2$ cells to iC3b depends on coating concentration of the ligand. In this experiment, the cell adhesion level reaches its maximum at iC3b concentration of 10 µg/mL. For inhibition experiments, usually, one uses the coating concentration, which allows 70–80% of maximal adhesion. The dashed line shows the level of nonspecific cell adhesion to polyvinylpyrrolidone in the absence of a ligand.

22 or 37°C are used. Cations should be tested individually, and EDTA should be tested as well to determine divalent ion dependence.

4. Different cell types will exhibit variable background adhesion. Plates may be washed multiple times until no visible attached cells are observed in the control wells.

5. Cell adhesion may be quantified as the relative fluorescence units (RFU) (**Fig. 2**). Alternately, values may be converted to cell number by comparing RFU with values extrapolated from a standard curve prepared from a known number of cells. To prepare the latter, dispense known amounts of the test cells (typically in the range 10^4 to 10^6 cells per tube) into separate tubes, pellet them by centrifugation, and freeze the cell pellets at –70°C for three or more hours. After thawing, add CyQuant reagent at 500 µL/pellet, incubate for 30 min at RT in the dark, transfer the entire contents into wells of a 48-well plate, and read the sample fluorescence as described previously.

6. For inhibition studies (e.g., blocking MAbs to candidate cellular receptors), at this step prepare a cell suspension with 10^6 viable cells/mL. Dispense the cells into 12 × 75 mm tubes in 400 µL/tube-aliquots and add as equal volume of the test inhibitor. Incubate the cells and inhibitor for 15–30 min at RT with gentle mixing, prior to adding to the 48-well ligand-coated plate. The described protocol is then followed. Inhibitory MAbs are typically used at final concentrations of 2–20 µg/mL.

7. Alternative methods for quantifying adherent cells. The most common of these

include labeling cells with radioactive [51]chromium; labeling cells with a fluorescent dye, such as Calcein AM; and fixing cells in the wells and then staining with Coomassie BB-R250. These methods are described next. Other methods, such as [35]sulfur-labeling *(16)*, colorimetric assay for acid phosphatase activity *(17)*, or staining with Crystal Violet *(18)* have been employed less frequently and details can be found in the references cited.

a. Cell labeling with [51]Cr *(19)*. This method is very reliable, but requires the *additional precautions and licensures for use of radioactive materials*. The method is based on labeling cells metabolically with water-soluble chromium salts. The protocol also requires the following *additional materials* and *equipment*: sodium chromate in saline, containing 10 mCi [51]Cr (e.g., Perkin Elmer), 5% sodium dodecyl sulfate (SDS) (w/v) in 2 *N* NaOH, scintillation counter (e.g., Beckman LC-6000 SC), scintillation mini-vials, scintillation cocktail.

Use the same procedures as described for the CyQuant method in **Subheading 3.1.**, **steps 1–7**, with the following modifications:

At **step 4** (cell preparation):
  i. Resuspend cell pellet in 1 mL HBSS, Ca^{2+}/Mg^{2+} and add 0.5 mCi ^{51}Cr saline.
  ii. Incubate 1 h at 37°C in the CO_2 incubator.
  iii. Wash cells three times with 50 mL HBSS and follow **steps 5–7** as described.

After **step 7**:

step 8: Rinse the plate three times with the 1 mL PBS and remove excess liquid from the wells.

step 9: Add 5% SDS in 2 *N* NaOH, 0.5 mL/well, cover the plate and incubate overnight at RT.

step 10: Using disposable plastic pipets, transfer the contents of each well into separate scintillation mini-vials, pipetting the liquid up and down several times to promote solubilization.

step 11: Add 5 mL of scintillation cocktail into each vial and count the samples in a scintillation counter.

b. Labeling cells with Calcein AM *(20)*. This method has the advantage of high sensitivity but the signal can vary greatly from experiment to experiment. Calcein AM is a specially designed nonfluorescent reagent, which converts to a fluorescent product intracellularly upon digestion with esterases. The method is based on the ability these fluorescent derivatives to accumulate intracellularly in a time-dependent manner.

The *additional reagent* required is Calcein AM (fluorescein-methylene-iminodiacetic acid) from Molecular Probes.

Use the same procedures described for CyQuant method (*see* **Subheading 3.1.**, **steps 1–7**) with the following modifications:

At **step 5**, add 100 μL of Calcein AM to the cell suspension and incubate in a CO_2 incubator at 37°C for 2 h.

At **step 8**, rinse the plate three times with 1 mL PBS and add 0.5 mL/well fresh HBSS, skip **steps 9–11**, and proceed directly to **step 12**.

If the fluorescence values are too low, allow the reaction to proceed in a CO_2 incubator at 37°C for additional time, up to 2–3 h, checking the fluorescence periodically.

c. Staining adherent cells with Coomassie BBR-250 *(21)*. This method is particularly suitable to examine adherent cells microscopically to determine the extent of cell spreading. Upon staining, adherent and spread cells are easily distinguishable under a microscope from cells, which are adherent, but not spread.

The following *additional reagents* will be needed: 3.7% paraformaldehyde (in PBS) or 70% ethanol, 0.25% Coomassie Brilliant Blue R-250 in 45% methanol/10% acetic acid, inverted optical microscope.

The same steps described for CyQuant method (*see* **Subheading 3.1.**, **steps 1–7**) are followed, with **steps 8–10** modified as follows:

step 8: Rinse the nonbound cells from the plate three times with 1 mL PBS and then fix attached cells with 3.7% paraformaldehyde or 70% ethanol for 10 min at RT.

step 9: Rinse the plate three times with PBS and stain cells with 0.25% Coomassie R-250 for 1 h at RT.

step 10: Wash the plate three times with 1 mL PBS and examine cells under a microscope.

8. Typical concentration range for migration experiments is 5–100 µg/mL. Transwell inserts by different manufacturers may vary in volumes. The volumes presented here are for Costar transwell inserts, 6.5 mm in diameter, in the 24-well format 3421, 3422, and 3415. For other inserts, refer to manufacturer's instructions.

9. Neutrophils, monocytes, or endothelial cells can be substituted, but inserts of different pore size are required and incubation times must be optimized.

10. Alternatively it is possible to assemble the migration unit (without filling upper chamber) at **Subheading 3.2.**, **step 1**. A frequently employed variation of the assay entails "precoating" of the membranes with ligand in order to form a concentration gradient of plastic-bound ligand across the membrane before cell loading. For such "precoating," add only 450 µL of the media to each well, reserving other 150 µL/well for addition just before filling the upper chamber and adding the cells. Some investigators believe that "membrane precoating" is essential for migration assays *(22)*, but we did not observe substantial differences using precoated or noncoated membranes in an overnight assay.

11. Cell migration may be expressed directly in RFU, or expressed as the number or percent of cells migrating, using a standard curve to convert RFU to cell number. To prepare standard curve, *see* **Note 5**.

12. For inhibition experiments, add dilutions of inhibitory MAbs (10–20 µg/mL) or test reagent to cell suspension and preincubate before proceeding to **Subheading 3.2.**, **step 5**. For such experiments, the accelerated method is especially suitable (*see* **Note 13b**).

13. There are several modifications of the described method for cell migration in Boyden chambers.

a. Staining cells with hematoxylin or Crystal Violet *(23)*. This method is suitable for photographing migrated cells that have adherent to membranes. It involves visualization of fixed with ethanol or formaldehyde cell with standard hystochemical techniques.

The following *additional reagents* will be needed: 3.7% paraformaldehyde or 70% ethanol, hematoxylin solution or 0.25% aqueous Crystal Violet, inverted optical microscope.

Perform **steps 1–7** as described under **Subheading 3.2.** Put inserts back into wells, and fix cells on the membrane with 1 mL 3.7% paraformaldehyde (for Crystal Violet, use 70% ethanol) at RT for 1 h. Remove fixing solution, wash inserts with dH$_2$O, and stain overnight with hematoxylin or Crystal Violet solutions.

Wash with dH$_2$O and examined stained cells microscopically.

b. Accelerated protocol. This method is particularly suitable for inhibition experiments, because during prolonged incubation blocking antibodies may be damaged by secreted cellular proteinases.

Substitute Costar Transwell 3422 with 8-μm pore size. Precoat for 30–60 min (*see* **Note 10**).

Use the same procedures as described in **Subheading 3.2.**, **steps 1–12** and **Note 10**, but reduce migration time at **step 6** to 6–8 h.

c. Using Calcein AM and Falcon HTS FluoroBlok Inserts (Becton-Dickinson). These inserts contain a light-opaque PET membrane specifically designed to absorb visible light within the 490 to 700 nm range, and block 99% of fluorescence of nonmigrated cells, which remain above the membrane. This design allows use of Calcein AM from Molecular Probes for cell labeling.

Use the same procedures as described under **Subheading 3.2.**, but 2–4 h before reading the assays, 100 μL of Calcein AM solution is added to lower chamber. Plates are covered with aluminum foil and returned to incubator. After 2–4 h, remove the plate and read the fluorescence.

d. Recently, a method was described using ATP-luminescence for cell quantitation *(22)*.

14. There are several methods that can be used to distinguish directional cell migration (chemotaxis) induced by specific attractants from nondirectional cell motility (chemotaxis or chemokinesis).

a. "Checkerboard assay" is a Boyden chamber-based method. If attractants are added to both chambers at various concentrations, the requirement of a gradient of the attractant can be plotted. For migration to be determined, the response is chemotactic; no migration will occur if there is no concentration gradient, i.e., if equal amounts of ligand are in upper and lower chamber. If the ligand induces a chemokinetic response, enhanced migration will occur even with the same amounts of ligand in the upper and lower chamber.

The checkerboard assay to discriminate between these possibilities is performed in the same way as described in **Subheading 3.2.**, but several concentrations of the attractant are added to the upper and the lower chambers while maintaining a constant total concentration.

b. Migration under agarose *(24)* is an alternative to Boyden chamber-based methods. This method is simple and can be used for a variety of cell types. Chemoattractant gradients are set up as the attractant diffuses through the agarose. Technically, the assay resembles the classical double immunodiffusion technique of Ouchterlony. No special supplies are required. The experiment is performed in 1% agarose/HBSS or DMEM plates. The agar plate has two or more round 0.5- to 1-mm wells, 2–10 mm apart. Chemoattractant, when loaded into one of the wells, begins to diffuse into the agar gel, forming a concentration gradient, which can be recognized by cells in a neighbored well and induce directional migration. The time of the migration depends on the diffusion rate of the tested ligand—larger molecules are slower to permeate into the gel and diffuse. To test effects on cell motility, the tested ligand is added directly to the wells containing the cells, and the distance that the cells diffuse is compared with that in the absence of ligand. To estimate the distance of cell migration, the simplest way is to photograph the agarose disc in an inverted microscope with ×200 magnification; the front of the migrated cells is visible without any special staining or other hystochemical methods. The migration distance may be expressed directly (in millimeters or even centimeters) as the migrated distance in the photoprints, or may be easy recalculated and examined over time to determine the migration rate. An advantage of the under agarose migration assay is that multiple chemoattractants can be studied simultaneously *(25)*.

References

1. Hynes, R. O. (2002) Integrins: bidirectional, allosteric signaling machines. *Cell* **110,** 673–687.
2. Xiong, J. P., Stehle, T., Zhang, R., et al. (2002) Crystal structure of the extracellular segment of integrin alpha Vbeta3 in complex with an Arg-Gly-Asp ligand. *Science* **296,** 151–155.
3. Harris, E. S., McIntyre, T. M., Prescott, S. M., and Zimmerman, G. A. (2000) The leukocyte integrins. *J. Biol. Chem.* **275,** 23,409–23,412.
4. Vetvicka, V., Thornton, B. P., and Ross, G. D. (1996) Soluble β-glucan polysaccharide binding to the lectin site of neutrophil or natural killer cell complement receptor type 3 (CD11b/CD18) generates a primed state of the receptor capable of mediating cytotoxicity of iC3b-opsonized target cells. *J. Clin. Invest.* **98,** 50–61.
5. Beller, D. E., Springer, T. A., and Schreiber, R. D. (1982) Anti-Mac-1 selectively inhibits the mouse and human type three complement receptor. *J. Exper. Med.* **156,** 1000–1010.
6. Arnaout, M. A., Todd, R. F., III, Dana, N., Melamed, J., Schlossman, S. F., and Colten, H. R. (1983) Inhibition of phagocytosis of complement C3- or immunoglobuoin G coated particles and of C3bi binding by monoclonal antibodies to a monocyte-granulocyte membrane glycoprotein (Mol). *J. Clin. Invest.* **72,** 171–179.

7. Vercellotti, G. M., Platt, J. L., Bach, F. H., and Dalmasso, A. P. (1991) Neutrophil adhesion to xenogeneic endothelium via iC3b. *J. Immunol.* **146,** 730–734.
8. Arnaout, M. A. (199) Leukocyte adhesion molecules deficiency: its structural basis, pathophysiology and implications for modulating the inflammatory response. *Immunol. Rev.* **114,** 145–180.
9. Ding, Z. M., Babensee, J. E., Simon, S. I., et al. (1999) Relative contribution of LFA-1 and Mac-1 to neutrophil adhesion and migration. *J. Immunol.* **163,** 5029–5038.
10. Vetvicka, V., Thornton, B. P., Wieman, T. J., and Ross, G. D. (1997) Targeting of natural killer cells to mammary carcinoma via naturally occurring tumor cell-bound iC3b and β-glucan-primed CR3 (CD11b/CD18). *J. Immunol.* **159,** 599–605.
11. Zhang, L. and Plow, E. F. (1996) A discrete site modulates activation of I domains: application to integrin $\alpha_M\beta_2$. *J. Biol. Chem.* **271,** 29,953–29,957.
12. Zhang, L. and Plow, E. F. (1996) Overlapping, but not identical sites, are involved in the recognition of C3bi, NIF, and adhesive ligands by the $\alpha_M\beta_2$ integrins. *J. Biol. Chem.* **271,** 18,211–18,216.
13. Solovjov, D. A., Pluskota, E., and Plow, E. F. (2005) Distinct roles for the α and β subunits in the functions of integrin $\alpha_M\beta_2$. *J. Biol. Chem.* **280,** 1336–1345.
14. Davis, G. E. (1992) The Mac-1 and p150,95 beta 2 integrins bind denatured proteins to mediate leukocyte cell-substrate adhesion. *Exp. Cell Res.* **200,** 242–252.
15. Wright, S. D. and Jong, M. T. (1986) Adhesion-promoting receptors on human macrophages recognize Escherichia coli by binding to lipopolysaccharide. *J. Exp. Med.* **164,** 1876–1888.
16. Charo, I. F., Nannizzi, L., Smith, J. W., and Cheresh, D. A. (1990) The vitronectin receptor $\alpha_v\beta_3$ binds fibronectin and acts in concert with $\alpha_5\beta_1$ in promoting cellular attachment and spreading on fibronectin. *J. Cell Biol.* **111,** 2795–2800.
17. Connolly, D. T., Knight, M. B., Harakas, N. K., Wittwer, A. J., and Feder, J. (1986) Determination of the number of endothelial cells in culture using an acid phosphatase assay. *Anal. Biochem.* **152,** 136–140.
18. Wennerberg, K., Lohikangas, L., Gullberg, D., Pfaff, M., Johansson, S., and Fässler, R. (1996) β1 integrin-dependent and -independent polymerization of fibronectin. *J. Cell Biol.* **132,** 227–238.
19. Elices, M. J., Urry, L. A., and Hemler, M. E. (1991) Receptor functions for the integrin VLA-3: Fibronectin, collagen, and laminin binding are differentially influenced by ARG-GLY-ASP peptide and by divalent cations. *J. Cell Biol.* **112,** 169–181.
20. Metelitsa, L. S., Gillies, S. D., Super, M., Shimada, H., Reynolds, C. P., and Seeger, R. C. (2002) Antidisialoganglioside/granulocyte macrophage-colony-stimulating factor fusion protein facilitates neutrophil antibody-dependent cellular cytotoxicity and depends on FcgammaRII (CD32) and Mac-1 (CD11b/CD18) for enhanced effector cell adhesion and azurophil granule exocytosis. *Blood* **99,** 4166–4173.
21. Retta, S. F., Ternullo, M., and Tarone, G. (1999) Adhesion to matrix proteins, in *Adhesion Protein Protocols, Methods in Molecular Biology,* (Dejana, E., Corada, M., eds.), Humana, Totowa, NJ, pp. 125–131.

22. de la Monte, S. M., Lahousse, S. A., Carter, J., and Wands, J. R. (2002) ATP luminescence-based motility-invasion assay. *Biotechniques* **33,** 98–104.

23. Forsyth, C. B., Solovjov, D. A., Ugarova, T. P., and Plow, E. F. (2001) Integrin αMβ2-mediated cell migration to fibrinogen and its recognition peptides. *J. Exp. Med.* **193,** 1123–1133.

24. Nelson, R., Quie, P. G., and Simmons, R. L. (1975) Chemotaxis under agarose: a new and simple method for measuring chemotaxis and spontaneous migration of human polymorphonuclear leukocytes and monocytes. *J. Immunol.* **115,** 1650–1656.

25. Heit, B., Tavener, S., Raharjo, E., and Kubes, P. (2002) An intracellular signaling hierarchy determines direction of migration in opposing chemotactic gradients. *J. Cell Biol.* **159,** 91–102.

18

Apoptosis Assays

Marcela Oancea, Suparna Mazumder, Meredith E. Crosby, and Alexandru Almasan

Summary

A large number of methods devoted to the identification of apoptotic cells and the analysis of the morphological, biochemical, and molecular changes that take place during this universal biological process have been developed. Apoptotic cells are recognized on the basis of their reduced DNA content and morphological changes that include nuclear condensation and which can be detected by flow cytometry (sub-G1 DNA content), Trypan Blue, or Hoechst staining. Changes in plasma membrane composition and function are detected by the appearance of phosphatidylserine on the plasma membrane, which reacts with Annexin V-fluorochrome conjugates. Combined with propidium iodide (PI) staining, this method can distinguish between the early and late apoptotic events. The best-recognized biochemical hallmarks of apoptosis are the activation of cysteine proteases (caspases), condensation of chromatin, and fragmentation of genomic DNA into nucleosomal fragments. Recognized by a variety of assays, activated caspases cleave many cellular proteins and the resulting fragments may serve as apoptosis markers. Finally, the mitochondria and the Bcl-2 family proteins play an important role in this process that can be recognized by translocation of apoptogenic factors, such as Bax and cytochrome c, in and out of mitochondria.

Key Words: Apoptosis; Bcl-2 family; caspase; Annexin V binding; microscopy; flow cytometry; methods; review.

1. Introduction

Apoptosis is a universal genetic program of cell death in higher eukaryotes that represents a basic process involved in cellular development and differentiation *(1,2)*. Alternative models of programmed cell death (PCD) have been proposed, which include autophagy, paraptosis, mitotic catastrophe, and the descriptive model of apoptosis-like and necrosis-like PCD. Cell morphology still remains an important criterion for distinguishing these various forms of cell death from classical apoptosis. Therefore, although individual features of

From: *Methods in Molecular Medicine, vol. 129:*
Cardiovascular Disease: Methods and Protocols, Volume 2: Molecular Medicine
Edited by: Q. K. Wang © Humana Press Inc., Totowa, NJ

apoptosis serve as useful markers, the mode of cell death should be confirmed by visual inspection of cells by light or electron microscopy.

The Bcl-2 family of proteins has been highly conserved during evolution; its members (24 to date) are critical regulators of apoptosis *(3)*. Pro-apoptotic members of this family, such as Bax, following their activation, promote apoptosis by causing the release of cytochrome c from mitochondria into the cytosol. Cytochrome c acts as a cofactor to stimulate the complexing of Apaf-1 with caspase-9, which then initiates activation of the caspase cascade *(4,5)*. Anti-apoptotic proteins, such as Bcl-2, prevent their release. Bax normally resides in the cytosol, but it is translocated to the mitochondria to promote apoptosis *(6)*. Genotoxic stressors, such as ionizing radiation, induce Bax expression and activation *(7,8)*.

Caspases are synthesized as inactive precursors, which are activated by proteolytic cleavage to generate active enzymes. The activation of caspases is a common and critical regulator of the execution phase of apoptosis, triggered by many factors, including treatment with radio- and chemotheraputic agents *(5,6,8–10)*. They further proteolytically cleave proteins that are essential for maintenance of cellular cytoskeleton, DNA repair, signal transduction, and cell cycle control. There are more than 300 in vivo caspase substrates *(11)*; among them are poly (ADP-ribose) polymerase (PARP)-1 and ICAD/DFF45, the cleavage of which results in liberation of a caspase-activated deoxyribonuclease (CAD) that is responsible for the oligucleosome-size DNA fragmentation characteristic of most apoptotic cells.

Numerous methods have been developed to identify apoptotic cells and analyze their morphological, biochemical, and molecular changes. Some simple methods, such as MTS, Trypan Blue, or Hoechst staining offer an initial indication for the occurrence of cell death. These initial observations must be followed-up by more specific assays. Changes in plasma membrane composition and function are detected by the appearance of phosphatidylserine on the plasma membrane, which reacts with Annexin V-fluorochrome conjugates. Apoptotic cells are recognized either on the basis of their reduced DNA-associated fluorescence as cells with diminished DNA content (sub-G1) or morphological changes. Activation of caspases can be examined through a variety of methods: colorimetric, immunoblot, or immunohistochemical. Activated caspases cleave many cellular proteins and the resulting fragments may also serve as useful markers. This chapter provides a few standard protocols that we have successfully used in our laboratory for a number of experimental systems, including cells grown in culture *(5,6,12,13)*, xenografts *(6)*, or patient-derived specimens following endomyocardial biopsy *(14)*. More detailed and additional protocols can be found in **ref.** *15*, our publications, or the extensive literature on apoptosis.

2. Materials

2.1. Preliminary Assays for Cell Death Detection

2.1.1. MTS Assay

MTS solution (CellTiter 96® AQueous One Solution Reagent, Promega).

2.1.2. Vital Dye Exclusion

1. Trypan Blue (0.4%, Sigma); store at room temperature.
2. Inverted microscope.

2.1.3. Hoechst Staining

1. 1X phosphate-buffered saline (PBS): 136.9 mM NaCl, 2.68 mM KCl, 8.1 mM Na$_2$HPO$_4$, 0.9 mM CaCl$_2$, 0.49 mM MgCl$_2$.
2. Hoechst 33258 dye (10 µg/mL, Sigma). Alternatively, Hoechst 33342 and 7-aminoactinomycin D (7-AAD) can be also used; all are stored in the dark, as they are light-sensitive.

2.2. Plasma Membrane Changes Detected by Annexin V Staining

1. Fluorescein (or other fluorophore)-conjugated Annexin V.
2. Propidium iodide (PI; Sigma): 50 µg/mL stock solution of PI in 1X PBS.
3. 1X binding buffer: 10 mM HEPES/NaOH, pH 7.4, 140 mM NaCl, 2.5 mM CaCl$_2$.
4. 5-mL polystyrene round-bottom tubes.

2.3. Flow Cytometry-Based Assays for Cellular Morphology and DNA Fragmentation

1. RNase A (1 mg/mL; Gentra Systems).
2. PI 50 µg/mL (final concentration); prepare a working concentration of 4 mg/mL that is stored at –20°C.
3. Absolute methanol (MeOH) chilled at –20°C. Ethanol (EtOH, alternative).
4. Pasteur pipets.
5. 5-mL polystyrene round-bottom tubes.
6. Flow cytometer (e.g., FACScan) and software for data analyses (e.g., CellQuest, Becton Dickinson).

2.4. Immunocytochemistry for Detecting Active Bax/Bak, Caspase-3, and Cytochrome c

1. Glass cover slips (22 × 22 mm) and slides (Fisher Scientific).
2. Formaldehyde: 4% in 1X PBS (dilute 37% formaldehyde stock in 1X PBS), make fresh each time.
3. Blocking buffer: 2% goat serum, 0.3% Triton X-100 in 1X PBS, sterile-filtered.
4. Primary antibodies: active-Bax (BD Pharmingen), active-Bak (Calbiochem), active caspase-3 (Cell Signalling), and cytochrome c (BD Pharmingen).
5. Secondary antibody, flourochrome-conjugated (Molecular Probes).

6. Vectashield, mounting medium for fluorescence (Vector Laboratories), with or without 4′,6′-diamidino-2-phenylindole hydrochloride (DAPI).
7. Nail polish.

2.5. Caspase-3 Activity Determination: Colorimetric Assay

1. Lysis buffer: 1% NP 40, 20 mM HEPES (pH 7.5), 4 mM EDTA. Just before use, add the following protease inhibitors: aprotinin (10 µg/mL), leupeptin (10 µg/mL), pepstatin (10 µg/mL), and phenylmethylsulfonyl fluoride (PMSF) (1 mM).
2. Reaction buffer: 100 mM HEPES (pH 7.5), 20% v/v glycerol, 5 mM dithiothreitol (DTT), 0.5 mM EDTA.
3. Caspase-3 substrate: acetyl-Asp-Glu-Val-Asp-*p*-nitroanilide (Ac-DEVD-pNA, Calbiochem), 20 mM stock in dimethylsulfoxide (DMSO) (stable for more than 1 yr at −20°C), 100 µM final concentration. Additional colorimetric as well as fluorometric substrates are available. The fluorometric substrates 7-amino-4-methylcoumarine (AMC) and 7-amino-4-trifluoromethylcoumarin (AFC) are more sensitive, but require a fluorometer capable of detecting the 380/460 and 405/500 excitation/emission spectra, respectively. AFC can be also detected colorimetrically at 380 nM.
4. Microtiter plate reader, spectrophotometer, or fluorometer.

2.6. Immunoblot Detection of Active Bax and Caspase-3

1. 1X PBS.
2. Lysis buffer: 20 mM HEPES, pH 7.5, 1 mM EDTA, 150 mM NaCl, 1% NP-40, 1 mM DTT with protease inhibitors (1 mM PMSF, 1 µg/mL leupeptin).
3. Protein assay reagent (Bio-Rad).
4. Bovine serum albumin (BSA).
5. Sodium dodecyl sulfate-polyacrylamide gel electrophoresis (SDS-PAGE).
6. Nitrocellulose membrane (e.g., Schleicher and Schull).
7. 1X PBST: 1X PBS with 1% Tween-20.
8. Milk (nonfat dry milk).
9. PARP-1 (Cell Signalling), active Bax (6A7; Pharmingen), or active caspase-3 (Cell Signalling) antibodies.
10. Secondary antibodies, anti-mouse or anti-rabbit (Amersham).
11. Chemiluminiscent reagents: Lumiglo (KPL) or ECL (Amersham).
12. Disuccinimidyl suberate (DSS), final concentration 2 mM.
13. Conjugation buffer: 20 mM sodium phosphate, pH 7.5 containing 0.15 M NaCl, 20 mM HEPES, pH 7.0, 100 mM carbonate/ bicarbonate, pH 9.0.
14. Quenching buffer: 1 M Tris-HCl, pH 7.5.

2.7. Cell Fractionation to Detect Protein Translocation to and From Mitochondria

1. Mitochondria isolation buffer: 20 mM HEPES-KOH, pH 7.2, 10 mM KCl, 1.5 mM MgCl$_2$, 1 mM EGTA, 1 mM EDTA, 250 mM sucrose, 1 mM EDTA, 1 mM EGTA, with protease inhibitors (1 mM PMSF, 5 µg/mL, aprotinin, 5 µg/mL, leupeptin, and 5 µg/mL pepstatin).

2. Trypan Blue dye.
3. Antibodies against cytochrome c Oxidase I (Molecular Probes), cytochrome c (Pharmingen), Bax (Santa Cruz), and as a control, β-actin (Sigma).

3. Methods
3.1. Preliminary Evidence for Cell Death Detection
3.1.1. MTS Assay

MTS assay is a colorimetric method to determine the number of viable cells in proliferation or chemosensitivity assays. MTS is a tetrazolium compound that is bioreduced by the cells into formazan, and the quantity of formazan produced is directly proportional to the number of living cells in culture. The absorbance of formazan at 490 nm can be measured directly from 96-well plates. Although very easy and amenable to a larger screen, the MTS data obtained alone are not a proof of apoptosis, as the assays measures changes in metabolic activity that could be also caused by a change in cell proliferation.

1. Use a 96-well plate containing cells cultured in a 100-μL volume of media.
2. Seed cells at a concentration of 2×10^4 cells/mL (2–3×10^3–10^4, depending on cell type and growth characteristics) in 100 μL medium.
3. Add 20 μL MTS solution to each well.
4. Incubate the plate for 1–4 h in a humidified 5% CO_2 atmosphere.
5. Record the absorbance at 490 nm using an ELISA plate reader.

3.1.2. Vital Dye Exclusion

The Trypan Blue exclusion assay provides a convenient and easy mean to obtain a preliminary assessment on cellular death. This represents the most practical method for assessing cell viability during routine cell culture maintenance, as cells undergoing apoptosis become permeable to the dye. However, this method may also score cells that undergo cell death through mechanisms other than apoptosis (e.g., autophagy).

1. Cells are mixed in equal volume with the Trypan Blue dye solution and are incubated for 5–10 min.
2. Cells are examined under an inverted microscope and scored for the number of dead cells (the blue-stained cells represent those that have taken up the dye) and the treated samples are compared with the untreated controls.

3.1.3. Hoechst Staining

Illuminating DNA-bound Hoechst results in blue-light fluorescence. Apoptotic cells appear first as brightly stained with condensed chromatin and are later partitioned into blue beads in a fragmented nucleus as a result of micronuclei formation. This assay allows examination of chromatin condensation of the apoptotic nuclei as a quick and easy way to differentiate between normal and apoptotic cells on the basis of their fluorescence (ultraviolet [UV] excitation <350 nm).

1. All cells (untreated and treated) are pooled by centrifugation and washed one time with 1X PBS.
2. Decant 1X PBS, mix the cells with Hoechst 33258 dye, and incubate for 5 min.
3. The fluorescence of the apoptotic cells is determined using a UV-equipped fluorescence microscope.
4. The number of apoptotic cells is scored in several fields.

3.2. Plasma Membrane Changes Detected by Annexin V Staining

During the early phases of apoptosis, Phosphatidyl serine (PS), a protein usually located on the inner leaflet of the plasma membrane in healthy cells, translocates to the outer layer where it is exposed at the external surface of the cells. Annexin V has a high affinity for PS, and fluorochrome-tagged Annexin V staining is used as an indicator of apoptosis. The staining is done in combination with PI, a nucleic acid-specific stain that is excluded from live and early apoptotic or necrotic cells but stains DNA and RNA once the plasma membrane is disrupted in these cells. Therefore, it is possible to distinguish live, healthy cells (negative for both Annexin V and PI) from early apoptotic cells (Annexin V positive/PI negative) and late apoptotic or necrotic cells (positive for both Annexin V and PI) by flow cytometry.

1. Remove medium and rinse cells with 1X PBS.
2. Trypsinize attached cells using Trypsin/EDTA. Only mild trypsinization should be used to get a single cell suspension, as trypsin may damage the PS on the plasma membranes. Alternative methods should be used (e.g., EDTA w/o trypsin) whenever these are effective to dissociate attached cells.
3. Wash cells twice with cold 1X PBS and resuspend 1×10^6 cells in 1 mL of 1X binding buffer.
4. Transfer 100 µL of the solution (1×10^5 cells) to a 5-mL polystyrene tube.
5. Add 5 µL of Annexin V and 10 µL of PI and gently vortex the cells.
6. Incubate at room temperature for 15 min in the dark.
7. Add 300 µL of 1X binding buffer to each tube.
8. Analyze by flow cytometry within 1 h.

3.3. Flow Cytometry-Based Assays for Cellular Morphology and DNA Fragmentation

The Sub-G1 method for detecting cell death relies on the principle that, because of DNA endonucleolytic cleavage, the fragmented low-molecular-weight DNA is released from cells during prolonged fixation. This will yield a population of cells that binds a quantitative DNA stain, PI, to a lesser degree than is characteristic for G1 cells; G1 represents the longest phase of the cell cycle, and therefore the largest fraction of cells are typically in G1. As a result, there will be a population of cells that appears to the left of the G1 peak (*see* **Note 1**).

Flow cytometry has the advantage of rapidly examining a large cell population. An analysis of the forward and side light-scatter signals of the cells provides an additional method for identification of apoptotic cells based on their physical properties. Thus, for example, as cells shrink during the early stages of apoptosis, the intensity of light that is scattered by these cells in a forward direction along the laser beam will also decrease. As chromatin condenses and apoptotic bodies are formed during the later stages of apoptosis, these cells reflect and refract more light, which can be determined by the increase in the intensity of light scattered at a 90° angle (side scatter).

1. Collect 1×10^6 cells by centrifugation at 500*g*.
2. Prepare a second set of 1-mL centrifuge tubes containing 900 µL of 100% (absolute methanol). MeOH must be chilled to –20°C.
3. Resuspend the cells in 100 µL of 1X PBS.
4. Add the cells drop-wise using a Pasteur pipet to the tubes containing the 100% MeOH, while gently vortexing to ensure that the cells are in a single-cell suspension.
5. Place the tubes in a –20°C freezer and allow fixation to proceed for at least 12 h.
6. Centrifuge the cells at 1000*g* and aspirate the MeOH.
7. Wash the fixed cells two times with 1 mL of cold 1X PBS, again centrifuging at 1000*g* and being careful to not aspirate cells.
8. Treat the cells with RNase A (use 100 µL of a 1 mg/mL solution per sample) for 20 min at 37°C.
9. Turn off the lights and stain cells with 50 µg/mL per sample of PI for at least 30 min at room temperature, or 15 min at 37°C.
10. Keep the samples in the dark and run the samples on the flow cytometer, measuring the emission wavelength (617 nm) using a 600- or 610-nm filter.

3.4. Immunocytochemistry to Detect Active Bax/Bak, Caspase-3, and Cytochrome c

Whenever Bax and Bak become activated, is a conformation change takes place when an internal epitope is exposed, which can be detected by specific antibodies. Whereas active Bax can be also detected by its mitochondrial translocation (below), Bak is present mostly in the mitochondria so immunocytochemistry is the only way to examine its activation. Following their activation, Bax and Bak permeabilize the mitochondrial outer membrane thus facilitating the release of cytochrome c into the cytosol.

1. For plating the cells, we use glass cover slips (sterilized by dipping in ethanol and passing through flame) that are placed into six-well plates. Cells (1×10^5 cells per well) are seeded and grown overnight.
2. Remove media and rinse cells with 1X PBS warmed up to 37°C.

3. To fix the cells, add 1–2 mL of 4% formaldehyde to each well. Leave cells to fix for 20 min at room temperature.
4. Wash each well with 1X PBS three times for 5 min.
5. Incubate cells in blocking buffer for 5–10 min at room temperature.
6. Dilute the primary antibody (two primary antibodies could be added at the same time, but they must be of different origin [e.g., one rabbit and the other mouse] in 100–200 µL blocking buffer, according to the recommended dilution).
7. Use a different six-well dish to incubate the antibodies. Soak filter paper (3-cm diameter circles) in 1X PBS and place them into the wells; this is necessary to maintain the humidity in the chamber. Put the cover slips on top of the soaked filter paper. Add the primary antibody carefully to cover the entire cover slip. Incubate at room temperature for 1–2 h.
8. Wash each well with 1X PBS three times for 5 min.
9. Add the secondary antibody (flourochrome-conjugated) in blocking buffer and incubate for 30–45 min at room temperature in the dark. For dual staining, the fluorophores must have different emissions spectra for each individual antibody (e.g., fluorescein isothiocyanate [FITC] at 525 and phycoerythrin at 578 n*M*). There is a set of very sensitive and stable Alexa dyes (Molecular Probes, now part of Invitrogen); consult *The Handbook: A Guide to Fluorescent Probes and Labeling Technologies* for a comprehensive resource for fluorescence technology and its applications (http://probes.invitrogen.com/handbook/).
10. Wash each well with 1X PBS three times for 5 min.
11. Pick up cover slips with a forceps and drain away excess 1X PBS.
12. For mounting, add a drop of Vectashield to a clean microscope slide and gently lay the cover slip on top.
13. Remove excess Vectashield by blotting with a Kimwipe, and seal with nail polish.
14. After adding the secondary antibody, it is important to keep the slides in the dark at all times. A similar protocol can be used for tissue sections (*see* **Note 2**).
15. Store slides in a –20°C freezer.

3.5. Caspase-3 Activity Determination: Colorimetric Assay

A simple colorimetric assay can measure the release of the chromogenic group from the synthetic substrate, most commonly *p*-nitroanilide (pNA) by activated caspases. Ac-DEVD-pNA is most frequently used, with the cleaved pNA being monitored colorimetrically through its absorbance at 405–410 nm. Although DEVD-based substrates are called caspase-3-specific, they are in fact cleaved by most caspases, with caspase-3 being the most efficient. In vitro titration experiments and/or the use of specific inhibitors may be required to distinguish the activity of various caspases *(8,15)*.

1. Wash cells (1 × 10⁶) with cold 1X PBS, resuspend them in 50 µL of cold lysis buffer, vortex, and keep on ice for 30 min.
2. Centrifuge the cell lysates at 12,000*g* for 10 min at 4°C, collect the supernatant in fresh tubes, and assay the protein concentration for each sample. Keep on ice.

3. To a 96-well, plate add reaction buffer, caspase substrate (100 µ*M* final concentration) and 20–50 µg cell lysates for a final 200-µL reaction volume.
4. Incubate samples at 37°C for 1–2 h and monitor the enzyme-catalyzed release of pNA at 405 nm using a microtiter plate reader.

3.6. Immunoblot Detection of Active Bax and Caspase-3

In case of Bax-mediated apoptosis, active Bax can be also detected by immunoblot using either active Bax antibody or by applying crosslinking agents. Moreover, in most of the cases, pro-caspase (inactive caspase)-3 is activated to active caspase-3 and it can be similarly detected by Western blot analysis. One of its many cellular substrates is PARP-1. In the apoptotic cells, PARP-1 (110 kDa) is cleaved to form two truncated fragments, most frequently the 86-kDa fragment being detected by the available commercial antibodies.

3.6.1. Immunoblot Analyses

1. Collect the treated and untreated cells (1×10^6) by centrifugation (500*g* for 5 min). Decant the medium and resuspend the cell pellet in cold 1X PBS very gently and spin it down (500*g* for 5 min). Decant the supernatant and repeat the process one more time. Remove 1X PBS carefully without disturbing the cell pellet.
2. Lyse the cells in a lysis buffer, with the cells incubated for 30 min on ice with occasional vortexing.
3. Centrifuge the cells for 15 min at 15,000*g* and collect the supernatants.
4. The protein estimation of these samples will be performed using a spectrophotometric method using the Bio-Rad Protein Assay reagent (working solution, 1:10 dilution) at 595 nm (1–2 µL of the sample will be mixed with 1 mL of diluted Bio-Rad protein assay reagent) and the concentration of unknown samples will be measured from the BSA standard curve (the curve can be drawn from the spectrophotometric readings of known concentrations of BSA).
5. Load 50–100 µg proteins as well as the protein standard marker on an 8% SDS-PAGE to separate the proteins under denaturing conditions.
6. Transfer the proteins to a nitrocellulose membrane either by the wet or semi-dry transfer method.
7. Block the membrane with 5% milk in PBS for 1 h at room temperature or overnight at 4°C.
8. Incubate the membrane with primary antibodies (PARP-1, active Bax, or active caspase-3) for 2 h at room temperature or overnight at 4°C (following the company's recommended dilution) (*see* **Note 3**).
9. Wash the blot three times with 1X PBST at room temperature at 10-min intervals.
10. Add the appropriate secondary antibody (anti mouse or anti rabbit depending on the primary antibody) with a 1:2000 dilution to the blot and incubate for 1–1.5 h at room temperature.
11. Wash the blot five times with 1X PBST at room temperature at 10-min intervals.
12. Wash the blot with double-distilled water for very short time to get rid of Tween-20

and develop it using Chemiluminiscent reagents, such as Lumiglo or ECL, following the company's suggested protocol.

3.6.2. Crosslinking Studies

1. Wash cells with conjugating buffer.
2. Add DSS to each sample to a final concentration of 2 mM and incubate for 30 min at room temperature.
3. Quench the crosslinker by the addition of 1 M Tris-HCl (pH 7.5) to a final concentration of 20 mM.
4. Separate proteins by SDS-PAGE and immunolbot, as described previously, with an anti-Bax antibody. Oligomerisation of Bax to dimers, trimers, or tetramers as detected by the size of Bax-immunoreactive bands is an indication of its activation in the mitochondria.

3.7. Cell Fractionation to Detect Protein Translocation To and From Mitochondria

During apoptosis, cytochrome c is released from the mitochondria into the cytosol. At the same time, Bax is activated and translocates to the mitochondria. The detection of these and other apoptosis-relevant proteins *(2,15)* in various subcellular compartments can be used as an important marker of apoptosis.

1. 5×10^7 cells (untreated and treated) are washed first with cold medium (without fetal bovine serum), then, with ice-cold mitochondria isolation buffer.
2. 5X volumes of the above buffer is added to the cell pellet and is left on ice for 30 min. The cell suspension is then homogenized gently with a Dounce homogenizer, with the extent of lysis being determined by means of Trypan Blue exclusion (80–90% of cells should be lysed; *see* **Note 4**). By this procedure, no or minimal cytochrome c should be present in the cytosolic extracts of healthy untreated cells.
3. The homogenate is centrifuged at 750g for 10 min to remove unbroken cells, large debris, and nuclei.
4. The supernatant is again centrifuged at 10,000g for 15 min.
5. The pellet containing mitochondria, designated as P10, is used for further experiments.
6. The supernatant is subjected to ultracentrifugation at 100,000g for 30 min.
7. The resulting pellet, designated as P100, represents the cellular membranes.
8. The supernatant consists of the cytosolic fraction, designated as S100.
9. The proteins in the cellular fractions are separated by SDS-PAGE and transferred to a nitrocellulose membrane.
10. Western blot analysis is performed using primary anti-cytochrome c and Bax antibodies. As controls, cytochrome c oxidase I is used as a mitochondrial marker with β-actin as a marker for the cytosol to indicate any possible mitochondrial or cytoplasmic contamination in the cellular fractions.

4. Notes

1. If cells enter apoptosis at phases other than G1, or if aneuploidy is present, there may not be a Sub-G1 peak. Additionally, microscopic examination should discern among debris, intact single cells, or doublets. Unless otherwise mentioned, keep the samples on ice throughout staining for flow cytometric studies.

2. Formalin-fixed and paraffin-embedded mouse *(6)* or patient-derived human *(14)* tissue sections can be also examined. The slides are deparaffinized with xylin and graded alcohol and treated with citrate buffer (pH 6.0) for 20 min for antigen retrieval before incubation with primary antibodies. Sections are counterstained with hematoxylin before being examined under the microscope. Immunohistochemistry for caspase-3 can be combined with the *in situ* detection of apoptotic cells by terminal deoxynucleotide transferase-mediated dUTP nick-end labeling (TUNEL) *(14)*. TUNEL or Comet assays are methods that detect DNA strand breaks that are associated with apoptosis. The samples are first immunostained for caspase-3 and, after washing in PBS, with a horseradish peroxidase (HRP)-linked secondary antibody. Immunoreactivity is visualized by a 10-min incubation with the HRP substrate diaminobenzidine. After staining for caspase-3, the same slides are then processed for *in situ* detection and localization of apoptosis at the level of single cells. Sections are then stained with antifluorescein antibodies linked with alkaline phosphatase, developed with Fast Red substrate, and counterstained with hematoxylin.

3. The molecular weight of native PARP-1 is 110-kDa and that of cleaved PARP-1 is 86 kDa. The molecular weight of pro-caspase-3 is 32 kDa, whereas active caspase-3 migrates at 17 as well as 10 kDa. Some antibodies recognize only the pro-form of caspase-3, some recognize only the active form, and some can recognize both. The primary antibodies can be reused for a couple of times if they are stored at 4°C in the presence of sodium azide (0.01%, w/v).

4. For cell fractionation protocols, kits from different companies (e.g., Qiagen, Pierce) are available that are practical and work well for separation of proteins from the various subcellular compartments. Optimal conditions for cell homogenization will depend on the cell type and Dounce homogenizer used, therefore, the number of strokes required to detect cytochome c in apoptotic but not in control cells will need to be determined.

Acknowledgments

This work was supported by research grants from the National Institutes of Health to AA (CA81504 and CA82858).

References

1. Green, D. R. and Evan, G. I. (2002) A matter of life and death. *Cancer Cell* **1,** 19–30.
2. Danial, N. N. and Korsmeyer, S. J. (2004) Cell death. Critical control points. *Cell* **116,** 205–219.

3. Cory, S. and Adams, J. M. (2002) The bcl2 family: regulators of the cellular life-or-death switch. *Nat. Rev. Cancer* **2**, 647–656.

4. Wang, X. (2001) The expanding role of mitochondria in apoptosis. *Genes Dev.* **15**, 2922–2933.

5. Chen, Q., Gong, B., and Almasan, A. (2000) Distinct stages of cytochrome c release from mitochondria: evidence for a feedback amplification loop linking caspase activation to mitochondrial dysfunction in genotoxic stress induced apoptosis. *Cell Death Differ.* **7**, 227–233.

6. Ray, S. and Almasan, A. (2003) Apoptosis induction in prostate cancer cells and xenografts by combined treatment with Apo2 ligand/tumor necrosis factor-related apoptosis-inducing ligand and CPT-11. *Cancer Res.* **63**, 4713–4723.

7. Gong, B. and Almasan, A. (1999) Differential upregulation of p53-responsive genes by genotoxic stress in hematopoietic cells containing wild-type and mutant p53. *Gene Expr.* **8**, 197–206.

8. Gong, B., Chen, Q., Endlich, B., Mazumder, S., and Almasan, A. (1999) Ionizing radiation-induced, Bax-mediated cell death is dependent on activation of serine and cysteine proteases. *Cell Growth Diff.* **10**, 491–502.

9. Gong, B. and Almasan, A. (2000) Apo2 ligand/TNF-related apoptosis-inducing ligand and death receptor 5 mediate the apoptotic signaling induced by ionizing radiation in leukemic cells. *Cancer Res.* **60**, 5754–5760.

10. Chen, Q., Chai, Y. -C., Mazumder, S., et al. (2003) The late increase in intracellular free radical oxygen species during apoptosis is associated with cytochrome c release, caspase activation, and mitochondrial dysfunction. *Cell Death Differ.* **10**, 323–334.

11. Fischer, U., Janicke, R. U., and Schulze-Osthoff, K. (2003) Many cuts to ruin: a comprehensive update of caspase substrates. *Cell Death Differ.* **10**, 76–100.

12. Mazumder, S., Gong, B., and Almasan, A. (2000) Cyclin E induction by genotoxic stress leads to apoptosis of hematopoietic cells. *Oncogene* **19**, 2828–2835.

13. Mazumder, S., Chen, Q., Gong, B., Drazba, J. A., Buchsbaum, J. C., and Almasan, A. (2002) Proteolytic cleavage of cyclin E leads to inactivation of associated kinase activity and amplification of apoptosis in hematopoietic cells. *Mol. Cell. Biol.* **22**, 2398–2409.

14. Masri, S. C., Yamani, M. H., Russell, M. A., et al. (2003) Sustained apoptosis in human cardiac allografts despite histologic resolution of rejection. *Transplantation* **76**, 859–864.

15. Reed, J. C. (2000) *Apoptosis.* Academic Press, San Diego, CA.

19

Preparation of Protein Crystals for X-Ray Structural Study

Soichi Takeda

Summary

The knowledge of accurate molecular structures obtained by X-ray protein crystallography is now inevitable for rational drug design and for understanding the molecular basis underlying genetic disorders found in patients. However, preparing protein crystals suitable for structural analysis is currently the bottleneck in structure determination by this method. The intent of this chapter is to present current methods of preparing protein crystals for structural studies for a wide range of biologists who have access to macromolecules but do not know how to handle them for crystallization. The chapter includes the pretreatment of a protein prior to the crystallization experiment, initial screens, and optimization of the crystallization conditions for further X-ray study. Finally, handling considerations that are important for a protein intended for crystallization experiments are discussed.

Key Words: X-ray crystallography; structural biology; crystallization; protein structure; rational drug design; synchrotron.

1. Introduction

The importance of solving protein structures continues to grow in fields ranging from basic biochemistry and biophysics to pharmaceutical development, medical science, and, of course, cardiovascular research. In order to obtain high-resolution, three-dimensional structural knowledge of proteins by X-ray crystallography, crystals diffracting at high resolution are needed. This chapter focuses on the essential principles and procedures involved in crystallization so as to provide a general understanding of what is entailed in this key step of solving X-ray protein structures. It is not our aim to convert biologists into X-ray crystallographers; complete explanation of the physical basis of the techniques and methods currently practiced is beyond the scope of this chapter.

From: *Methods in Molecular Medicine, vol. 129:*
Cardiovascular Disease: Methods and Protocols, Volume 2: Molecular Medicine
Edited by: Q. K. Wang © Humana Press Inc., Totowa, NJ

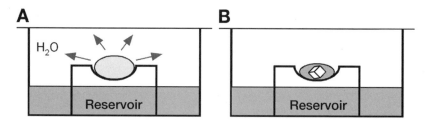

Fig. 1. Principle of the vapor diffusion (sitting drop) method for crystallization. The concentration of the reservoir is initially twice that in the droplet (**A**), and the two become equal to that of the reservoir that has a volume several orders of magnitude larger than the droplet. The drop decreases volume during the process so that the concentration of all components in the drop, including the protein, rise significantly. If the variables are right, this results in protein crystallization (**B**).

This chapter includes neither protein expression and purification protocols nor methods associated with X-ray diffraction data collection and structural analysis; rather, it simply focuses on the basis of crystallization experiments. If one needs further information as well as more detailed protocols on crystallization, please see the textbooks listed in the references *(1–7)*.

Although there are a variety of methods for setting up protein samples for crystallization, the most widely used method is crystallization by vapor diffusion. In this method, vapor diffusion occurs in a closed system because of a difference in concentration between a small droplet of protein, typically 0.3–10 µL, and a larger body of liquid, typically 0.1–1 mL (*see* **Fig. 1**). The protein drop is made by diluting protein twofold with liquid from the larger body, usually referred as the reservoir solution; therefore, the protein drop starts at half the concentration of the contents in the reservoir solution. This concentration gradient drives vapor diffusion, resulting in the gradual concentration of protein and, if the variables are right, protein crystallization. Reservoir solutions can contain a wide range of chemical variables, including buffers for pH control, salts (NaCl, ammonium sulfate, and so on), precipitating agents (polyethylene glycol, organic solvents), reducing agents (dithiothreitol and so on), and detergents.

As the variability of conditions required for crystallizing proteins is too large for exhaustive searches, more practical approaches for initial searches are employed. This is termed "sparse matrix" screening. The sparse matrix design was first introduced in 1991 by Jancarik and Kim *(8)* (*see* **Table 1** and **Note 1**). Various ready-made kits, some are the extensions of the original one and the others are based on different strategies, are currently commercially available and are used effectively for initial crystallization screens of large numbers of proteins.

Table 1
Fifty Solutions for the Original Sparse Matrix Screen *(7)*

No.	Salt	Buffer	Precipitant
1	0.02 *M* Ca chloride	0.1 *M* Na acetate pH 4.6	30% MPD
2	None	None	0.4 *M* K/Na Tartrate
3	None	None	0.4 *M* ammonium phosphate
4	None	0.1 *M* Tris-HCl pH 8.5	2.0 *M* ammonium sulfate
5	0.2 *M* Na citrate	0.1 *M* HEPES/NaOH pH 7.5	30% MPD
6	0.2 *M* Mg chloride	0.1 *M* Tris/HCl pH 8.5	30% PEG4000
7	None	0.1 *M* Na cacodylate pH 6.5	1.4 *M* Na acetate
8	0.2 *M* Na citrate	0.1 *M* Na cacodylate pH 6.5	30% iso-propanol
9	0.2 *M* ammonium acetate	0.1 *M* Na citrate pH 5.6	30% PEG 4000
10	0.2 *M* ammonium acetate	0.1 *M* Na acetate pH 4.6	30% PEG 4000
11	None	0.1 *M* Na citrate pH 5.6	1.0 *M* ammonium phosphate
12	0.2 *M* Mg chloride	0.1 *M* HEPES-Na pH 7.5	30% iso-propanol
13	0.2 *M* Na citrate	0.1 *M* Tris-HCl pH 8.5	30% PEG 400
14	0.2 *M* Ca chloride	0.1 *M* HEPES/NaOH pH 7.5	28% PEG 400
15	0.2 *M* ammonium sulfate	0.1 *M* Na cacodylate pH 6.5	30% PEG 8000
16	None	0.1 *M* HEPES/NaOH pH 7.5	1.5 *M* Li sulfate
17	0.2 *M* Li sulfate	0.1 *M* Tris/HCl pH 8.5	30% PEG 4000
18	0.2 *M* Mg acetate	0.1 *M* Na cacodylate pH 6.5	20% PEG 8000
19	0.2 *M* ammonium acetate	0.1 *M* Tris-HCl pH 8.5	30% iso-propanol
20	0.2 *M* ammonium sulfate	0.1 *M* Na acetate pH 4.6	25% PEG 4000
21	0.2 *M* Mg acetate	0.1 *M* Na cacodylate pH 6.5	30% MPD
22	0.2 *M* Na acetate	0.1 *M* Tris-HCl pH 8.5	30% PEG 4000
23	0.2 *M* Mg chloride	0.1 *M* HEPES/NaOH pH 7.5	30% PEG 400
24	0.2 *M* Ca chloride	0.1 *M* Na acetate pH 4.6	20% iso-propanol
25	None	0.1 *M* imidazole pH 6.5	1.0 *M* Na acetate
26	0.2 *M* ammonium acetate	0.1 *M* Na citrate pH 5.6	30% MPD
27	0.2 *M* Na citrate	0.1 *M* HEPES/NaOH pH 7.5	20% iso-propanol
28	0.2 *M* Na acetate	0.1 *M* Na cacodylate pH 6.5	30% PEG 8000
29	None	0.1 *M* HEPES/NaOH 7.5	0.8 *M* K/Na tartrate

(Continued)

Table 1 *(Continued)*
Fifty Solutions for the Original Sparse Matrix Screen *(7)*

No.	Salt	Buffer	Precipitant
30	0.2 *M* ammonium sulfate	None	30% PEG 8000
31	0.2 *M* ammonium sulfate	None	30% PEG 4000
32	None	None	2.0 *M* ammonium sulfate
33	None	None	4.0 *M* Na formate
34	None	0.1 *M* Na acetate pH 4.6	2.0 *M* Na formate
35	None	0.1 *M* HEPES/NaOH 7.5	0.8 *M* Na/K phosphate
36	None	0.1 *M* Tris-HCl pH 8.5	8% PEG 8000
37	None	0.1 *M* Na acetate pH 4.6	8% PEG 4000
38	None	0.1 *M* HEPES/NaOH pH 7.5	1.4 *M* Na citrate
39	2.0 *M* ammonium sulfate	0.1 *M* HEPES/NaOH pH 7.5	2% PEG 400
40	None	0.1 *M* Na citrate pH 5.6	20% iso-propanol, 20% PEG 4000
41	None	0.1 *M* HEPES/NaOH pH 7.5	10% iso-propanol, 20% PEG 4000
42	0.05 *M* K phosphate	None	20% PEG 8000
43	None	None	30% PEG 1500
44	None	None	0.2 *M* Mg formate
45	0.2 *M* Zn acetate	0.1 *M* Na cacodylate pH 6.5	18% PEG 8000
46	0.2 *M* Ca acetate	0.1 *M* Na cacodylate pH 6.5	18% PEG 8000
47	None	0.1 *M* Na acetate pH 4.6	2.0 *M* ammonium sulfate
48	None	0.1 *M* Tris-HCl pH 8.5	2.0 *M* ammonium phosphate
49	1.0 *M* Li sulfate	None	2% PEG 8000
50	0.5 *M* Li sulfate	None	15% PEG 8000

PEG, polyethylene glycol; MPD: 2-methyl-2,4-pentanediol.

Because good-quality crystals are not usually obtained in the first screen, once crystals (most often microcrystals) have been observed in trial experiments, crystallization conditions must be improved for crystal size and quality. At this stage, we usually perform a "grid screen." For each condition, two variables (such as pH and polyethylene glycol [PEG] concentration) are altered in a two-dimensional (x, y) grid. After fine-tuning of all the parameters,

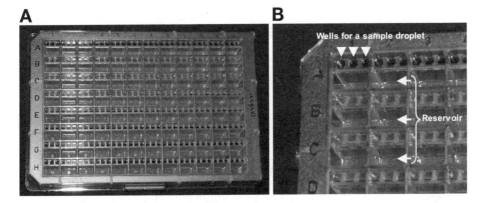

Fig. 2. Greiner CrystalQuick 96-well sitting drop crystallization plate. The plate has 8 vertical wells and 12 horizontal wells. Within each well is a rectangular reservoir with 0.1 mL of fill volume. Adjacent to the reservoir is a ledge containing three drop-support wells for each sample.

crystals suitable for X-ray study are obtained. If the crystals have appropriate size and are really made of protein, not salt, then this is the time to start characterizing them by X-ray diffraction with the help of a protein crystallographer.

2. Materials

2.1. Preparation of Proteins for Crystallization

1. Tris-buffer(TB): 10 mM Tris-HCl, pH 7.5 (*see* **Note 2**). Prepared by diluting 100X stock solution (1 M Tris-HCl, pH 7.5) with deionized water.
2. Dialysis tubes: Spectra/Por 7 or its equivalent, whose membrane has been treated to minimize the content of heavy metals that can affect crystallization of the protein. Rinse with TB prior to use to remove sodium azide that has been added as a preservative when shipped.
3. Centrifugal filter device: Amicon Ultra-4 (Millipore). There are five devices with different nominal molecular weight limits (NMWLs; 5000, 10,000, 30,000, 50,000, and 100,000). For higher recovery, use a NMWL device with a cutoff range a bit smaller than the molecular weight (MW) of the protein of interest. Prerinse the devices with TB prior to use.

2.2. Initial Screening of Crystallization Conditions

1. Crystal screen: Crystal Screen (Hampton Research) or Crystal Screen Basic (Sigma-Aldrich) containing 50 solutions (*see* **Table 1** and **Note 1**) described in the original sparse matrix by Jancarik and Kim *(8)*.
2. Crystallization plate: Greiner CrystalQuick 96-well sitting drop crystallization plate (Hampton Research; *see* **Fig. 2** and **Note 3**).

3. Sealing tape: a roll of 4-in. wide Crystal Clear Sealing Tape (Hampton Research) or its equivalents. Tapes or films used for sealing crystallization plate should be optically transparent for viewing with a microscope.

3. Methods

Crystallization experiments start with "crystal quality" protein (*see* **Note 4**). Prior to a crystallization experiment, the protein sample should be concentrated in a low-ionic-strength buffer. The crystallization of the protein can be divided into the following two stages: (1) initial screening to obtain any kind of crystals or promising precipitates and (2) optimization to improve the crystals for X-ray diffraction data collections. Ninety-six-well crystallization plates (*see* **Fig. 2** and **Note 2**), which have been developed for sitting drop vapor diffusion to facilitate high-throughput crystallization, are used for both for screens and optimizations. Commercially available "sparse matrix" screens are currently the best choice for initial trials (*see* **Table 1** and **Note 1**). The crystallization experiments are examined daily by observation of the protein droplets using a stereo microscope. The conditions that produce microcrystals should be optimized by "grid screening" to grow high-quality (free of cracks and defects) single crystals of appreciable size (0.05–0.1 mm at least for the dimensions of a face) suitable for X-ray study.

3.1. Preparation of the Proteins for Crystallization

1. Prepare several milligrams of the protein of interest with appropriate purity (*see* **Note 5**).
2. If the protein is lyophilized, dissolve the protein in approx 1 mL of TB (*see* **Note 6**). If the protein is hard to dissolve, then incrementally increase the salt (50, 100, 150, and 200 m*M* NaCl) until it is fully in solution.
3. Dialyze the protein against 1 L of TB (*see* **Note 7**). If the protein is already in solution, start from this step. Change the dialysis solution twice at 6-h intervals. If the sample precipitates, add NaCl in the dialysis solution in order to prevent precipitation, and repeat the step. The salt concentration of the protein sample should be as low as possible. Ideally, it is best to prepare samples in a lower buffer concentration without salt.
4. Remove undisclosed particles by centrifugation (20,000g for 10 min).
5. Concentrate the protein solution with a centrifugal filter device Amicon Ultra-4. In general, 10 mg/mL is a good starting protein concentration for initial crystallization trials (*see* **Note 8**). Add the sample to the Amicon Ultra filter unit and spin at a maximum 4000g for approx 10–60 min in a swinging-bucket rotor.
6. Recover the concentrated protein by inserting a pipet into the bottom of the filter unit.
7. Store the protein at 4°C until it is used in the crystallization experiment. For longer storage, –70°C is better; however, freezing and rethawing of the sample should be avoided. Therefore, aliquot the protein into several tubes (100–200 μL each) and quick-freeze each one in a liquid nitrogen bath before placing at –70°C.

8. Do not mix different purification batches in crystallization trials. Because it is not uncommon for one batch of protein to crystallize whereas the next will not, it is vital to keep a history of each sample and to track each batch separately.

3.2. Setting Up Protein Drops for Initial Crystallization Screening

1. These instructions assume the use of a Greiner CrystalQuick 96-well sitting drop crystallization plate (**Fig. 2**). Depressions in the plate may be sprayed with pressurized air or some inert gas to blow away dust just before dispensing reservoir solutions. Pipet 0.1 mL of each crystallizing solution of the screen in each of the 96 reservoirs.
2. Pipet 0.5 µL of the protein solution onto the drop-support well of A1 (*see* **Notes 9** and **10**). To carry out crystallization experiments on such a submicroliter scale, it is recommended to use Pipetman P2 (Gilson) or its equivalent.
3. Pipet 0.5 µL of reagent from the reservoir onto the drop-support well of A1 and mix with the protein solution.
4. Repeat **steps 2** and **3** for the remaining reservoirs.
5. Seal the plate with a strip of clear sealing tape.
6. Leave the plate in an incubator, and maintain a fairly constant temperature. Crystallization trials should be performed at a minimum of two temperatures, usually 20 and 4°C, because most protein crystals have been obtained at these temperatures. If possible, try another temperature between 10 and 15°C.
7. The crystallization plates are examined using a stereo microscope (1) immediately after setup, (2) once a day for the first week, and (3) once a week for several weeks (*see* **Note 11**).
8. In wells in which the protein precipitated immediately after making the drop, repeat the setup with modification. Halve the reservoir solution concentration with deionized water and repeat **steps 2–5**. It may slow crystal nucleation.
9. If enough protein sample is left, repeat **steps 1–8** with other screening kits, e.g., Crystal Screen II, PEG/ION Screen, INDEX, SALTRx (Hampton Research), Extension Kit, Low Ionic Kit, PEG Grid Screening Kit (Sigma-Aldrich), Wizard Screens (Emerald BioStructures), and so on. Different screens consist of solutions designed based on different strategies, thus they may compensate for gaps in the original sparse matrix screen (8).

3.3. Observation of the Drops by a Stereo Microscope

1. Scan the drops at about ×20–40 magnification, and when something suspicious appears, increase the magnification to ×80 or ×100 for a better view (*see* **Notes 12** and **13**). Scan the entire depth of the drop, because crystals will form at different levels.
2. Crystals occur in a great variety of shapes such as needles, blades, walnuts, plates, and various geometric shapes and in various sizes (hardly observable 10 µ to 1 mm). An example is shown in **Fig. 3**.
3. Crystals are often distinguished from amorphous substances by their flat faces with sharp edges and by their anisotropy. Anisotropy of the crystals is examined by putting them between a crossed polarizer attached to a stereo microscope. They

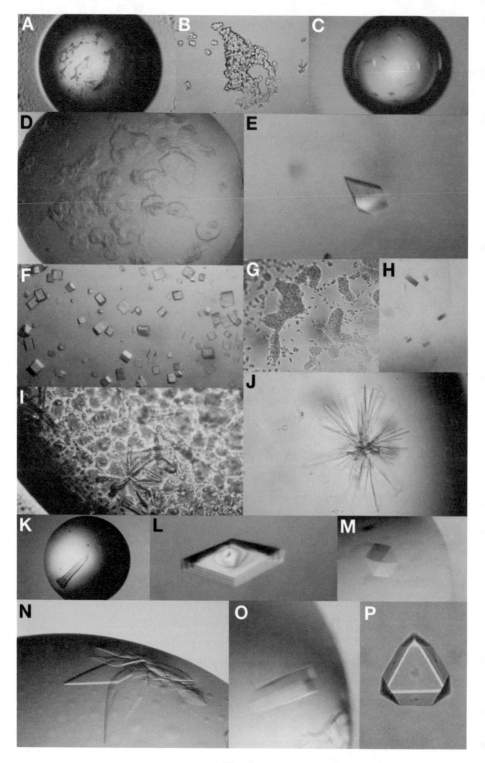

Fig. 3.

sometimes display beautiful colors, because the crystals are birefringent (*see* **Fig. 3C,E,H,L**).

4. Carefully observe everything to be familiar with the differences between microcrystals, amorphous aggregates, and sweater fuzz. If something suspicious is found, make new drops under the same conditions and check its reproducibility. True crystals should be reproduced if the protein is not degraded.

5. When either crystals or micro crystals are found, it is important to verify that the crystals are protein and not salt. IZIT (Hampton Research) is an example of a protein-binding dye. If the crystals obtained are suspected to be salts, a grain of the dye can be added to the drop. Salt crystals will not absorb the dye (*see* **Note 14**).

6. Another method of verifying protein crystals is to take a needle and try to crush the crystals. Salt crystals are so hard to break that one can often hear them snap. Protein crystals are much more fragile and easier to smash.

3.4. Optimization of the Crystallization Conditions

1. Once the crystals (most often microcrystals or suspicious crystals) are obtained in trial experiments, crystallization conditions must be improved for crystal size and quality. pH and precipitant concentration are two of the most important determinants of protein solubility; therefore, they will be the first parameters optimized by a grid screen.

2. Prepare reservoir solutions for the grid screen with variations in pH (in steps of 0.5 pH units initially, then 0.1 pH units finally) vs precipitant concentrations (decreasing in steps of 5%, initially), beginning around the pH value and the precipitant concentration that was found in the initial screen (*see* **Note 15**). Refine those parameters until the optimal crystallization conditions are found.

3. Protein concentration, temperature, and droplet size should also be optimized.

4. Add inhibitors, substrate, or co-factors to the protein drop using the optimized well conditions. Repeat the initial screen with the additive compound if an effect is found (*see* **Note 16**).

Fig. 3. (*Opposite page*) Photo micrographs of the results of crystallization. Crystals or microcrystals of various morphologies obtained from various proteins, including troponin complexes (*9,10*), in initial crystallization screens are shown in **A**, **B**, **D**, and **F–J**. Transparent spherulite clusters made of tiny crystals were observed (**B**) in a close up view of **A**, suggesting that the well condition was a good starting point for optimization. After optimization of the conditions, single crystals with sharp edges were obtained (**C**) and successfully used for X-ray study. Crystals grown too quickly without edges (**D**) were improved by lowering both the protein and the precipitant concentrations (**E**). Single separated crystals (**K–M**, **O**, and **P**) or single crystals in the cluster of plates (**N**) were obtained after refining the crystallization conditions and were used for diffraction studies. Some crystals, not all, show birefringence (**C**, **E**, **H**, and **L**). Sometimes crystals eventually appear in the oil phase of a drop of salt-polyethylene glycol (PEG)-protein (**I**), because the protein may preferentially partition into the PEG-rich oily phase, thereby becoming locally concentrated enough to nucleate.

5. Repeat **steps 2–4** for other conditions that were not optimized before.
6. Once crystals with the appropriate size are obtained, start to characterize them by X-ray diffraction. For structural studies, it is not morphology but the diffraction quality of the crystals that is important.

4. Notes

1. Although sparse matrix screens are a biased sampling of crystallization parameters, selected from known or published successful crystallization conditions, they are an efficient method to screen a large number of parameters with a limited amount of protein. In our experiences, the first crystals from nearly half of the proteins tested in the initial screens were obtained using such sparse matrix-based ready-made kits. For example, the first crystals of the complexes of troponin, TnC/TnI(1-47) dimer *(9)* and TnT/TnC/TnI trimer *(10)*, were obtained from the solutions no. 38 and no. 17 of Crystal Screen (Hampton Research), respectively.
2. The solution in which the protein is finally dissolved should be as simple as possible (*see* **Note 7**), and 10 m*M* HEPES/NaOH, pH 7.0 is also a common example. It is better not to use phosphate buffers for proteins intended for crystallization even during the preparation procedure, because they often give rise to salt crystals. For proteins susceptible to oxidation, one often needs to add an excess amount of dithiothreitol (~20 m*M*) both in the drop and in the reservoir in order to keep the sample homogeneous (*see* **Note 10**).
3. 96-well plates are much more compact and use less material than 24-well plates, which have been conventionally used. In our experience, there are no obvious differences between the two systems in the results from the initial screens.
4. The protein should be at least 90–95% pure by sodium dodecyl sulfate-polyacrylamide gel electrophoresis (SDS-PAGE) *(11)* and staining with Coomassie Brilliant Blue. Always consider further purification of the protein (1) if the initial screen does not produce any promising results or (2) to improve crystal quality when optimizing. It is our belief that poor purity is the most common cause of unsuccessful crystallization, and the purity requirements of macromolecules must be higher than in other fields of molecular biology. On the other hand, it is not always true that proteins with high purity are easily crystallized. In our case, before truncating the fragile portion of the troponin complex *(10)*, full-length molecules that are extremely pure (more than 99% on SDS-PAGE) would never crystallize. In such cases, try screens with different constructs of varying lengths, different isoforms, or the protein from different sources. Small changes in the physical properties of the proteins can substantially affect its ability to crystallize. Isolated structural domains of proteins are very often easily crystallized with high quality, and limited proteolysis is one of the best methods to figure out which structural domains are suitable for crystallization experiments *(12)*.
5. The initial gels prior to the crystallization experiments are important for documentation of the homogeneity of the protein, possible batch variations, and for verification of protein stability. As proteins degrade with time, comparison of the gels from failed crystallization drops with the original ones will establish if the protein

has deteriorated. Aging results from the action of contaminants either already present or introduced into the samples or from modifications generated by oxidants. In some cases, changes in crystal formation are owing to the presence of fungi or mold that multiply in the stored protein solutions. Store solutions in airtight bottles to prevent contamination by airborne micro-organisms and wear gloves during manipulations; fingers are always contaminated by proteases and bacteria that may degrade the proteins.

6. Handle the protein solution gently. When mixing a lyophilized sample into solution or thawing a sample, one should take care not to make foam, because foam can be a sign of denaturation.

7. Dialysis will remove nonvolatile buffers and other chemicals that may have been present either before lyophilization or in the solution of the final purification step. Sometimes trace amounts of impurities can affect the ability of proteins to crystallize. The buffer concentration of the sample solution (10 mM) is 10 times lower than the buffer concentration in the reservoir solutions of the screens, which usually contain 100 mM of buffer. Hence, the pH of the crystallization drops becomes closer to that of the reservoirs, which allows the screens to be more effective.

8. For obtaining the protein concentration, spectrophotometry is an accurate and easy method. Theoretical molar absorption coefficients ε of polypeptides can be calculated from the content of tryptophan and tryrosine using:

$$\varepsilon_{280nm} = 5500n_x + 1490n_y,$$

where 5500 and 1490 are the good estimates of the molecular absorption coefficients for tryptophan and tyrosine residues in proteins at 280 nm (*13*), and n_x and n_y are the numbers of those residues, respectively. Thus, protein concentration is obtained from:

$$c \ (mg/mL) = A_{280nm} \times \varepsilon_{280nm}/M_r \ (M_r; \ \text{molecular weight of the protein})$$

9. Before a crystallization experiment, solid particles such as dust, denatured proteins, and solid contaminants from purification columns should be removed. This can be achieved simply by centrifugation (20,000g for 5 min) immediately prior to setting up the crystallization trials.

10. It is better to make drops as small as possible. Saving the sample allows screening of more conditions. In addition, there is a great advantage in that a smaller drop reaches equilibrium faster, resulting in faster crystallization. One of our proteins crystallizes within a day from a drop consisting of 0.3 μL of protein and 0.3 μL of reservoir solution, however is never crystallizes from the larger drops. After solving structure, it turned out that the protein was oxidized to form a disulfide bond between two of three neighboring cysteine residues within a few days, resulting in sample heterogeneity that prevented crystallization (*see* **Note 2**).

11. When the storage space is large enough for the plates, the experiment may be continued for as long as 1 yr. Because the crystallization plates are made of polystyrene that allows for some evaporation overtime, this long-term storage can eventually result in crystallization.

12. The stereomicroscope should have an observation platform large enough to support the crystallization plate when looking at all the drops. It is better to have transmitted light with a separate light source connected with an optical fiber in order to prevent heating the base, because crystals can be dissolved easily by temperature variation.

13. It is highly recommended to use a microscope with a higher magnification lens (~×100) because it is sometimes very difficult to distinguish microcrystals and amorphous precipitates using microscopes with lower magnification (~×50). We use the Leica MZ-16 stereo microscope for viewing drops. If a stereo microscope with a high magnification lens is not available, a standard microscope with a ×10 objective lens and ×10 eyepieces for a better view may be used.

14. In protein crystals, the molecules are loosely packed with large solvent-filled channels that normally occupy 40–60% of the crystal volume. This is an advantage when reacting the protein with small reagent molecules such as dyes or heavy metal compounds to be used for phasing, because they can diffuse through these channels and reach reactive sites in the all the protein molecules in the crystal.

15. It is important to find the threshold at which the protein starts to precipitate, because nucleation of crystals usually occurs close to this point, and crystals grow under the supersaturated condition.

16. Inhibitors, substrates, or co-factors (coenzymes) induce some conformational changes in proteins upon binding, and this might result in a more compact and stable state. The apoprotein and protein–ligand complex may be sufficiently different in solubility and physical behavior in many cases. Thus, this may provide a second or third chance at growing crystals unless one does not have any crystals from the apoprotein. In addition, such a complex is inherently more interesting than the apoprotein alone when the structure is eventually determined.

References

1. Drenth, J. (1994) *Principles of Protein X-Ray Crystallography.* (Cantor, C.R., ed.), Springer-Verlag, New York.
2. Blundell, T. L. and Johnson, L. N. (eds.) (1976) *Protein Crystallography.* Academic, Inc., San Diego.
3. Blow, D. (ed.) (2002) *Outline of Crystallography for Biologists.* Oxford University Press, New York.
4. Ducruix, A. and Giege, R. (eds.) (1999) *Crystallization of Nucleic Acids and Proteins: A Practical Approach.* Oxford University Press, New York.
5. McPherson, A. (ed.) (1999) *Crystallization of Biological Macromolecules.* Cold Spring Harbor Laboratory, New York.
6. Terese, M. B. (ed.) (1999) *Protein Crystallization: Techniques, Strategies, and Tips.* International University Line, La Jolla.
7. McRee, D. E. (ed.) (1999) *Practical Protein Crystallography.* Academic, San Diego.
8. Jancarik, J. and Kim, S. H. (1991) Sparse matrix sampling: a screening method for crystallization of protein. *J. Appl. Cryst.* **24,** 409–411.

9. Vassylyev, D. G., Takeda, S., Wakatsuki, S., Maeda, K., and Maeda, Y. (1998) Crystal structure of troponin C in complex with troponin I fragment at 2.3-A resolution. *Proc. Natl. Acad. Sci. USA* **95,** 4847–4852.

10. Takeda, S., Yamashita, A., Maeda, K., and Maeda, Y. (2003) Structure of the core domain of human cardiac troponin in the Ca(2+)-saturated form. *Nature* **424,** 35–41.

11. Laemmli, U. K. (1970) Cleavage of structural proteins during the assembly of the head of bacteriophage T4. *Nature* **227,** 680–685.

12. Takeda, S., Kobayashi, T., Taniguchi, H., Hayashi, H., and Maeda, Y. (1997) Structural and functional domains of the troponin complex revealed by limited digestion. *Eur. J. Biochem.* **246,** 611–617.

13. Pace, C. N., Vajdos, F., Fee, L., Grimsley, G., and Gray, T. (1995) How to measure and predict the molar absorption coefficient of a protein. *Protein Sci.* **4,** 2411–2423.

20

Structural Elucidation of Integrin $\alpha_{IIb}\beta_3$ Cytoplasmic Domain by Nuclear Magnetic Resonance Spectroscopy

Jun Qin

Summary

Integrin $\alpha_{IIb}\beta_3$ is a heterodimeric (α/β) cell surface receptor critical for platelet aggregation, and its dysfunction is linked to thrombosis and a number of other vascular diseases. Upon agonist stimulation, which leads to platelet aggregation, $\alpha_{IIb}\beta_3$ is activated via a distinct inside-out signaling pathway, i.e., the short α_{IIb}/β_3 cytoplasmic tails receive intracellular signals, which trigger the conformational change of the extracellular domain for the high-affinity ligand binding. The structural basis for how the $\alpha_{IIb}\beta_3$ cytoplasmic face regulates the inside-out activation of the receptor has been extensively studied over the past decade. We have recently used nuclear magnetic resonance (NMR) spectroscopy to characterize and determine the structural features of the $\alpha_{IIb}\beta_3$ cytoplasmic domain. This chapter describes detailed practical procedures for performing these NMR studies, which have provided key atomic insights into the mechanism of the $\alpha_{IIb}\beta_3$ function, especially its inside-out signaling.

Key Words: Integrin; cytoplasmic domain; platelet aggregation; NMR.

1. Introduction

Integrins are a major class of heterodimeric cell surface receptors that play a key role in cell–cell and cell–extracellular matrix interactions *(1,2)*. The $\alpha_{IIb}\beta_3$ is the major integrin on platelets and is required for platelet aggregation. Dysfunction/mutation of this receptor is linked to several cardiovascular diseases, such as thrombosis, Glanzmann's thrombasthenia, and atherosclerosis *(3)*. Therefore, understanding the mechanism of the $\alpha_{IIb}\beta_3$ function is of both physiological and pathological significance. The α_{IIb}- and β_3-subunits are type I transmembrane receptors, each consisting of a single transmembrane domain, a large extracellular domain of several hundred amino acids, and a short cytoplasmic tail. The extracellular domains of the subunits are known to form a binding site

From: *Methods in Molecular Medicine, vol. 129:*
Cardiovascular Disease: Methods and Protocols, Volume 2: Molecular Medicine
Edited by: Q. K. Wang © Humana Press Inc., Totowa, NJ

for soluble ligands such as fibrinogen and von Willebrand factor, whereas the intracellular cytoplasmic tails anchor to the cytoskeletal/signaling proteins (1,2). In this manner, the inside and outside of the cells are physically linked, allowing a cooperative regulation of platelet adhesive functions.

A unique feature of the $\alpha_{IIb}\beta_3$ and other integrin receptors is their bidirectional signaling (4). Similarly to nonintegrin receptors, $\alpha_{IIb}\beta_3$ transduces signals to the cytoplasm upon binding to the extracellular ligands (outside-in signaling), which regulate cascades of intracellular responses and signaling such as phosphorylation and dephosphorylation reactions, calcium mobilization, and cytoskeleton assembly and reorganization. However, unlike other nonintegrin receptors, ligand binding to $\alpha_{IIb}\beta_3$ is not generally constitutive but is tightly modulated by intracellular signals through a process known as "inside-out" signaling (5), i.e., agonist stimulation induces an inside-out signal from the cytoplasmic face to the extracellular domain, transforming it from a low- to a high-affinity ligand-binding state (integrin activation). Extensive mutational/biochemical studies have indicated that a major conformational change occurs throughout the receptor during the inside-out signaling process (for a review, see ref. 6). The studies also revealed that although it is small and devoid of enzymatic activity, the cytoplasmic face of $\alpha_{IIb}\beta_3$ plays a central role in the control of the inside-out signaling process (6). This is evidenced by abundant biochemical/mutational data as highlighted next: (1) although intact $\alpha_{IIb}\beta_3$ can remain latent both in unstimulated cells and in a purified state, deletion of the cytoplasmic and transmembrane region activates the receptor (7); (2) point mutations in the membrane-proximal regions of the cytoplasmic tails or deletion of either can result in constitutive activation of integrin (8–10); (3) replacement of the cytoplasmic–transmembrane regions by an artificial clasp inactivates the receptor, whereas disruption of the clasp activates the receptor (11,12); (4) fluorescence resonance energy transfer (FRET) experiments in vivo demonstrated that there is a clasping/unclasping process of cytoplasmic tails during integrin activation (13). These results not only demonstrated that the $\alpha_{IIb}\beta_3$ cytoplasmic face imposes a long-range negative structural constraint on receptor activation but also led to a widespread proposition that the cytoplasmic tails of integrin α_{IIb}- and β_3-subunits interact with each other to maintain the receptor in the latent state. Biochemical (14–16) and nuclear magnetic resonance (NMR) structural (17,18) studies showed that such interaction indeed occurs.

This chapter describes the detailed practical procedures by which the NMR studies were performed to characterize the structural features of the $\alpha_{IIb}\beta_3$ cytoplasmic tails both in aqueous solution (17) and in a membrane environment (19), which have provided key atomic insights into the mechanism of the $\alpha_{IIb}\beta_3$ function, especially its inside-out signaling pathway during integrin activation.

2. Materials

2.1. Peptide Synthesis and Preparation of Bacterial Expression Vectors

1. The unlabeled cytoplasmic tails of α_{IIb} (989–1008) and β_3-N (719–739) (C-terminal D740-T762 is truncated) are synthesized by Lerner Research Institute Biotechnology Core. The peptides are HPLC-purified and verified by mass spectroscopy.
2. The α_{IIb} cytoplasmic tail is subcloned into the pET31b vector (Novagen, Inc.), which expresses small peptides in *Escherichia coli* into the inclusion bodies by fusing to an insoluble protein, ketosteroid isomerase (KSI).
3. The β_3 cytoplasmic tail is subcloned into the pET15b vector (Novagen, Inc.), which expresses proteins/peptides in *E. coli* by fusing to a linker containing His-tag, GSS(H)$_6$SSGLVPRGSHM. The linker is cleavable by CNBr.
4. α_{IIb} and β_3 cytoplasmic tails are subcloned into the pMAL-c2x vector (MBP-α_{IIb} and MBP-β_3) containing a highly soluble N-terminal maltose-binding protein (MBP) as the fusion (New England Biolabs, Inc.) (*see* **Note 1**).

2.2. Protein Expression and Purification

1. Standard LB medium for preparing bacterially produced unlabeled proteins/peptides.
2. M9 minimal medium containing ^{15}NH4Cl (1.1 g/L) and/or ^{13}C glucose (3 g/L) and/or ^{2}H$_2$O. The detailed protocols for making the medium are shown in **Tables 1** and **2**. To make a 70% deuterated sample (average percentage), 70% ^{2}H$_2$O and 30% H$_2$O are mixed as the water medium.
3. French press for lysing large volume of cells (<40 mL lyse buffer).
4. Nickel resin (Novagen, Inc.) and Amylose resin (Amsham Bioscience, Inc.) for affinity-based protein purification.
5. Superdex-75 Column for gel-filtration experiment.
6. Fast protein liquid chromatography (FPLC) purification system.

2.3. NMR Instruments, Computers, and Software

1. Greater than 500 MHz NMR spectrometer equipped with a triple-resonance (^{1}H/^{15}N/^{13}C) probe or triple-resonance cryogenic probe.
2. Silicon graphics (SGI) workstation.
3. NMRPipe *(20)* for NMR data processing and analysis, PIPP *(21)* for data analysis.
4. Xplor-NIH *(22)* installed on SGI for structure calculation.
5. Insight II (Accelrys, Inc.) and MolMol *(23)* installed on SGI for structural analysis and display.

3. Methods

3.1. Bacterial Expression and Purification of α_{IIb} and β_3 Tails

The α_{IIb} tail is expressed in *E. coli* into the inclusion bodies using the pET31b construct. Purification of the peptide including the CNBr cleavage of KSI was performed according to the standard procedures provided by the manufacturer (Novagen, Inc.). The β_3 tail (K716-T762) is expressed in *E. coli* using the pET15b

Table 1
Composition of Minimal Medium[a]

Compound	Amount	Comments
K_2HPO_4	10.0 g/L	
KH_2PO_4	13.0 g/L	
Na_2HPO_4	9.0 g/L	
K_2SO_4	2.4 g/L	
$^{15}NH_4Cl$	1.1 g/L	
^{13}C Glucose[c]	2–5 g/L	Amount variable and must be optimized to reduce the cost (~$100/g)
Trace element solution[b,c]	10 mL/L	*See* **Table 2**
1 *M* $MgCl_2 \cdot 6H_2O$[c]	10 mL/L	
Thiamine (Vit. B_1), 5 mg/mL[c]	6 mL/L	
Antibiotics[c]	~0.1 mg/L	

[a]The media must be sterilized.
[b]Trace element solution is a combination of trace elements shown in **Table 2**.
[c]Sterilized using a 0.2-μM filter (no autoclaving).

Table 2
Composition of Trace Element Solution[a]

Compound	g/100 mL[b]
$CaCl_2 2H_2O$	0.600
$FeSO_4 7H_2O$	0.600
$MnCl_2 4H_2O$	0.115
$CoCl_2 6H_2O$	0.080
$ZnSO_4 7H_2O$	0.070
$CuCl_2 2H_2O$	0.030
H_3BO_3	0.002
$(NH_4)_6Mo_7O_{24} 4H_2O$	0.025
EDTA	0.500

[a]Add ingredients one at a time, waiting 5–10 min before they fully dissolve. After adding EDTA and stirring for a few hours, the color of the solution should be golden brown (if it is greenish, then leave stirring overnight). Sterilize afterwards by filtering through a 0.2-μM filter.
[b]A fresh stock of 100–200 mL is usually made and sterilized using a 0.2-μM filter (no autoclaving).

construct and purified using a denaturation-renaturation protocol (Novagen, Inc.) followed by HPLC (*see* **Note 2**). Expression and purification of the α_{IIb} and β_3 tails each fused to MBP were performed according to the protocols from New England Biolabs, Inc. followed by gel-filtration (*see* **Note 3**). All purified peptides and proteins are verified by sodium dodecyl sulfate-polyacrylamide gel electrophoresis (SDS-PAGE). To make isotope-labeled α_{IIb} tail, β_3 tail, MBP-α_{IIb} tail, and MBP-β_3 tail, cells were grown in M9 minimal medium containing $^{15}NH4Cl$ (1.1 g/L) and/or ^{13}C glucose (3 g/L) and/or ^2H_2O.

3.2. Sample Preparation of Isotope-Labeled and Unlabeled α_{IIb} Tail, β_3 Tail, and α_{IIb}/β_3 Tail Complex in Solution

1. Samples for ^1H–^{13}C heteronuclear single quantum coherence (HSQC) titration experiments: to examine the α_{IIb}/β_3 tail interaction, HSQC titration experiments are performed by keeping the ^{15}N-labeled α_{IIb} at 80 μM mixed with 1–3 concentration of unlabeled β_3 or vice versa (*see* **Note 4**).

2. Samples for structural analyses of the α_{IIb}/β_3 tail complex in aqueous solution: to detect intermolecular nuclear Overhauser effects (NOEs) and to analyze the structures of the unlabeled bound peptides, 1 mM $^{15}N/^{13}C$-labeled MBP-β_3 is mixed with 1–3 mM unlabeled α_{IIb} peptide in 20 mM phosphate buffer, pH 6.3, 5 mM Ca^{2+} (*see* **Note 5**). To examine the transferred NOE, a solution of 1 mM unlabeled α_{IIb} tail is prepared in the absence or presence of 0.1 mM MBP-β_3 in 20 mM phosphate buffer, 5 mM Ca^{2+}, pH 6.3. Similarly, a solution of 1 mM unlabeled β_3-N (K716–K738) is prepared in the absence or presence of 0.1 mM MBP-α_{IIb} in 20 mM phosphate buffer, 5 mM Ca^{2+}, pH 6.3 (*see* **Note 5**). A 1 mM mixture of α_{IIb} tail and β_3-N in 1:1 ratio is also made for a two-dimensional (2D) nuclear Overhauser enhancement spectroscopy (NOESY) experiment as compared with the free α_{IIb} and β_3-N.

3. Samples for structural analyses of α_{IIb} tail and β_3 tail in membrane-mimic dodecylphosphocholine (DPC) micelles. To characterize the structures and membrane-binding properties of α_{IIb} and β_3 tails, 1 mM ^{15}N- and/or ^{13}C-labeled α_{IIb} or β_3 tail is dissolved in 50, 100, 150, 300, and 500 mM deuterated DPC in 20 mM phosphate buffer, 5 mM Ca^{2+}, pH 6.3. The 300 mM DPC is chosen as the optimal condition for binding (spectra no longer change when adding more DPC). To detect the intermolecular NOEs between $^{15}N/^{13}C$-labeled α_{IIb}/β_3 tails and DPC, nondeuterated DPC is used (*see* **Note 6**).

3.3. NMR Experiments and Structural Analysis of α_{IIb}/β_3 Complex in Aqueous Solution

All heteronuclear NMR experiments in aqueous solution are performed as described in **refs.** *24* and *25*. These experiments obtain two types of information: (1) through-bond connectivities on which all the individual $^1H/^{15}N/^{13}C$ nuclei could be assigned (*17*) and (2) through-space connectivities on which proton–proton contacts within less than 5 Å can be identified and assigned based on the assignments from (1) (*17*). All experiments are performed at 25°C. All of the spectra are processed with NMRPipe (*15*) and visualized with Pipp (*16*).

1. α_{IIb}/β_3 tail interaction as examined by HSQC experiments: once the resonance assignments of free ^{15}N-α_{IIb} and ^{15}N-β_3 tails are assigned, HSQC experiments can

be performed to examine the interaction of ^{15}N-labeled α_{IIb} with unlabeled β_3 or vice versa using the samples prepared under **Subheading 3.2.** (*see* **Note 7**).

2. α_{IIb}/β_3 tail interaction as examined by NOESY experiments: 2D NOESY experiments (mixing time 400 ms) are performed on the free form of α_{IIb} tail, β_3-N, and the mixture of α_{IIb}/β_3-N. As a result of the binding-induced folding, the mixture of α_{IIb}/β_3-N should give a much larger amount of NOEs as compared with the sum of NOEs obtained from free α_{IIb} and β_3-N *(18,19)*.

3. α_{IIb}/β_3 tail interaction as examined by transferred NOE experiments: to increase the solubility of the α_{IIb}/β_3 tail complex in water and to obtain additional structural information for the α_{IIb}/β_3 tail interaction, the highly soluble MBP was used and found to be highly effective *(17)*. In particular, MBP fused to the β_3 dramatically increases the solubility of the β_3 tail at pH greater than 6.0. Further, MBP artificially increases the size of the weakly bound peptide complex, which makes it feasible to perform high-sensitivity transferred NOE experiments *(26)* (*see* the sample preparation in **Subheading 3.2.**). Transferred NOESY experiments are performed with mixing times of 100, 200, 300, and 400 ms to analyze NOE build-up in order to eliminate spin-diffusion artifacts (*see* **Note 8**). A control NOESY experiment (mixing time 400 ms) is always performed, e.g., on the 1 m*M* α_{IIb} tail mixed with 0.1 m*M* MBP (obtained by cleaving β_3 tail from MBP-β_3 followed by gel-filtration) (*see* **Note 8**). Double-quantum-filtered (DQF)-correlation spectroscopy (COSY), total correlated spectroscopy (TOCSY) (mixing time 60 ms), and NOESY (mixing time 300 ms) are performed to assign resonances in both free and bound peptides using the conventional 2D NMR method *(27)*. Because the chemical shift changes of either α_{IIb} or β_3 tails are small upon their interactions, the assignments are transferable between free and bound forms.

4. *Filtered* NOESY experiments to detect intermolecular NOEs between α_{IIb} and β_3 tails: as a result of the high solubility of the α_{IIb}/β_3 complex fused to MBP (>1 m*M*), intermolecular NOEs between the α_{IIb} and ^{15}N/^{13}C-labeled MBP-β_3 could be obtained using 2D/three-dimensional (3D) ^{15}N/^{13}C-filtered NOESY *(28)* (mixing time 150 ms; *see also* the sample preparation in **Subheading 3.2.**). A control experiment is performed on ^{15}N/^{13}C-labeled MBP mixed with an unlabeled α_{IIb} tail, which should yield no intermolecular NOEs. The resonance assignments of the unlabeled α_{IIb} peptide in complex with ^{15}N/^{13}C-labeled MBP-β_3 are made using 2D ^{14}N/^{12}C filtered TOCSY and NOESY spectra *(29)*. These assignments are transferable to those in MBP-β_3 *(17)*.

5. Structure determination of α_{IIb}/β_3 tail complex. Structure determination of the α_{IIb}/β_3 tail complex can be performed based on a combination of the transferred NOEs, 2D ^{14}N/^{12}C-filtered NOEs of the bound peptides, and intermolecular NOEs between the peptides. The structure of the α_{IIb}/β_3 complex can be calculated on the SGI workstation using X-PLOR-NIH *(22)*. The individual subunit structures of α_{IIb} and β_3 tails are first calculated separately based on a combination of 2D ^{14}N/^{12}C-filtered NOEs of the bound peptides and transferred NOEs. The complex is then calculated afterward by including intermolecular NOEs. The distance restraints were grouped into four distance ranges, 1.8–2.5, 1.8–3.5, 1.8–5.0, and 1.8–6.0 Å, corresponding to strong, medium, weak, and very weak NOEs.

3.4. NMR Experiments and Structural Analysis of α_{IIb}/β_3 Tails in DPC Micelles

The resonance assignments and NOE analyses (τ_m = 150 ms) of $^{15}N/^{13}C$-labeled α_{IIb}/β_3 tails in DPC are made using the same set of standard triple-resonance experiments as in **Subheading 3.3.**, but at the temperature of 40°C to reduce DPC-induced line-broadening. Intermolecular NOEs between DPC and $^{15}N/^{13}C$-labeled β_3 are obtained using 3D $^{15}N/^{13}C$ filtered (F1) NOESY with mixing time of τ_m = 100 ms. Structure calculations of α_{IIb}/β_3 tails in DPC are performed as described previously for individual α_{IIb}- or β_3-subunits.

4. Notes

1. There is a long linker between MBP and the β_3 tail: S(N)$_{10}$LGIEGRISEFGS, which is cleavable by factor Xa (New England Biolabs, Inc). Importantly, although MBP dramatically increases the solubility of β_3 tail and its complex with α_{IIb} tail, it exerts little effect on the structural properties of the fused β_3 tail and its interaction with the α_{IIb} tail *(17)*.

2. The β_3 cytoplasmic tail peptide is easy to precipitate at greater than 1 m*M* and pH greater than 6.0 in pure water. The precipitation occurs more easily when there is salt in the solution. In contrast, the α_{IIb} cytoplasmic tail is highly soluble at pH greater than 6.0, and is tolerable with salt. We often keep the α_{IIb} peptide in a 10 m*M* stock solution at pH 6.2, 5 m*M* CaCl$_2$, 20 m*M* phosphate buffer.

3. The quality of amylase resin purchased from the company varies time to time, which affects the purification yield of the MBP-β_3 or MBP-α_{IIb} tail. Keep in mind that the affinity between MBP and the resin is low (~3 μ*M*), and thus one may see a substantial amount of unbound MBP-α_{IIb} or MBP-β_3 tails in the wash fractions. Remember to run gel filtration after the elusion of the MBP-α_{IIb} and MBP-β_3 from the amylase resin. This is especially important for MBP-β_3, because some fraction of MBP-β_3 is aggregated during the purification. It is strongly recommended that protease cocktail inhibitors be added throughout the purification.

4. It is very easy to induce precipitation when mixing α_{IIb}/β_3 peptides, possibly as a result of the formation of unstable complex. Our experience indicates that is important to keep the α_{IIb} and β_3 peptides in a very low-salt condition for the HSQC titration experiments. The more salt the solution contains, the more precipitation can occur while mixing the α_{IIb}/β_3 peptides. The α_{IIb}/β_3 tail interaction is noticeable only when the pH of the mixture is greater than 6.0. We normally keep the pH at 6.2–6.5. Higher pH (>6.5) can induce large precipitation for the α_{IIb}/β_3 peptide mixture. Also, less precipitation occurs when adding excess of α_{IIb} into ^{15}N-labeled β_3 than vice versa, because the β_3 tail is much less soluble than the α_{IIb} peptide.

5. Divalent cations, including Ca^{2+}, bind to the C-terminal of the α_{IIb} tail in a 1:1 stoichiometry, which stabilizes the α/β complex *(15–17)* and stabilizes the α_{IIb} structure *(30)*. Hence, 5 m*M* Ca^{2+} is used to saturate or nearly saturate the 1 m*M* peptides. Although a high concentration of calcium phosphate may lead to some precipitation, we found that 5 m*M* CaCl$_2$ dissolved in 20 m*M* phosphate buffer did

not induce precipitation. Because α_{IIb} is highly soluble, its excess can be mixed with $^{15}N/^{13}C$-labeled MBP-β_3 for detecting intermolecular NOEs.

6. Because of a high concentration of DPC (300 mM), the NOE intensities may be too high. We found that adding some fraction (200 mM) of deuterated DPC to non-deuterated DPC (100 mM) helps to reduce the NOE intensity without losing the intermolecular NOE information.

7. These experiments take a few hours or overnight because they must be performed at low concentration (<0.1 mM) as a result of the low solubility of the mixture *(17)*. Small yet definitive chemical shift changes could be observed for ^{15}N-labeled α_{IIb} in the absence and presence of unlabeled β_3 or vice versa *(17)*.

8. Although spin diffusion might occur at a higher mixing time, our experience indicated that 400 ms mixing time was fine to generate a well folded α_{IIb} tail structure bound to MBP-β_3. Among all the NMR experiments we have used to detect α_{IIb}/β_3 tail interaction, this transferred NOE experiment is the most sensitive and efficient way. However, care must be taken to avoid some aggregation-induced NOE. In other words, if a peptide is mixed with any aggregated proteins, one may observe some nonspecific binding between the peptide and the aggregate. Hence, it is important to run gel filtration to eliminate the aggregated component and also run a control experiment in which MBP alone is mixed with the target peptide for the study.

Acknowledgments

The author would like to thank Olga Vinogradova, Thomas Haas, Edward Plow, Julie Vaynberg, and Xiangming Kong for useful discussions. This work was supported by National Institutes of Health grants to J. Q.

References

1. Hynes, R. O. (1987) Integrins: a family of cell surface receptors. *Cell* **48,** 549–550.
2. Schwartz, M. A., Schaller, M. D., and Ginsberg, M. H. (1995) Integrins: emerging paradigms of signal transduction. *Annu. Rev. Cell. Biol.* **11,** 549–599.
3. Shattil, S. J. and Ginsberg, M. H. (1997) Integrin signaling in vascular biology. *J. Clin. Invest.* **100,** S91–S95.
4. Giancotti, F. G. and Ruoslahti, E. (1999) Integrin signaling. *Science* **285,** 1028–1032.
5. Hughes, P. E. and Pfaff, M. Integrin affinity modulation. (1998) *Trends Cell Biol.* **8,** 359–364.
6. Woodside, D. G., Liu, S., and Ginsberg, M. (2001) Integrin activation. *Thromb. Haemost.* **86,** 316–323.
7. Peterson, J. A., Visentin, G. P., Newman, P. J., and Aster, R. H. (1998) A recombinant soluble form of the integrin alpha IIb beta 3 (GPIIb-IIIa) assumes an active, ligand-binding conformation and is recognized by GPIIb-IIIa-specific monoclonal, allo-, auto-, and drug-dependent platelet antibodies. *Blood* **92,** 2053–2063.
8. O'Toole, T. E., Mandelman, D., Forsyth, J., Shattil, S. J., Plow, E. F., and Ginsberg, M. H. (1991) Modulation of the affinity of integrin alpha $_{IIb}$beta$_3$ (GPIIb-IIIa) by the cytoplasmic domain of alpha$_{IIb}$. *Science* **254,** 845–847.

9. O'Toole, T. E., Katagiri, Y., Faull, R. J., et al. (1994) Integrin cytoplasmic domains mediate inside-out signal transduction. *J. Cell Biol.* **124,** 1047–1059.

10. Hughes, P. E., Diaz-Gonzalez, F., Leong, L., et al. (1996) Breaking the integrin hinge. A defined structural constraint regulates integrin signaling. *J. Biol. Chem.* **271,** 6571–6574.

11. Lu, C., Takagi, J., and Springer, T. A. (2001) Association of the membrane proximal regions of the alpha and beta subunit cytoplasmic domains constrains an integrin in the inactive state. *J. Biol. Chem.* **276,** 14,642–14,648.

12. Takagi, J., Erickson, H. P., and Springer, T. A. (2001) C-terminal opening mimics 'inside-out' activation of integrin alpha5beta1. *Nat. Struct. Biol.* **8,** 412–416.

13. Kim, M., Carman, C. V., and Springer, T. A. (2003) Bidirectional transmembrane signaling by cytoplasmic domain separation in integrins. *Science* **301,** 1720–1725.

14. Muir, T. W., Williams, M. J., Ginsberg, M. H., and Kent, S. B. (1994) Design and chemical synthesis of a neoprotein structural model for the cytoplasmic domain of a multisubunit cell-surface receptor: integrin alpha IIb beta 3 (platelet GPIIb-IIIa). *Biochemistry* **33,** 7701–7708.

15. Haas, T. A. and Plow, E. F. (1996) The cytoplasmic domain of α$_{IIb}$β$_3$: a ternary complex of the integrin α and β subunits and a divalent cation. *J. Biol. Chem.* **271,** 6017–6026.

16. Vallar, L. and Kieffer, N. (1999) Divalent cations differentially regulate integrin α$_{IIb}$ cytoplasmic tail binding to β$_3$ and to Calcium- and integrin-binding protein. *J. Biol. Chem.* **274,** 17,257–17,266.

17. Vinogradova, O., Velyvis, A., Velyviene, A., et al. (2002) A structural mechanism of integrin alpha(IIb)beta(3) "inside-out" activation as regulated by its cytoplasmic face. *Cell* **110,** 587–597.

18. Weijie, A. M., Hwang, P. M., and Vogel, H. J. (2002) Solution structures of the cytoplasmic tail complex from platelet integrin alpha IIb- and beta 3-subunits. *Proc. Natl. Acad. Sci. USA* **99,** 5878–5883.

19. Vinogradova, O., Vaynberg, J., Kong, X., Haas, T. A., Plow, E. F., and Qin, J. (2004) Membrane-mediated structural transitions at the cytoplasmic face during integrin activation. *Proc. Natl. Acad. Sci. USA* **101,** 4094–4099.

20. Delaglio, F., Grzesiek, S., Vuister, G. W., Zhu, G., Pfeifer, J., and Bax, A. (1995) NMRPipe: a multidimensional spectral processing system based on UNIX pipes. *J. Bio. NMR* **6,** 277–293.

21. Garrett, D. S., Powers, R., Gronenborn, A. M., and Clore, G. M. (1991) A common sense approach to peak picking in two- three- and four-dimensional spectra using automatic computer analysis of contour diagrams. *J. Magn. Res.* **95,** 214–220.

22. Schwieters, C. D., Kuszewski, J. I., Tjandra, N., and Clore, G. M. (2003) The Xplor-NIH NMR molecular structure determination package. *J. Magn. Res.* **160,** 65–73.

23. Koradi, R., Billeter, M., and Wuthrich, K. (1996) MOLMOL: a program for display and analysis of macromolecular structures. *J. Mol. Graph.* **14,** 51–55, 29–32.

24. Clore, G. M. and Gronenborn, A. M. (1998) Determining the structures of large proteins and protein complexes by NMR. *Trends Biotechnol.* **16,** 22–34.

25. Ferentz, A. E. and Wagner, G. (2000) NMR spectroscopy: a multifaceted approach to macromolecular structure. *Q. Rev. Biophys.* **33,** 29–65.

26. Clore, G. M. and Gronenborn, A. (1983) Theory of the time-dependent nuclear overhauser effect–applications to structural analysis of ligand-protein complexes in solution. *J. Magn. Res.* **53,** 423–442.

27. Wüthrich, K. (1986) *NMR of Proteins and Nucleic Acids.* John Wiley and Sons, New York.

28. Zwahlen, C., Legault, P., Vincent, S. J. F., Greenblatt, J., Konrat, R., and Kay, L. E. (1997) Methods for measurement of intermolecular NOEs by multinuclear NMR spectroscopy: application to a bacteriophage (N-peptide/box B RNA complex. *J. Am. Chem. Soc.* **119,** 711–721.

29. Ikura, M. and Bax, A. (1992) Isotope-filtered 2D NMR of a protein-peptide complex: study of a skeletal muscle myosin light chain kinase fragment bound to calmodulin. *J. Am. Chem. Soc.* **114,** 2433–2440.

30. Vinogradova, O., Haas, T., Plow, E. F., and Qin, J. (2000) A structural basis for integrin activation by the cytoplasmic tail of the α_{IIb} subunit. *Proc. Natl. Acad. Sci. USA* **97,** 1450–1455.

21

Applications of Electron Cryo-Microscopy to Cardiovascular Research

Ashraf Kitmitto

Summary

Electron cryo-microscopy (cryo-EM) techniques have wide applications for the study of biological structures. The focus of this chapter is the use of cryo-EM and associated methods for the analysis of the three-dimensional (3D) structure of proteins and multicomponent macromolecular assemblies. Data evolving from these methods pertaining to the quaternary organization of proteins and protein–protein interactions, bridges an important gap between linear genomic information and understanding physiological function. This chapter provides general methods for examining two-dimensional crystalline arrays of proteins as well as single, randomly oriented protein complexes. It is significant that single-particle analysis of electron microscopy images has provided the only 3D data to-date for the two principal components of muscle excitation contraction coupling in the heart, namely the L-type voltage-gated calcium channel and the ryanodine receptor. This chapter describes approaches for identifying the extracellular and intracellular domains of the 3D structure of the L-type voltage-gated calcium channel and also incorporates general details for labeling and visualizing His-tagged proteins.

Key Words: Cryo-electron microscopy; electron crystallography; single particle analysis; L-type voltage-gated calcium channels; cardiac calcium cycling.

1. Introduction

The imaging of biological specimens by electron microscopic methods provides a means to determine the three-dimensional (3D) structure of large macromolecular complexes, as well as relatively small proteins, with wider applications for capturing conformational states and protein–protein interactions (for examples, *see* **refs.** *1* and *2*). Electron cryo-microscopy (cryo-EM) involves the quick freezing of a biological sample in an aqueous environment. The sample is plunged into liquid ethane with vitrification of the specimen by rapid cooling preventing evaporation of the surrounding water molecules. The

From: *Methods in Molecular Medicine, vol. 129:*
Cardiovascular Disease: Methods and Protocols, Volume 2: Molecular Medicine
Edited by: Q. K. Wang © Humana Press Inc., Totowa, NJ

freezing velocity (>10,000 Ks^{-1}) is at such a speed that the water molecules have no time to crystallize. The specimen is therefore imaged in its frozen-hydrated state close to native conditions free of chemical stains or fixatives. Advantages of this cooling process are that radiation damage by the electron beam is limited and thermal vibrations are minimized.

Cryo-EM has, over the last 10–15 yr, made a significant impact toward studying macromolecules not readily amenable to nuclear magnetic resonance (NMR) and X-ray crystallography methods. One approach is the analysis of two-dimensional (2D) crystals of proteins termed *electron crystallography*. However, not all protein complexes are amenable to 2D crystallization methods or are available in sufficient quantities to undertake crystallization trials. Techniques have therefore been developed for the study of randomly orientated nonordered single protein complexes in solution using a technique called *single-particle analysis* (SPA). Both electron crystallography and SPA have been applied to the study of proteins in the heart. Analysis of 2D crystals of the cardiac gap junctions provided structural details that enabled an understanding at the molecular level of current flow in the heart *(3)*. Examples of 3D structures of cardiac proteins determined using SPA include the intact ATP synthase from bovine heart mitochondria *(4)* and bovine cardiac NADH:ubiquinone oxidoreductase (complex I) *(5)*. Calcium homeostasis in the heart is regulated by the synergistic action of a series of proteins, many of which are membrane proteins such as the L-type voltage-gated calcium channels (VGCC), the ryanodine receptor, sodium/calcium exchanger, sarcoplasmic recticulum Ca^{2+}ATPase, and the plasma membrane calcium pump; for review, *see* **ref. 6**. It is noteworthy that with the exception of the skeletal muscle isoform of the Ca^{2+}ATPase *(7)*, there are no high-resolution structures currently available for the aforementioned channels, pumps, and transporters; this is probably due in part to difficulties in overexpressing and purifying these poly-topic integral membrane proteins. SPA methods, typically only requiring micro-gram amounts of protein, have led to the determination of the only 3D structures for the ryanodine receptor *(8)* and the cardiac L-type calcium channel *(9)* to-date. Cryo-EM and SPA methods have also advanced our understanding of the molecular basis of ryanodine receptor regulation through small ligand and protein binding (for examples, *see* **refs. 2** and *10*). Other exciting developments in cryo-EM techniques include time-resolved studies whereby transient states are freeze-trapped on a millisecond time scale *(11)*.

Other applications of cryo-EM include electron tomography for mapping complex multicomponent assemblies and cells with the potential to provide information to span the gap between molecular and cellular studies. However, this chapter will focus on general approaches and considerations for specimen preparation for the study of either 2D crystals or single particles together with techniques for identifying particular functional groups and protein domains. Methods for labeling the extracellular and intracellular polypeptides of the L-type VGCC are described as well as a general method for labeling His-tagged proteins.

2. Materials

2.1. Negative Staining

1. 2% (w/v) uranyl acetate in Milli-Q water.
2. Parafilm.
3. Whatman 50 filter paper.
4. A selection of tweezers: fine-tip, curved, straight-tipped, and self-gripping cross-over type.
5. Grid storage box.

2.2. Cryo-EM

1. Dewar flask.
2. Liquid nitrogen.
3. Ethane gas and vessel for holding liquid ethane slurry in liquid nitrogen bath. **Safety note:** if liquid ethane comes in contact with skin, it will cause burning; therefore, wear appropriate protective clothing and safety glasses.
4. Freeze-plunger unit.
5. Whatman 50 filter paper.
6. Grid box for storage in liquid nitrogen.

2.3. Cryo-Negative Staining

1. 10% (w/v) ammonium molybdate in Milli-Q water. Using concentrated HCl, adjust the pH to between pH 6.5 and 7.0.
2. 2% (w/v) trehalose in Milli-Q water.
3. Parafilm.
4. Whatman 50 filter paper.
5. A selection of tweezers: fine-tip, curved, straight-tipped, and self-gripping cross-over type.
6. Grid storage box.

2.4. Lectin-Gold Labeling of the Extracellular Glycosylated Moieties of the α_2-Subunit of the L-Type VGCC

1. Wheat germ agglutinin (WGA)-5 nm gold (British Biocell Ltd.).
2. Protease inhibitors added to buffers for final concentrations of 0.1 mM phenylmethylsulfonyl fluoride (PMSF), 1 µM pepstatin A, and 1 mM benzamidine.
3. Eppendorf tubes (1.5 mL).

2.5. Immuno-Labeling of the Intracellular β-Subunit of the L-Type VGCC

1. Eppendorf tubes (1.5 mL).
2. 10-mL screw-top ultracentrifuge tubes (Beckman) for 70.1 Ti rotor (Beckman).

3. Anti-β polyclonal antibody a gift from Professor Annette C. Dolphin, University College London, UK *(12)*.

Several antibodies against the individual L-type VGCC subunits are available commercially and can be used in place of the antibody employed in this method.

2.6. Labeling of His-Tagged Proteins Using Ni-NTA Gold

1. Ni-NTA gold-1.8 nm (Nanoprobes Inc.).
2. Copper (400 mesh) carbon-coated glow discharged grid.
3. Milli-Q water.
4. 2% (w/v) uranyl acetate in Milli-Q water.
5. Whatman 50 filter paper.
6. Parafilm.
7. A selection of tweezers: fine-tip, curved, straight-tipped, and self-gripping cross-over type.

3. Methods

For the examination of a biological sample in a microscope, the sample must be supported. In transmission electron microscopy, the sample is mounted on a grid commonly made from a copper mesh (diameter of 3.05 mm). For negative staining purposes, copper grids (400 mesh) with a carbon support film overlaid (typically 5–10 nm thick) are suitable in most cases. However, for high-resolution cryo-EM studies, the choice of grid type is more critical; therefore, before providing details of methods for sample preparation, the types of grids available are discussed briefly as follows. Bare grids (i.e., devoid of support film) may be purchased and support films produced in-house. However, this requires substantial expertise and specialist equipment, and because a wide variety of grids are available commercially, these methods will not be described here.

3.1. EM Grids

3.1.1. Grids for 2D Crystals

The flatness of the carbon support film is critical. If the film is not flat, then this can lead to a nonuniform ice layer. Furthermore, the presence of irregularities in the carbon support film can lead to crystalline areas at slightly different tilt angles, leading experimentally to blurring of diffraction spots of merged data and loss of high-resolution data (*see* **Note 1**).

3.1.2. Holey Grids

For studies of randomly oriented individual complexes in solution (single particles), holey grids are routinely used. The carbon is deposited on the grid so that it is punctuated by holes, with the application of the sample leading to the protein occupying the holes and thereby eliminating any noise contribution from the carbon film (*see* **Note 2**).

3.2. Sample Preparation

The following methods are general procedures applicable to a protein sample in solution.

3.2.1. Negative Staining

This is a rapid method for fixing the biological sample on an EM grid and is advised as a first step in order to check the sample homogeneity, or the size and order of 2D crystalline arrays and the conditions and concentrations required for adherence to the EM grid with and without glow discharging (*see* **Note 3**), prior to undertaking the more technically demanding methods for sample vitrification.

1. Pipet a 10- to 20-µL aliquot of the protein sample (protein concentration ~100 µg/mL^{-1}) on a sheet of Parafilm (*see* **Note 4**).
2. Float a glow discharged carbon-coated grid shiny side (the side with the carbon support film overlaid) in contact with the surface of the droplet for 30 s (*see* **Note 5**).
3. Blot the grid at 90° to a filter paper continuously for a minimum of 10 s. Hold the grid at right angles to the filter paper so that only the edge of the grid is in contact with the filter paper (*see* **Note 6**).
4. Float the grid on a 20-µL droplet of Milli-Q water for 5–10 s (*see* **Note 7**).
5. Blot the grid after each wash by holding it at 90° to a filter paper continuously for a minimum of 10 s (*see* **Note 8**).
6. Float the grid on a 20-µL droplet of 2% (w/v) uranyl acetate for 30 s (*see* **Notes 9 and 10**).
7. Blot the grid at 90° to a filter paper continuously for 15 s, then blot the back (dull side) of the grid (i.e., not the side on which the carbon film and sample has been applied) for at least 15 s.
8. Transfer the grid to another pair of tweezers and repeat the blotting regimen several times.
9. Allow the grid to air-dry and place in a grid box until required.

3.2.2. Sample Vitrification (Cryo-EM)

Much of the sample preparation for cryo-EM can be automated, e.g., Vitroblot™. The advantages of using an automated system are that conditions are reproducible but with the flexibility of the user being able to define both the physical and mechanical conditions. It is important to regulate temperature, relative humidity, blotting conditions (number and duration), and freezing velocity. However, the various steps can be broken down as follows, with a freeze-plunger as a minimum requirement.

1. Fill a large dewar flask with liquid nitrogen.
2. Ethane gas is applied into a metal cup seated in the bath of liquid nitrogen (*see* **Note 11**).
3. Pick up an EM grid with tweezers with a clamping ring (straight with fine tips) to grip the grid.
4. Insert the tweezers and grid into the plunger and position directly above the liquid ethane.
5. Using a 0.5- to 10-µL pipet, apply a small volume of the sample. e.g., 3–5 µL, at a suitable dilution to the grid (*see* **Note 12**).
6. With a filter paper, touch the face of the grid (with the sample loaded) with the filter paper to produce a thin film over the grid (*see* **Notes 13** and **14**). **Note:** as the filter paper is taken away and loses contact with the grid, the plunger plunges the grid into the liquid ethane with a high velocity.
7. Detach the tweezers from the plunger, and make sure to keep the grid in the surrounding liquid nitrogen.
8. Transfer the grid into a storage box maintained in the surrounding liquid nitrogen bath (*see* **Notes 15** and **16**).

3.2.3. Cryo-Negative Staining

A method that is rapidly gaining in popularity is a combination of cryo-EM and negative staining, aptly termed cryo-negative staining *(13,14)*. The methods described here have been optimized for the examination of single protein complexes in solution.

3.2.3.1. METHOD 1

1. Pipet a 20-µL aliquot of the protein sample (protein concentrations ~100–150 µg/mL) on a sheet of Parafilm (*see* **Note 12**).
2. Float a carbon-coated holey grid on the surface of the droplet for 30 s.
3. Blot the grid at 90° to a filter paper continuously for a minimum of 10 s (*see* **Note 6**).
4. Mix equal volumes (e.g., 250 µL of each) of freshly prepared 2% (w/v) trehalose and 10% (w/v) ammonium molybdate, vortex, and centrifuge the mixture for 5 min at 5000*g* (Eppendorf centrifuge 5415C, precooled).
5. Aliquot 20 µL of the ammonium molybdate/trehalose mix onto a sheet of Parafilm.
6. Float the blotted grid from **step 4** on the 20-µL droplet of the ammonium molybdate/trehalose mix for 30 s.
7. Blot the grid at 90° to a filter paper continuously for 15 s, and then blot the back of the grid so that the dull side, i.e., not the side on which the carbon coat and sample have been deposited, is in full contact with the filter paper for about 15 s. Repeat this blotting regimen several times.

3.2.3.2. METHOD 2

This method is particularly recommended when preferred orientations of the sample are observed in preliminary studies, and is used in conjunction with holey grids.

1. Pipet a 20-µL droplet of the protein sample (at 150–200 µg/mL) in a 1.5-mL Eppendorf tube.
2. To the sample add an equal volume, i.e., 20 µL, of 10% (w/v) ammonium molybdate and 20 µL of 2 % (w/v) trehalose solution.
3. Vortex the mixture for 5 s.
4. Aliquot a 20-µL drop of the protein/molybdate/trehalose mix on to a sheet of Parafilm.
5. Float a holey carbon grid on the droplet for 1 min (*see* **Note 17**).
6. Blot as in **Subheading 3.2.3.1., step 7**.

In both Methods 1 and 2, the grid is then placed in a specimen cryo-holder cooled in liquid nitrogen, which is then inserted into the microscope. Wait until the temperature drops to less than –180°C and stabilizes before examining the grid. If the grid is examined under room temperature conditions, this is then negative staining.

3.3. Labeling of Purified Proteins for Identification of Domains and Subunits

An important step in terms of characterising a protein complex in three dimensions is the identification of domains, or subunits within the complex. Methods for labeling the extracellular and intracellular polypeptides of the L-type VGCC are described. Labeled protein was visualized using negative-staining methods, giving high contrast for illustration purposes as shown in **Fig. 1**.

3.3.1. Lectin-Gold Labeling

The α_2-subunit of the L-type VGCC found in both skeletal and cardiac muscle is heavily glycosylated and has been shown to bind WGA *(Triticum vulgaris)* **(15)**. In studies to characterize the 3D structure of the VGCCs and identify the extracellular α_2-subunit, we employed WGA conjugated to 5 nm colloidal gold **(16)**. Upon negative staining, the gold is visualized as an electron-dense (black) particle and the protein is white.

1. Add an excess of WGA-gold (5 nm), 100 µL (100 µg/mL concentration) of purified VGCC.
2. Incubate at 4°C for 24 h.
3. Remove aggregated gold by centrifugation of the sample mix at 13,000g (Eppendorf centrifuge 5415C, precooled) for 10 min at 4°C. Keep the supernatant.
4. Take a 20-µL aliquot from the supernatant for examination by EM as described under **Subheading 3.2.3.1.**

Skeletal muscle VGCCs labeled with a single WGA-gold are shown in **Fig. 1A** after negative staining with ammonium molybdate/trehalose. Dual-labeled complexes, reflecting the dimeric nature of the isolated complex, were also observed.

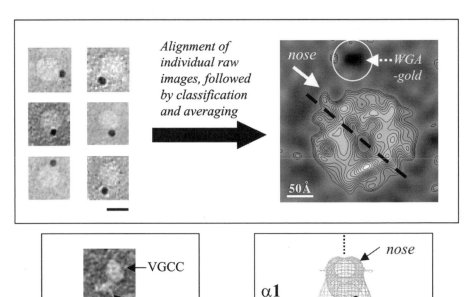

Fig. 1. Labeling of the extracellular and intracellular subunits of the L-type voltage-gated calcium channel (VGCC) and characterization of the three-dimensional structure. (**A**) A montage of purified VGCC dimers (skeletal muscle) labeled with wheat-germ agglutinin (WGA)-gold (5 nm) (protein is visualized as white and gold as black; scale bar = 200 Å). A selection of labeled particles were aligned, subjected to hierarchical ascendant classification and then averaged to calculate the projection map on the left (no symmetry constraints applied). The twofold symmetry of the complex is apparent, with the dotted line indicating the symmetry axis. The projection map shows a putative side-view of the complex, i.e., perpendicular to the membrane normal. The WGA-gold binds close to a density termed the nose. This feature was observed in the three-dimensional (3D) structures of both cardiac and skeletal muscle VGCCs, and therefore could be assigned as the extracellular portion of the complex and allowed orientation of the complex with respect to the t-tubular membrane. Scale bar = 50 Å. (**B**) Top: image of a VGCC dimer with an IgG (anti-beta subunit) bound, thereby labeling the intracellular domain of the complex. Bottom: A VGCC dimer labeled with an IgG binding to the β polypeptide localized to the cytosol and a single WGA-gold binding to the extracellular glycosylated moieties of the α_2 subunit. Scale bar = 200 Å. (**C**) The 3D structure of the cardiac VGCC determined

3.3.2. Combining Antibody and WGA-Gold Labeling of the L-Type VGCC

Immuno-labeling of the β-subunit of the skeletal L-type VGCC (*see* **Fig. 1B**).

1. Add an excess of antibody (anti-β: VGCC molar ratio of ~40:1) to 150 µL (corresponding to ~7.5 µg protein) of the WGA-gold labeled purified skeletal muscle VGCC prepared in **Subheading 3.3.1.**
2. Incubate the WGAgold-VGCC: antibody mix on ice for 3 h.
3. Transfer the WGAgold-VGCC-antibody mix to a 10-mL ultracentrifuge tube (Beckman) and centrifuge at 4°C for 15 min at 100,000*g* (Beckman Optima Ultracentrifuge) (*see* **Note 18**).
4. Take a 20-µL aliquot from the supernatant and load onto a glow discharged carbon grid for sample preparation as described in **Subheading 3.2.2.1.**

3.3.3. Ni-NTA-Gold

This is a relatively new product from Nanagold® for labeling of His-tagged proteins. As well as having applications to label transfected cells with His-tagged proteins, this label has the potential for use in high-resolution EM studies. In this way, it may be used to identify a domain, or N-terminus of a His-tagged protein (for examples, *see* **refs. *17*** and ***18***). The size of the gold label is 1.8 nm, and the Ni-NTA group is quite small in comparison with, for example, an antibody. In addition, there is the added advantage that because there are no additional proteins attached, the label has the potential of binding closely to the 6X-His-tag, giving higher-resolution labeling.

1. Aliquot 20 µL of the His-tag protein (concentration ~100 µg/mL) onto a piece of Parafilm.
2. Float a glow-discharged grid on the sample drop for 30 s.
3. Blot the grid on filter paper by touching the edge of the grid to the filter paper as described in **Subheading 3.2.1., step 3**.
4. Float the grid on a 20-µL aliquot of the Ni-NTA gold (30 nmol) for 30 s (*see* **Note 19**).
5. Blot the grid on filter paper (as described in **Subheading 3.2.1., step 3**).

Fig. 1 *(Continued)* at 23 Å resolution *(9)* determined using single particle analysis methods is presented using light grey meshing (XtalView) and displayed at thresholds (3σ above the mean density), highlighting only the principal protein densities as viewed perpendicular to the membrane plane (i.e., side view). In one-half of the dimmer, an X-ray crystallographic structure for the β core (1T3L.pdb) shown in dark grey is matched to the electron microscopy structure, with the crystal structure of the tetrameric voltage-dependent potassium channel from *Aeropyrum pernix,* KvAP, (1ORS.pdb), analogous to the (1 subunit, displayed in black) Scale bar = 50 Å. TM, transmembrane (putative position of the lipid bilayer); in, intracellular side; ex, extracellular side.

6. Wash the grid twice on a droplet of Milli-Q water as described in **Subheading 3.2.1., step 4** to remove any unbound Ni-NTA gold.
7. Blot the grid between washes as described in **Subheading 3.2.1., step 4**.
8. Initially examine the labeled protein using negative staining following **Subheading 3.2.1., steps 6** and **7**.

4. Notes

1. As a result of the different thermal expansion coefficients of copper and carbon, cryo-crinkling can occur. Titanium and molybdenum grids have been determined to lead to less wrinkling of the carbon support film and, therefore, maintenance of high-resolution information. There are several reviews that discuss these issues in detail (for an example, *see* **ref. *19***).
2. Problems may be encountered using holey grids, e.g., the sample does not occupy the holes but associates with the carbon film. This phenomenon has been observed with positively charged proteins and is exacerbated if the grids have been glow-discharged. If this happens, try not glow-discharging; however, because of the slightly negative charge of the carbon film, this effect may be difficult to eliminate. One approach has been developed using a secondary thin carbon layer deposited over the holey grid to which the sample is then applied. Alternatively, use grids with a flat carbon coat.
3. Glow-discharging involves the formation of negatively charged ions in the glow-discharge chamber which are deposited on the carbon film, providing a hydrophilic surface for adsorption of the protein sample.
4. If sample volume is limited, then between 2 and 5 μL can be directly pipeted onto the carbon-coated grid held by tweezers (self-gripping crossover tweezers type recommended).
5. The way in which a protein associates with an EM grid is influenced by inherent physiochemical properties of the sample. Therefore, some experimentation with protein concentration and incubation time will be required when working with an uncharacterized protein to determine optimal protein loading. For SPA, at least 50–100 well separated particles per micrograph should be aimed for.
6. Curved nonself-gripping tweezers are recommended to minimize capillary action, which will interfere with the blotting.
7. If the sample buffer contains high concentrations of cryo-protectants, e.g., glycerol, or salts, then repeat this step.
8. The edge of the grid should be lightly in contact with filter paper with no force applied, or the grid will bend, leading to breakage of the grid mesh.
9. Centrifuge the uranyl acetate solution for 5 min at 5000*g* (Eppendorf centrifuge 5415C) to pellet undissolved uranyl acetate crystals, taking the aliquot from the supernatant. If uranyl acetate is not blotted from the grid or crystals are not spun down, then black patches of stain will cover the grid and obscure the sample.
10. Uranyl acetate is acidic (pH ~4.0) and therefore may not be suitable for pH-sensitive proteins.
11. A slurry of liquid ethane forms in the cup. Stir with a pair of tweezers to help slightly melt it.

12. If the grid is first glow-discharged, then initially try protein concentrations similar to that for negative staining, i.e., approx 100 µg/mL, but more concentrated samples may be required if the grid has not been glow-discharged.

13. In order to get a firm blotting motion, cut the filter paper in half, then fold into quarters so that it is triangular in shape.

14. To determine conditions for the correct thickness of ice may take some practice (typically between 1000 and 2000 Å thick).

15. All tweezers used for handling the grids and cryo-holder should be cooled in liquid nitrogen. At this stage, it is critical that temperature does not arise above approx −150 to −140°C, or ice crystals will form in the sample, making it unsuitable for cryo-EM.

16. The addition of low concentrations trehalose and glucose (e.g., 3–5% w/v) to protein samples have been found to help maintain the integrity of the structure and reduce water evaporation during the vitrification *(20)*.

17. The grids were not glow-discharged for studies of the PilQ *(14)*.

18. There are several different approaches to isolate protein–antibody complexes, including size-exclusion chromatography and ultrafiltration. However, size-exclusion was not possible in this case, as asolecithin would need to be omitted (it absorbs ultraviolet), which it was found to lead to the dissociation of the VGCC dimer complex *(9)*. Therefore, ultracentrifugation was employed. For some proteins, it may be prudent to first examine the sample mix directly by EM, i.e., without separation of aggregated and unbound antibody before embarking on a separation method, as there are reports of protein stability being compromised (for an example, *see* **ref.** *21*).

19. This method may result in preferred orientations of the protein, and, therefore, full occupancy will not be achieved despite the high affinity of the Ni-NTA for the His-tag. In order to optimize the binding conditions and increase occupancy, experimentation with parameters such as incubation time and label concentration is recommended.

Acknowledgments

The author would like to acknowledge Dr. Richard Collins (Faculty of Life Sciences, Manchester University) for discussions regarding optimization of cryo-negative staining and Dr. Robert C. Ford (Faculty of Life Sciences, Manchester University) for proofreading this chapter.

References

1. Sharma, M. R., Jeyakumar, L. H., Fleischer, S., and Wagenknecht, T. (2000) Three-dimensional structure of ryanodine receptor isoform three in two conformational states as visualized by cryo-electron microscopy. *J. Biol. Chem.* **275,** 9485–9491.

2. Samso, M. and Wagenknecht, T. (2002) Apocalmodulin and Ca^{2+}-calmodulin bind to neighboring locations on the ryanodine receptor. *J. Biol. Chem.* **277,** 1349–1353.

3. Unger, V. M., Kumar, N. M., Gilula, N. B., and Yeager, M. (1999) Electron cryo-crystallography of a recombinant cardiac gap junction channel, in *Gap Junction-Mediated Intercellular Signalling in Health and Disease*. pp. 22–37.

4. Rubinstein, J. L., Walker, J. E., and Henderson, R. (2003) Structure of the mito-chondrial ATP synthase by electron cryomicroscopy. *EMBO* **22**, 6182–6192.

5. Grigorieff, N. (1998) Three-dimensional structure of bovine NADH: ubiquinone oxidoreductase (Complex I) at 22 angstrom in ice. *J. Mol. Biol.* **277**, 1033–1046.

6. MacLennan, D. H., Abu-Abed, M., and Kang, C. (2002) Structure-function rela-tionships in Ca²⁺ cycling proteins. *J. Mol.Cell. Cardiol.* **34**, 897–918.

7. Toyoshima, C., Nakasako, M., Nomura, H., and Ogawa, H. (2000) Crystal struc-ture of the calcium pump of sarcoplasmic reticulum at 2.6 angstrom resolution. *Nature* **405**, 647–655.

8. Sharma, M. R., Penczek, P., Grassucci, R., Xin, H. B., Fleischer, S., and Wagenknecht, T. (1998) Cryoelectron microscopy and image analysis of the cardiac ryanodine receptor. *J. Biol. Chem.* **273**, 18,429–18,434.

9. Wang, M. C., Collins, R. F., Ford, R. C., Berrow, N. S., Dolphin, A. C., and Kitmitto, A. (2004) The three-dimensional structure of the cardiac L-type voltage-gated calcium channel—comparison with the skeletal muscle form reveals a com-mon architectural motif. *J. Biol. Chem.* **279**, 7159–7168.

10. Sharma, M. R., Jeyakumar, L. H., Fleischer, S., and Wagenknecht, T. (2002) Three-dimensional visualization of FKBP12.6 binding to cardiac ryanodine receptor (RyR2) in open buffer condition. *Biophys. J.* **82**, 3145.

11. Berriman, J. and Unwin, N. (1994) Analysis of transient structures by cryomicroscopy combined with rapid mixing of spray droplets. *Ultramicroscopy* **56**, 241–252.

12. Brickley, K., Campbell, V., Berrow, N., et al. (1995) Use of site-directed antibod-ies to probe the topography of the alpha(2) subunit of voltage-gated Ca²⁺ channels. *FEBS Lett.* **364**, 129–133.

13. Adrian, M., Dubochet, J., Fuller, S. D., and Harris, J. R. (1998) Cryo-negative staining. *Micron.* **29**, 145–160.

14. Collins, R. F., Frye, S. A., Kitmitto, A., Ford, R. C., Tonjum, T., and Derrick, J. P. (2004) Structure of the Neisseria meningitidis outer membrane PilQ secretin com-plex at 12 angstrom resolution. *J. Biol. Chem.* **279**, 39,750–39,756.

15. Florio, V., Striessnig, J., and Catterall, W. A. (1992) Purification and reconstitution of skeletal-muscle calcium Channels. *Methods Enzymol.* **207**, 529–546.

16. Wang, M. C., Dolphin, A., and Kitmitto, A. (2004) L-type voltage-gated calcium channels: understanding function through structure. *FEBS Lett.* **564**, 245–250.

17. Buchel, C., Morris, E., Orlova, E., and Barber, J. (2001) Localisation of the PsbH subunit in photosystem II: a new approach using labeling of His-tags with a Ni²⁺-NTA gold cluster and single particle analysis. *J. Molec. Biol.* **312**, 371–379.

18. Hainfeld, J. F., Liu, W. Q., Halsey, C. M. R., Freimuth, P., and Powell, R. D. (1999) Ni-NTA-gold clusters target his-tagged proteins. *J. Struct. Biol.* **127**, 185–198.

19. Vonck, J. (2000) Parameters affecting specimen flatness of two-dimensional crys-tals for electron crystallography. *Ultramicroscopy* **85**, 123–129.

20. De Carlo, S., Adrian, H., Kallin, P., Mayer, J. M., and Dubochet, J. (1999) Unexpected property of trehalose as observed by cryo-electron microscopy. *J. Microscop. Oxford* **196,** 40–45.
21. Benacquista, B. L., Sharma, M. R., Samso, M., Zorzato, F., Treves, S., and Wagenknecht, T. (2000) Amino acid residues 4425-4621 localized on the three-dimensional structure of the skeletal muscle ryanodine receptor. *Biophy. J.* **78,** 1349–1358.

22

Stem Cells in Cardiovascular Disease

Methods and Protocols

Marc S. Penn and Niladri Mal

Summary

Stem cells are cells capable of proliferation, self-renewal, and differentiation into various organ-specific cell types. Stem cells are subclassified based on their species of origin (mice, rat, human), developmental stage of the species (embryonic, fetal, or adult), tissue of origin (hematopoietic, mesenchymal, skeletal, neural), and potential to differentiate into one or more specific types of mature cells (totipotent, pluripotent, multipotent). Embryonic stem (ES) cells are totipotent, primitive cells derived from the embryo that have the potential to become all specialized cell types. Conversely, adult stem cells are undifferentiated cells found in differentiated tissue that retain the potential to renew themselves and differentiate to yield organ-specific tissues. Stem cells are attractive candidates for novel therapeutics for patients with different heart diseases, including congestive heart failure, most commonly caused by myocardial infarction. The remarkable proliferative and differentiation capacity of stem cells promises an almost unlimited supply of specific cell types including viable functioning cardiomyocytes to replace the scarred myocardium following transplantation.

Key Words: Stem cells; myocardial infarction; heart failure; therapeutics.

1. Introduction
1.1. Embryonic Stem Cells

Embryonic stem (ES) cells are derived from the inner cell mass of an early embryo called the blastocyst. ES cells are highly expandable in culture, have the capacity to differentiate into cells derived from all three primary germ layers (*1*), and have far-reaching implications for potential use in treating cardiovascular disease as a result of their capability to (1) spontaneously differentiate into multiple lineages including cardiomyocytes, endothelial cells, and vascular smooth

From: *Methods in Molecular Medicine, vol. 129:*
Cardiovascular Disease: Methods and Protocols, Volume 2: Molecular Medicine
Edited by: Q. K. Wang © Humana Press Inc., Totowa, NJ

muscle cells; and (2) release several cardioprotective factor and angiogenic factors such as vascular endothelial growth factor (VEGF) and stromal cell-derived factor (SDF)-1. Unfortunately, their utility may be limited because of their potential for tumorigenicity, including teratomas, concern related to immune rejection, and ethical, moral, and political issues surrounding their applications.

1.2. Adult Stem Cells

Recently, stem cells with remarkable proliferation and differentiation potential have been isolated from bone marrow, skeletal muscle, liver, and brain, and accumulating reports demonstrating the differential potentials of tissue-specific adult stem cells are more versatile than had previously been thought. Recent studies have shown that transplantation of stem cells directly into the region of infracted myocardium or intravenously in the peri-infarct period improves cardiac function. However, many of the findings in this new field are controversial, including the frequencies in which these cells are detected in the recipient organ, the capacity of these stem cells to differentiate into organ-specific cells, and the origin of these cells. The optimal cell type and dose, delivery route, delivery catheter, timing, and frequency of stem cell injections are still being defined. Question arises as to whether tissue injury is necessary for the differentiation and homing of these cells and the mechanisms by which differentiation occurs. It is also unclear how this phenomenon can be safely and reasonably exploited for clinical use in humans.

1.3. Adult Stem Cell Use in Cardiovascular Research

A variety of adult stem cells may be utilized in cardiovascular research. However, isolation, enrichment, and in vitro and in vivo differentiation potential will significantly vary with different stem cell populations.

1.3.1. Bone Marrow-Derived Stem Cells

Adult bone marrow contains hematopoietic stem cells, which differentiate into all types of mature blood cells, and endothelial progenitor cells, which differentiate to form new vessels and mesenchymal stem cells, which in turn are capable of differentiation into mature cells of multiple mesenchymal origins.

1.3.1.1. Hematopoietic Stem Cells

Hematopoietic stem cells (HSCs) are defined by their ability to regenerate all of the hematopoietic lineages in the transplanted host. Multiple approaches have been used to isolate and characterize HSCs. Isolation protocol differs with species of origin and age of the animal at the time of isolation. HSCs do not express surface markers associated with the terminal maturation of specific blood cell types. These mature markers are utilized to negatively select for HSCs.

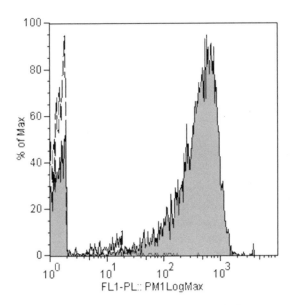

Fig. 1. Flowcytometric analysis of enriched hematopoietic stem cells from murine bone marrow; fluorescent intensity (*x*-axis) and percentages of c-Kit positive (shaded area) cell number (*y*-axis) vs negative control.

Markers commonly used to isolate human *lin*-HSC are glycophorin A, CD2, CD3, CD4, CD8, CD14, CD15, CD16, CD19, CD20, CD56, and CD66b *(2)*. HSCs in several species have been identified as positive for Sca-1, Thy-1, and C-kit (CD117) **(Fig. 1)**. Adult bone marrow of many species also contain a rare population of cells designated as side population (SP) cells, a purified CD34- c-kit+ Sca-1+ subpopulation of HSCs that actively efflux Hoechst dye 33342 and can be isolated by flow sorting on the basis of their dim fluorescent signal relative to other cells. SP cells highly express a transmembrane transporter protein "P-glycoprotein," which allows them to actively exclude Hoechst dye and fluoresce in this particular manner *(3)*. SP cells are also present in other tissues, including skeletal muscle.

1.3.1.2. MESENCHYMAL (MARROW STROMAL) STEM CELLS

Adult mesenchymal stem cells (MSCs) **(Fig. 2)** are pluripotent cells derived from bone marrow that can be expanded to large numbers in vitro while maintaining their potential to differentiate into various somatic cell types of all three germ layers. The in vitro differentiation of MSCs provides new perspectives for studying the cellular and molecular mechanism of early development and the generation of donor cells for transplantation therapies. MSCs derived in different laboratories use different techniques that share common features, including that

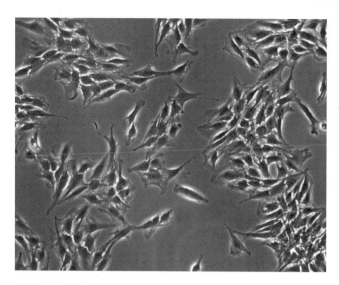

Fig. 2. Differential interference contrast (DIC) microscopic picture of Lewis rat mesenchymal stem cells in culture with typical adherent morphology (×10).

they grow in culture as adherent cells that preferentially attach to a polystyrene flask surface, that they have a finite life span, and that they uniformly lack antigens such as CD45 and CD34 that typically identified in HSCs. A wide array of cytokines and surface markers have been used to identify, isolate, and expand MSCs. MSCs are attractive candidates for cellular therapy after myocardial infarction because they are easy to isolate, have a broad differentiation potential, and proliferate in vitro. There is also accumulating evidence that MSC are hypoimmunogenic *(4)*, a characteristic that has broad implications in terms of allogenic therapy. Several groups have demonstrated the ability of cultured MSCs to differentiate into neural cells, skeletal muscle cells, smooth muscle cells, and possibly cardiomyocytes. MSC also have a paracrine affect due to the release of several cytokines such as VEGF and SDF-1, which can favorably alter that microenvironment of injured tissue. Unfortunately, the variations in the isolation techniques and culture media used to grow MSCs in different laboratories may have lead to variable findings in the literature, in turn leading to the controversial differential potential of these cells.

1.3.1.3. Multipotent Adult Progenitor Cells

Multipotent adult progenitor cells (MAPCs) **(Fig. 3)** are a population of bone marrow-derived cells that co-purify initially with MSCs and grow as adherent cells ex vivo. However, unlike MSCs, MAPCs can be cultured indefinitely in a relatively nutrient-deficient medium. MAPCs express telomerase and maintain

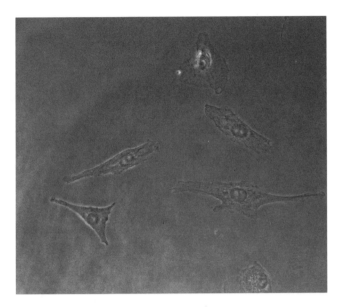

Fig. 3. Differential interference contrast microscopic picture of Lewis rat multipotent adult progenitor cells in culture with typical adherent morphology (×40).

telomere length after many cell doublings, consistent with their ability to grow indefinitely in vitro and self-renew in vivo *(5)*. These cells also differ from MSCs in the expression of CD44 and, unlike MSCs, MAPCs can differentiate into cells from all three germ layers. Because the cell culture conditions of MSCs and MAPCs are substantially different, a comparison of these cells under identical culture conditions has yet to be performed. Whether MAPCs represent a rare subpopulation of MSCs or whether their differential potential developed under unique in vitro cell culture conditions is still uncertain.

1.3.1.4. ENDOTHELIAL PROGENITOR CELLS

Endothelial progenitor cells (EPCs) are defined as cells that are positive for both HSC markers, such as CD34, CD133, and an endothelial marker protein such as VEGFR2, and that incorporate *Dil-Ac-LDL (6)*. EPCs are isolated from peripheral blood and bone marrow as well as from different sources; tissue-resident stem cells from the heart *(7)* can be isolated by cultivation in medium favoring endothelial differentiation. EPCs that have been transplanted or that have migrated to the infarct area improve cardiac function and prevent ventricular remodeling after myocardial infarction. Potential mechanisms for this improvement include neovascularization after differentiation into mature endothelial cells; inhibition of apoptosis of cardiac myocytes in the infarct border zone leading to salvage of hibernating myocardium; and release of other

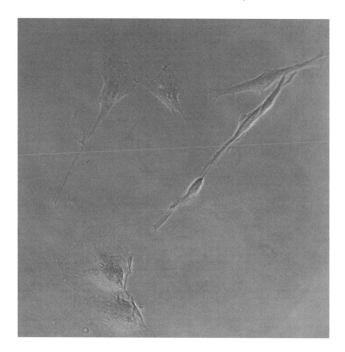

Fig. 4. Differential interference contrast microscopic picture of Lewis rat skeletal muscle satellite stem cells in culture with characteristic adherent morphology (×40).

stem cells, including HSCs, in the infarct area via newly formed vessels. However, controversy exists with respect to the identification and the origin of EPCs. EPCs are difficult to isolate, purify, and expand ex vivo; may change their differential potential during ex vivo expansion; and are unavailable in adequate quantities from a single animal for therapeutic intervention.

1.3.2. Skeletal Myoblast

Skeletal myoblasts (**Fig. 4**) are satellite cells that reside within skeletal muscle tissue and have the potential for self renewal and differentiation into skeletal muscle. Skeletal myoblasts have been used as a possible replacement tissue in infracted myocardium because they are resistant to ischemia, they are fatigue-resistant as a result of slow twitch fibers, they have high proliferative potential in culture, and autologous muscle stem cells could be isolated by muscle biopsy thereby circumventing graft rejection. However, future application of skeletal myoblasts may be limited, as they downregulate expression of major adherence junction proteins (i.e., N-cadherin) and gap junction proteins (i.e., connexin 43) after terminal differentiation and myotube formation *(8)*, leading to failure of successful electromechanical coupling with the host myocardium which increases arrythmogenic potential of recipient heart after transplantation.

1.3.3. Cardiac Stem Cells

Cardiac myocytes have been traditionally regarded as terminally differentiated cells. However, in recent years, compelling evidence has accumulated suggesting that the heart has regenerative potential, perhaps as a result of the presence of cardiac stem cells in the heart. Cardiac stem cells may be considered clones of adult stem cells that can be isolated from the adult mammalian heart based exclusively on the expression of a stem cell-related surface antigen such as c-kit or Sca-1 in the mouse *(9,10)*. The relevant surface makers in humans are still under investigation.

2. Methods
2.1. Considerations of Study Design
2.1.1. Approaches for Identifying Donor-Derived Cells in Target Recipient Organs

Researchers have used a donor-specific marker absent in the recipient to track and determine the fate of transplanted stem cells. Commonly used donor-specific markers are the Y-chromosome (in sex-mismatched transplantation), transgenes (green fluorescent protein [GFP], yellow fluorescent protein [YFP], and red fluorescent protein [RFP]; chemiluminesent-luciferase), nucleotides (BrdU), membrane staining dye (Dil), and Nanomolecules (quantum dots). Each of these approaches has advantages and disadvantages.

2.1.1.1. Y-CHROMOSOME

In male-to-female transplantation, use of Y-chromosome as donor-specific marker has several advantages, namely, that Y-chromosome is present in every intact donor cell and that whole-chromosome paint probes make it relatively easy to image the Y-chromosome. However, Y-chromosome may not be visible in all donor-derived cells, particularly in thin tissue sections that only partially sample the nuclei being assessed. Complicating the technique is that it is technically difficult to interpret Y-chromosome fluorescence *in situ* hybridization (FISH) on thicker sections that contain the full thickness of many cells. In addition, Y-chromosome staining potentially may cause false-positive results because of nonspecific binding of probe.

2.1.1.2. TRANSGENE

Cells from transgene donor animals that express transgenes such as luciferase or GFP are transplanted into recipients lacking the transgene. In experiments using a transgenic model, data must be interpreted with caution because transgene silencing *(11)* can occur and because promiscuous multilineage gene expression, commonly known as "gene priming," can potentially cause transgene expression in a wide variety of cells in which the cell type-specific promoter may not generally be active *(12)*.

1. Fluorescent reporter gene: GFP was initially recognized as a protein involved in the bioluminescence of the jellyfish *Aequorea victora*. The GFP transgene produces a green fluorescent product when expressed in stem cells, without the need for exogenous substrate, cofactors, or chemical staining. GFP fluorescence is species-independent, stable in vivo and even after tissue fixation, and is suitable for a variety of applications such as in monitoring gene expression, protein localization, and stem cell homing, and in migration studies Several GFP mutants have been developed, including enhanced GFP (EGFP), YFP, and RFP, that fluoresce more intensely than the wild-type GFP or have shifted excitation maxima, and are useful for fluorescence microscopy and multicolor fluorescence-activated cell sorting (FACS) analysis.

2. Chemiluminence reporter gene: firefly luciferase, renila luciferase: the cDNA encoding luciferase (*luc*) cloned from firefly *Photinus pyralis* is used for in vitro and in vivo reporting of transcriptional activity in eukaryotic cells. Luciferase generates luminescence through mono-oxygenation of luciferin, utilizing O_2 and ATP as cosubstrates. Luminescence correlates directly to expression of the *luc* reporter gene in transfected cells or cell lysates. However, the utility of luciferase as a reporter of in vivo gene regulation has been controversial because of confusion about whether luciferin can penetrate cell membrane. At neutral pH, luciferin carries a single negative charge and could not cross the hydrophobic lipid bilayer. Acidic buffers such as dimethylsulfoxide (DMSO), nigericin, ionic detergents, or combinations can be used to facilitate the intracellular accessibility of luciferin in vitro *(13)*.

3. Other reporter genes: β-galactosidase is an enzyme that splits lactose into glucose and galactose. This enzyme is an excellent marker for the *lac*Z gene, which encodes β-galactosidase and is frequently used as a reporter gene in animals and yeast cells. X-Gal (5-Bromo-4-chloro-3-indolyl-β-D-galactopyranoside) is a substrate for chromogenic detection of target sequences and produces a dark blue precipitate on enzymatic hydrolysis in the presence of β-galactosidase activity.

2.1.1.3. Nucleotides Incorporation

5-bromo-2'-deoxyuridine (BrdU) is a uridine derivative that, selectively incorporated into DNA at the S phase of cell cycle, can be used for identification of DNA synthesis in suspensions of cells, cell smears, and tissue sections. For the incorporation of BrdU to occur in DNA in place of thymidine, the BrdU must be phosphorylated in the cell by thymidine kinase. BrdU is used for studies of the cell cycle, to track stem cells, and to determine stem cell proliferation in the presence of inhibitors (cytotoxic drugs) and stimulators (growth factors). Fluorescent-conjugated second antibodies can be used with antibodies specific for BrdU that cause BrdU-incorporated DNA to fluoresce. However, anti-BrdU also identifies BrdU in single-stranded DNA, free BrdU, and BrdU coupled to a protein carrier, and cross-reacts with iodouridine and chlorodeoxyuridine.

2.1.1.4. INCORPORATION OF CELL MEMBRANE DYE

Fluorescent dye such as *Dil* (1,1'-dioctadecyl3, 3,3,3'-tetra-methylind-carbocyanine percholate) may be used for in vitro imaging of live *(14)* and dead cells and for in vivo imaging of a live whole animal or cells. *Dil* is utilized in studies of tracing transplanted cells and to get critical information about location, histology, and the number of transplanted cells, as this dye does not spread from labeled to unlabeled cells, nor does it appear to have any major adverse effects on living cells. However, the intensity of the dye will eventually be diluted to an undetectable level by the division of dye-labeled cells. Therefore, this technique particularly suits short-term cell linage tracing. In order to confirm whether the *Dil* fluorescence is present in living cells, Hoechst 33258 dye is use to stain tissue sections.

2.1.1.5. NANOCRYSTALS

Nanocrystals, such as fluorescent quantum dots (Qdots), are crystals in the quantum-confined size range that can be fine-tuned to emit light at a variety of wavelengths, including near-infrared and infra-red spectrum, simply by altering the size of the core, and, therefore, constitute a set of multicolored molecular beacons for use in imaging living cells. Qdot nanocrystals may be delivered into the cytoplasm of live cells using a custom targeting peptide. Once inside the cells, Qdots are not transferred to adjacent cells and may be used as a tool for a variety of studies of live cells, including migration, motility, and morphology studies. Unlike regular fluorescence dyes that tend to fade away over time, Qdots provides stable fluorescent signal for long time *(15)*.

2.2. Markers Used for Identification of Stem Cells and Their Different Characteristics (Stem Cell Surface Markers)

Researchers have yet to find a single molecular marker that is expressed exclusively in a particular category of stem cells. However, by targeting various combinations of markers, it is possible to isolate different populations of stem cells. Although functions have yet to be ascertained for many of these markers, their expression is gained (lineage markers) or lost as stem cells differentiate, which provides a useful tool to identify as well as isolate stem cells from differentiated cells. Regulation of a particular stem cell marker gene may be different in different species; therefore, markers must be characterized in each species independently. For example CD34, the most commonly used marker to enrich human HSCs, is expressed among only 10% of the adult mouse HSCs *(16)*. The following are examples of a few stem cell surface markers utilized to isolate and characterize different populations of stem cells.

2.2.1. c-kit (CD117, Stem Cell Factor Receptor)

c-kit is a transmembrane receptor with tyrosine kinase activity. It binds to stem cell factor (SCF). It is expressed in many tissues and cells and involved in development of several lineages of stem cells, such as germ cells, neural crest-derived melanocytes, and hematopoietic precursor cells. Cell differentiation caused a loss of c-kit surface receptors.

2.2.2. Stem Cell Antigen-1

Stem cell antigen (Sca)-1 is a GPI-linked surface protein of the Ly-6 family (Ly-6A/E). Sca-1 is the most recognized HSC marker in mice.

2.2.3. CD34

CD34 is a critical marker for human HSCs. CD34 expression on primitive cells is downregulated as they differentiate into mature cells. However, HSCs may be CD34+ or CD34–, and the selection of cells expressing CD34 might result in exclusion of more primitive stem cells.

2.2.4. CD133

CD133 a glycosylated protein containing five transmembrane domains expressed in majority of, but not all, CD133+ progenitor cells from peripheral blood that can be induced to differentiate into endothelial cells in vitro. Using an anti-CD133 antibody can also directly isolate human neural stem cells.

2.2.5. CD105 (Endoglin)

CD105 is a component of the transforming growth factor (TGF)-β receptor. It is expressed in mesenchymal stem cells, endothelial stem cells, mature monocytes, and in about 20% of mouse bone marrow SP cells.

2.2.6. CD201 (Endothelial Protein C Receptors)

CD201 is expressed in endothelial cells and involved in the regulation of coagulation and inflammation. It is also expressed at high levels in murine and human HSCs.

2.2.7. ATP-Binding Cassette Superfamily G Member 2

ATP-binding cassette superfamily G member (ABCG)2 is a member of the family of ABC transporters and found in a wide variety of stem cells, including CD34– HSCs a Hoechst-negative phenotype of SP, mouse skeletal muscle, and ES cells. The expression of ABCG2 appears to be downregulated with the acquisition of CD34 on the cell surface.

2.2.8. Oct-4

Oct-4 is the first and most recognized marker used for the identification of totipotent ES cells and germ cells. Oct-4 is a DNA-binding transcription protein that activates gene transcription via a *cis*-element containing octamer motif. Differentiation of ES cells results in downregulation of Oct-4.

2.2.9. Stage-Specific Embryonic Antigens

Stage-specific embryonic antigens (SSEAs) are used as an ES cell marker in different species. SSEAs were typed initially as SSEA-1, -3, and -4 based on three different monoclonal antibodies recognizing defined carbohydrate epitopes associated with lacto- and globo-series glycolipids. Undifferentiated primate and human ES cells express SSEA-3 and SSEA-4 but not SSEA-1. Undifferentiated mouse ES cells express SSEA-1, but not SSEA-3 or SSEA-4. However, the oviduct epithelium, endometrium, and epididymis as well as some areas of the brain and kidney tubules in adult mice have also been shown to be reactive with SSEA-1 antibodies make it less specific.

2.2.10. Proliferation Markers

In human and comparative mammalian stem cell research, proliferation markers use to evaluate stem cell replication in different stages.

1. Ki67. Ki-67 antigen is expressed during the G1, S, G2, and early mitosis phases, providing a quantitative estimate of the fraction of cells in the cell cycle at the time of observation, but is not expressed during the G0 (resting) phase. Because Ki-67 antigen has a short half-life, it can be used as a marker of actively proliferating stem cells.
2. Proliferating cell nuclear antigen (PCNA). PCNA is a highly conserved 36 kD acidic nuclear protein that is expressed during cell replication and DNA repair. PCNA interacts with DNA polymerase and with RF-C protein to bind at DNA primer–template junctions. Immunostaining of S-phase nuclei will detect PCNA in sites of DNA synthesis. However, PCNA has a longer half-life than Ki 67 and thus persists in cells that are already in the resting G-phase of the cell, makes PCNA less specific as a proliferation marker and has been largely supplanted by Ki 67.
3. Minichromosome maintenance protein (MCM)5. MCM5 is a protein with an important role in the control of DNA replication. MCM5 is expressed throughout G1 and S phase, becomes undetectable in G2 and early mitosis, and is present again in anaphase and telophase.

2.3. Stem Cells Transplantation in Heart

Stem cells may improve heart function after infarction by increasing vascularity by differentiation into endothelial cells, by myogenic repair owing to their differentiation into cardiac myocytes, and through the release of cytokines and other factors that promote myogenic repair and prevent fibrosis. However, the optimal cell type and dose, delivery route, delivery catheter, timing, and frequency of stem cell injections are still undefined and controversial.

2.4. Route of Stem Cell Delivery to Heart

2.4.1. Intravenous Route

The intravenous route is the simplest and least invasive method of transplantation of stem cells. The femoral vein can be surgically isolated and exposed; the tail vein is commonly used in animal model. However, there may be potential for embolization when a large quantity of cells is delivered, and homing of stem cells to extracardiac organs (lung, liver, spleen) may limit the number of cells reaching the infarct region. Most importantly, studies have demonstrated the critical need to be sure that the harvested cells are well distributed.

2.4.2. Intramyocardial Injection

Direct myocardial injection of stem cells needs smaller numbers of stem cells to achieve engraftment compared with intravenous administration and allows for direct visualization of the potential target zone. However, this mode of delivery is invasive and associated with well-known surgical risk, and may lead to islands of cells in the infracted myocardium, providing a substrate for electrical instability and ventricular arrhythmias.

2.4.3. Intracoronary Artery Injection

Injecting stem cells directly to the clamped aorta, with subsequent migration of the cells through the coronary arteries to the infarction scar, allows stem cells to home and engraft homogenously; delivers the maximum concentration of cells to the site of infarct and peri-infarct tissue; and is a less-invasive mode of delivery compared with intracardiac route. However, they may adversely effect coronary perfusion and may induce myonecrosis.

2.5. Stem Cell–Host Interactions

There are several aspects of the implanted stem cell–host interaction that must to be addressed as we attempt to understand the mechanisms underlying stem cell therapies: first, the host immune response to transplanted cells; second, the homing mechanisms that guide delivered stem cells to the site of injury; and third, differentiation of transplanted stem cells under the influence of local signals.

2.6. Host Immune Response to Transplanted Stem Cells

Autologous transplantation of stem cells is the safest approach from immunological perspective; however, adult stem cells are limited in supply in each patient, and, therefore, are difficult to isolate and purify. Nonetheless, the stem cells from the patient's body must be isolated and expanded in culture to obtain a sufficient amount for transplantation, and this necessitates a long lead time to start therapy. The major obstacle with xenogenic transplantation includes immune rejection due to tissue incompatibility at the human leukocyte antigen (HLA) level. The requirement for strong immunosuppression to prevent destruction of the xenogenic cellular transplant deters the researcher. Allogenic transplantation of stem cells is advantageous because of less immunoreactivity compared with xenografting and due to the reduced expression of immune-related cell-surface proteins in stem cells compared with mature differentiated tissues. However, severity of immunoreactivity varies with stem cell type and differentiation stage. Recent studies have demonstrated that MSCs are capable of suppressing mixed lymphocyte reactions (MLRs) involving autologous or allogenic T-cells or dendritic cells, which opens the possibility of allogenic mesenchymal stem cell transplantation as a new therapeutic avenue that obviates the need for immunosuppression.

2.7. Factors That Play a Role in the Mobilization, Organ-Specific Homing, Engraftment, and Differentiation of Stem Cells

Stem cell homing requires a number of factors such as cytokines, transcription factors, cell–cell interaction, and cell–matrix interaction. It seems clear that stem cells such as HSCs and MSCs, when delivered by intravenous infusion, are capable of specific migration to a site of injury. The mechanisms that guide homing, chemotaxis, and migration of implanted cells in the infarct zone are unclear; however, several factors may play roles; first, chemoattractant released from local tissue injury, such as VEGF, SDF-1, granulocyte colony-stimulating factor (G-CSF), and SCF; second, increased vascular permeability; third, expression of adhesion proteins such as integrin and intercellular adhesion molecule (ICAM)-1; fourth, along with homing receptors such as CXCR4, C-C chemokine receptors (CCRs) that facilitate their attachment, which is mediated by cell-to-cell contact; fifth, release of matrix metalloproteinase in the infarct area which degrades extracellular tissue matrix and enhances stem cell mobilization; and sixth, a neovasculature and fibrillar collagen scaffolding.

2.7.1. Chemokines

Chemokines are a low-molecular-weight, large family of structurally and functionally related proteins that, in association with adhesion molecules, play a pivotal role in inflammatory and immunological processes such as chemotaxis, leukocyte adhesion, leukocyte trafficking, and angiogenesis. Most chemokines have four conserved cysteine residues that, based on the amino-terminal cysteine motif, are classified into four superfamilies: CXC, CC, C, and CX3c chemokines. Chemokines are transducer of their biological signals through interaction with seven-transmembrane G protein-coupled receptors. Several chemokines have been thought to play an important role in stem cell mobilization and homing.

2.7.2. Stromal Cell-Derived Factor-1

SDF-1 is a member of CXC chemokines. SDF-1 and its receptor, CXCR4, are essential for cardiogenesis, hematopoiesis, and vasculogenesis during embryonic development, in addition to involvement in chemotaxis of leukocytes subsets and endothelial cells. Unlike other chemokines characterized by their inducible expression, SDF-1 appears to be constitutively expressed. Mice with SDF-1–/– or CXCR4–/– conditions die either in the uterus or within 1 h of birth with defects in cardiac ventricular septal formation, impaired liver B-cell lymphopoiesis, organ-specific vasculogenesis, and cerebellar neuronal patterning *(17)*.

2.7.3. Monocyte Chemotactic Protein-3

Monocyte chemotactic protein (MCP)-3 is a member of the CC or β-chemokine subfamily chemokine. Similarly to other CC chemokines, such as MCP-1 and macrophage inflammatory protein (MIP), MCP-3 demonstrates chemotactic preference for monocytes, lymphocytes, eosinophils, and basophils *(18)*. MCP-3 interacts with two primary CC chemokine receptors, i.e., CCR2 and CCR3, and is involved in cell recruitment in inflammation and carcinogenesis. Recent data have also shown that MCP-3 may play a role as a regulator in cellular differentiation.

2.7.4. Vascular Endothelial Growth Factor

VEGF is a glycoprotein, and several variants of VEGF have been described that arise by alternative mRNA splicing. The receptors for VEGF and related ligands include VEGFR-1 (Flt-1), VEGFR-2 (KDR/Flk-1), and VEGFR-3 (Flt-4); neuropilin-1; and neuropilin-2.

2.7.5. Stem Cell Factor

SCF is a glycoprotein that plays a key role at the early stages of hematopoiesis. SCF stimulates the proliferation of myeloid, erythroid, and lymphoid progenitors in bone marrow cultures and has been shown to act synergistically with colony-stimulating factors (CSFs). It also plays a key role in mast cell development, gametogenesis, and melanogenesis.

2.7.6. Colony-Stimulating Factors

CSFs are cytokines that stimulate the proliferation of specific pluripotent stem cells of the bone marrow in adults. G-CSF is specific for cells of the granulocytic lineage, macrophage CSF (M-CSF) is specific for cells of the macrophage lineage, and granulocyte/macrophage CSF (GM-CSF) has proliferative effects on both classes of lymphoid cells.

2.7.7. Cell–Cell Junction Proteins

For any stem cell to become an effective member of myocardium, it is necessary to form an effective electromechanical junction with surrounding cardiac myocytes to trigger synchronous calcium-dependent contractions in heart. Different stem cells have varied level of expression of adherent (cadherins) and gap junction proteins (connexins) in vivo, which makes them coordinate electromechanical activity in the myocardium differently. Stem cells expressing junction proteins or the genetic manipulation of stem cells to induce junctions is necessary to make stem cell graft beat synchronously with the host myocardium.

2.8. In Vivo Differentiation

The fundamental principle behind stem cell therapy is that, after undifferentiated cells are delivered to the site of injury, they will differentiate under the influence of local signals into cells of appropriate phenotype. These undifferentiated cells then contribute to the repair of the injured tissue. There is ample evidence indicating that this is the case; however, there are little or no data concerning the specifics that give rise to differentiation *in situ*.

2.9. Markers Used for Identification of Differentiated Cardiomyocyte Derived From Stem Cells

2.9.1. Transcription Factors

Transcriptional activators are proteins that regulate the expression of tissue specific genes and are required for maintaining the differentiated phenotypes of various lineages. In the heart, myocyte enhancer factor (MEF)2 proteins are recruited by GATA-4 to activate synergistically the promoters of several cardiac genes, such as myocin light chain, α-myosin heavy chain, α-actin, troponin T, troponin I, desmin, and atrial natriuretic factor. Csx/Nkx2.5 is a transcription factor restricted to the initial phase of myocyte differentiation.

2.9.1.1. GATA-4

Members of the GATA family share a conserved zinc finger DNA binding. Both GATA-4 and GATA-6 are found in heart, pancreas, and ovary; lung and liver tissues exhibit GATA-6, but not GATA-4, expression *(19)*. Although expression patterns of the various GATA transcription factors may overlap, it is not yet apparent how the GATA factors are able to discriminate in binding their appropriate target sites.

2.9.1.2. GATA 5

GATA 5 is a member of GATA family transcription factors and contains two GATA-type zinc fingers. GATA 5 is required for endothelial and endocardial cell differentiation. GATA-5 expressions have been observed in differentiated heart and gut tissues and are present throughout the course of development in the heart *(19)*.

2.9.1.3. Nkx 2.5

Nkx2.5 is a homeodomain containing nuclear transcription proteins. During cardiomyogenesis, expression of Nkx 2.5 is required for cardiac septation, in which a single atrium and ventricle are separated into four chambers *(20)*. Mutations that disrupt Nkx2.5 can result in atrial-septal defect, embryonic lethality, and congenital heart disease *(21)*.

2.9.1.4. MEF-2

MEF-2 is a muscle-specific DNA-binding protein. MEF-2 expression is ubiquitous, but preferential in skeletal and cardiac muscle cells *(22)*.

2.9.2. Cytoskeletal Proteins

2.9.2.1. Ventricular Myosin (Light Chain, Heavy Chain), α-Sarcomeric Actin, α-Sarcomeric Actinin

Actin and myosin are two major, highly conserved cytoskeletal proteins that are expressed in all eukaryotic cells, are implicated in a myriad of cellular processes such as locomotion, secretion, cytoplasmic streaming, phagocytosis, and cytokinesis, and are crucial components of the contractile apparatus of muscle cells. Myosin interacts with actin to generate the force for cellular movements. A variety of specific antibodies against cardiac cytoskeletal proteins are available to identify newly formed cardiacmyocytes, such as cardiac myosin heavy chain α/β, cardiac myosin light chain I, α-sarcomeric actin, and α-sarcomeric actinin.

2.9.2.2. Troponin

Troponin facilitates interactions between actin and myosin by binding to calcium. Troponin contains three subunits, troponin I, C, and T. Troponin C, the calcium-binding subunit, is expressed in cardiac and slow skeletal muscle and is involved in regulating excitation–contraction coupling in the cardiac muscle. Troponin I is the inhibitory subunit of troponin and exists as fast and slow skeletal muscle isoforms and cardiac troponin I, which is exclusively expressed in cardiac muscle *(23)*. Troponin T, the tropomyosin-binding subunit of troponin, plays a role in conferring calcium sensitivity to actomyosin ATPase activity, and exists as fast and slow skeletal and cardiac isoforms *(24)*.

2.9.2.3. Desmin

Desmin is the main intermediate filament in mature skeletal, cardiac, and smooth muscle cells. The antibody that does not cross-react with other intermediate filament proteins is useful for the identification of myodifferentiation in stem cells.

2.9.3. Natriuretic Peptides

The natriuretic peptides (NPs) constitute a family of polypeptide hormones, potent vasoactive substances that exert vasorelaxant, natriuretic, and antigrowth activities and that are thought to play a key role in cardiovascular homeostasis.

Atrial natriuretic factor, or atrial natriuretic peptide (ANP) belongs to the natriuretic peptide family hormone secreted primarily by atrial myocytes in response to local wall stretch.

B-type natriuretic peptide (BNP) is from same family of hormones and has structural similarity and some biological actions in common with ANP, such as natriuresis in vivo and dilatation of preconstricted blood vessels in vitro. BNP is also derived predominantly from heart tissue.

2.9.4. Junction Proteins

2.9.4.1. N-CADHERIN

The cadherin superfamily of proteins is a group of calcium-mediated cell–cell adhesion molecules. Cadherins are responsible for a whole range of processes including development, wound healing, cell–cell signaling, and cell growth and differentiation. The major adherens junction protein in the mammalian heart is N-cadherin.

2.9.4.2. GAP JUNCTION PROTEINS

Gap junctional channels are essential for action potential propagation from the sinoatrial node to the working myocardium and, thereby, for coordinating cardiac contraction. These proteins are structural subunits of gap junctions, intracellular channels that provide a pathway between cells for the exchange of ions, metabolites, second messengers, and small molecules up to 1 KDa. Several roles have been attributed to this form of cellular communication, including the regulation of early events during development, cell differentiation, cell growth and proliferation.

The most abundantly expressed connexin in the mammalian heart is connexin *(Cx)43*, which is apparent in cell cytoplasm and at the surface of closely aligned cells. This protein is responsible for intracellular connections and electrical coupling through the generation of plasma-membrane channels between myocytes.

Cx40 is a gap junction protein expressed specifically in developing and mature atrial myocytes *(25)* and is the major isoform present in the conduction system in the mammalian heart. Cx40-deficient mice display pronounced sinoatrial and atrioventricular conduction disturbances with increased atrial vulnerability to arrhythmogenesis *(26)* and display high incidence of cardiac malformations *(27)*.

Cx45 protein is reported to have a widespread distribution in the heart and to be a component of the gap junctions of all types of myocytes (working, conductive, and nodal myocytes). However, expression its level varies with developmental stage of the heart.

Cx37 is widely distributed in multiple compartments of cardiovascular system. Cx37 is mostly expressed in endothelial cells in the intima and in the tunica media of actively growing vessels in heart.

2.10. Stem Cells as a Vehicle of Gene Therapy

Stem cells are easily transduced by a variety of viral and nonviral vectors and therefore can be envisioned as vehicles for either long-term (stable) or short-term (transient) gene transfer, and this could facilitate the therapeutic effect of stem cells, as in SDF-1 overexpressions in MSCs to enhance homing and survival *(28)*, or *Akt* overexpression in MSCs to enhance survival *(29)*. Stem cells also could be used as "factories" for sustained production and delivery of a transgenic protein to cure systemic deficiency disorders such as hemophilia, type I diabetes mellitus, and hypothyroidism and their consequent deleterious effect on the cardiovascular system.

3. Controversial Issues in Stem Cell-Based Therapeutic Approaches

3.1. Cell Overlay

Cell overlay is of particular concern when the recipient cell overlies the donor-derived stem cell and might be incorrectly identified as donor cell. Several approaches can be taken to rule out cell overlay, including analysis of serial sections and detection of a single-cell layer using techniques such as confocal microscopy.

3.2. Tissue Autofluorescence

Autofluorescence, either intrinsic or induced by fixation media and tissue processing, may either mask specific fluorescent signals or be mistaken for fluorescent labels, such as in formalin fixed-paraffin sections of myocardium, lipofuscin granules shown as autofluorescent particles at all three wavelengths. Blood-derived pigments, other intrinsic fluors such as riboflavin and flavin coenzymes and reduced nicotinamide adenine dinucleotide (NADH) are another source of unwanted fluorescence that necessitate to analyze photographic documentation of fluorescent microscopic finding critically *(30)*.

3.3. Irreproducibility of Research Data

Many of the finding in this new field are controversial and irreproducible and challenge our existing paradigms of cell differentiation. However, significant differences in the study designs used may be responsible for the differences in findings. The primary differences are in the donor stem cell subpopulations used, the age of the donor and recipient subject, and the different methods of isolation and detection of donor-derived stem cells.

3.4. Differentiation Vs Fusion as a Possible Mechanism for Stem Cell Plasticity

The underlying mechanism by which adult stem cells cross the linkage barrier may be speculated to be either through transdifferentiation or fusion. Transdifferentiation refers to the ability of one committed cell type to change its gene expression pattern to that of a completely different cell type. An alternative mechanism could be fusion of a stem cell with a recipient cell to form a heterokaryon *(31)*, thereby converting the gene expression pattern of the original stem cell type to that of fusion partner. The concern, of course, would be that resultant cells carry high potential for malignant transformation and require extensive follow-up investigations to understand the paradigms.

4. Untoward Effect of Stem Cell Therapy

4.1. Stem Cell Therapy and Arrhythmia

The ideal stem cell must be compatible both mechanically and electrically with the host myocardium in order for stem cell therapy to be widely applicable therapeutically. Transplanted stem cells might be proarrythmogenic as a result of: heterogeneity of action potentials between the recipient and the transplanted stem cells; intrinsic arrhythmic potential of injected stem cells; local injury, fibrosis, or edema induced by intramyocardial injection or immunoreactions; or increased nerve sprouting induced by stem cell injection, which exposes a potential serious limitation of stem cell therapy. Cultured stem cells may exhibit one or all of the three arrythmogenic mechanisms: re-entry, automaticity, and triggered activity. The proarrythmogenic effect of stem cell therapy may be transient or long-term, and the incidence, type, and time course of arrhythmias varies with the type of transplanted stem cells. Nonetheless, the occurrence of cardiac arrhythmia is highly unpredictable, which necessitates further research and careful long-term follow-up studies to understand the mechanism and natural course of stem cell-induced arrhythmia.

4.2. Immunoreactivity and Inflammatory and Toxic Effects of Stem Cells

Immunoreactivity of allogenic and xenogenic stem cells is a major limitation of current stem cell transplantation research.

4.3. Malignant Potential and Stem Cell Therapy

There is concern that stem cells may have malignant potential because of telomerase maintenance, fusion, or other mechanisms. Currently, there is increasing evidence of stem cells stably expressing transgenes. One challenge will be maintaining stable gene expression while minimizing the risk of vector-associated malignancies.

4.4. Undesirable Paracrine and Endocrine Effects

Stem cells may liberate a variety of cytokines, inflammatory mediators, and growth factors that may have a deleterious effect on the host.

4.5. Unwanted Site-Specific Differentiation of Stem Cells

Recent studies have demonstrated that injection of a certain type of bone marrow cells into ischemic zones in the rat heart triggered an unexpected intramyocardial calcification with potentially serious consequences *(32)*. This demands careful consideration in the selection of candidate stem cells and better understanding of the molecular mechanism governing their site-specific differentiation.

5. Biological and Molecular Techniques Specifically Relevant to Stem Cell Research

A series of biological and molecular techniques are in use in stem cell research. Outcomes may vary among researchers depending on variability in the methods used in different laboratories, such as differences in culture techniques, stem cell isolation and selection techniques, methods utilized in mRNA or DNA amplification, and extraction of protein or nucleic acid. A lot of stem cell populations may differ with another set due to different growth phases, and there may be intracellular fluctuations in different biological molecules in stem cells and nutrient and temperature differences in the stem cell microenvironment. The confluency of stem cells in culture media can also cause a variation in results. Each technique also has its benefits and limitations when applied to the investigation of stem cell biology.

5.1. Determining Viability of Stem Cells Before Transplant by Dye Exclusion Test

A test to determine cell viability in which a dilute solution of certain dyes (e.g., Trypan Blue, eosin Y, nigrosin, Alcian blue) is mixed with a suspension of live cells; cells that exclude dye are considered to be alive whereas cells that stain are considered to be dead. However, this is not always an accurate test because it indicates only the structural integrity of the cell membrane and has a greater binding efficiency for protein in solution than in injured cells; therefore, it should only be used for protein-free solutions. Cells should not be left in the dye for a long period of time, because viable cells may also begin to take up the dye.

5.2. Flow Cytometry

A flow cytometer is an instrument used for automated analysis of cells or subcellular components by detection of the fluorescence or light scatter of sample fractions passing in narrow-stream droplets through a laser beam. Sample data must be acquired on flow cytometer as soon as possible after staining, as stem cells may lose viability or disintegrate rapidly. To preserve cell integrity, paraformaldehyde fixation may be used; however, it is possible that the quality of staining may be diminished by such fixation. When performing multicolor labeling, directly conjugated monoclonal antibodies can be added simultaneously, rather than sequentially. Every experiment must include controls. Negative controls are samples of the same cell population treated exactly as the test sample, but with the omission or modification of one of the staining steps. Examples of negative controls are unstained cells, cells exposed to the conjugated secondary antibody alone, or cells exposed to isotype controls, which are the same isotype and format (e.g., purified, biotin or fluorochrome) as the primary antibody and titrated in parallel. For multicolor staining, single-color-stained controls should be included. To identify markers on an unknown or novel cell type, positive controls (i.e., cells that are known to express the antigen of interest) should be included in each experiment and should be handled exactly as the test samples. To identify intracellular protein and cytokine expression in stem cells, permeabilization of the cells is necessary. However, the permeabilization increases the amount of protein available for nonspecific interaction, which increases false-positive results. Paraformaldehyde fixation following the permeabilization step is necessary; however, it may cause nonspecific trapping of antibodies leading to increased autofluorescence. Careful titration of staining antibody and use of a species-specific *FcR* blocking step may reduce the nonspecific staining.

6. Conclusions

Substantial early evidence points to the therapeutic utility of stem cells in a variety of preclinical and clinical studies. Precisely, the potential clinical applications of stem cells are limited only by our imagination and by the potential of the stem cell types. However, there is a wide variation in the characteristic surface markers and the expandability and multipotentiality of the stem cells isolated by different investigators. There is a need for universally acceptable characterization of stem cells, and it is critical that researchers optimize and standardize experiment during selection of the cell source and cell phenotype and assessment of cell function and fate. A degree of caution is necessary, because the functional and electrophysiological properties and tissue-specific differential potential of different stem cells are not well characterized. Additional critical studies are necessary to determine the most effective and safe stem cell type to treat cardiovascular disorders with a focus on myocardial repair and the clinical significance of cell therapy-induced arrhythmias.

References

1. Pera, M. F., Reubinoff, B., and Trounson, A. (2000) Human embryonic stem cells. *J. Cell. Sci.* **113,** 5–10.
2. Wognum, A. W., Eaves, A. C., and Thomas, T. E. (2003) Identification and isolation of hematopoietic stem cells. *Arch. Med. Res.* **34,** 461–475.
3. Scharenberg, C. W., Harkey, M. A., and Torok-Storb, B. (2002) The ABCG2 transporter is an efficient Hoechst 33342 efflux pump and is preferentially expressed by immature human hematopoietic progenitors. *Blood* **99,** 507–512.
4. Di Nicola, M., Carlo-Stella, C., Magni, M., et al. (2002) Human bone marrow stromal cells suppress T-lymphocyte proliferation induced by cellular or nonspecific mitogenic stimuli. *Blood* **99,** 3838–3843.
5. Morrison, S. J., Prowse, K. R., Ho, P., and Weissman, I. L. (1996) Telomerase activity in hematopoietic cells is associated with self-renewal potential. *Immunity* **5,** 207–216.
6. Urbich, C. and Dimmeler, S. (2004) Endothelial progenitor cells: characterization and role in vascular biology. *Circ. Res.* **95,** 343–353.
7. Beltrami, A. P., Barlucchi, L., Torella, D., et al. (2003) Adult cardiac stem cells are multipotent and support myocardial regeneration. *Cell* **114,** 763–776.
8. MacCalman, C. D., Bardeesy, N., Holland, P. C., and Blaschuk, O. W. (1992) Noncoordinate developmental regulation of N-cadherin, N-CAM, integrin, and fibronectin mRNA levels during myoblast terminal differentiation. *Dev. Dyn.* **195,** 127–132.
9. Messina, E., De Angelis, L., Frati, G., et al. (2004) Isolation and expansion of adult cardiac stem cells from human and murine heart. *Circ. Res.* **95,** 911–921.
10. Oh, H., Bradfute, S. B., Gallardo, T. D., et al. (2003) Cardiac progenitor cells from adult myocardium: homing, differentiation, and fusion after infarction. *Proc. Natl. Acad. Sci. USA.* **100,** 12,313–12,318.
11. Jakobsson, J., Rosenqvist, N., Thompson, L., Barraud, P., and Lundberg, C. (2004) Dynamics of transgene expression in a neural stem cell line transduced with lentiviral vectors incorporating the cHS4 insulator. *Exp. Cell Res.* **298,** 611–623.
12. Hu, M., Krause, D., Greaves, M., et al. (1997) Multilineage gene expression precedes commitment in the hemopoietic system. *Genes Dev.* **11,** 774–785.
13. Gould, S. J. and Subramani, S. (1988) Firefly luciferase as a tool in molecular and cell biology. *Anal. Biochem.* **175,** 5–13.
14. Fraser, S. E. (1996) Lontophoretic dye labeling of embryonic cells. *Methods Cell Biol.* **51,** 147–160.
15. Jaiswal, J. K., Mattoussi, H., Mauro, J. M., and Simon, S. M. (2003) Long-term multiple color imaging of live cells using quantum dot bioconjugates. *Nat. Biotechnol.* **21,** 47–51.
16. Osawa, M., Hanada, K., Hamada, H., and Nakauchi, H. (1996) Long-term lymphohematopoietic reconstitution by a single CD34-low/negative hematopoietic stem cell. *Science* **273,** 242–245.
17. Zou, Y. R., Kottmann, A. H., Kuroda, M., Taniuchi, I., and Littman, D. R. (1998) Function of the chemokine receptor CXCR4 in haematopoiesis and in cerebellar development. *Nature* **393,** 595–599.

18. Combadiere, C., Ahuja, S. K., Van Damme, J., Tiffany, H. L., Gao, J. L., and Murphy, P. M. (1995) Monocyte chemoattractant protein-3 is a functional ligand for CC chemokine receptors 1 and 2B. *J. Biol. Chem.* **270,** 29,671–29,675.

19. Laverriere, A. C., MacNeill, C., Mueller, C., Poelmann, R. E., Burch, J. B., and Evans, T. (1994) GATA-4/5/6, a subfamily of three transcription factors transcribed in developing heart and gut. *J. Biol. Chem.* **269,** 23,177–23,184.

20. Schott, J. J., Benson, D. W., Basson, C. T., et al. (1998) Congenital heart disease caused by mutations in the transcription factor NKX2-5. *Science* **281,** 108–111.

21. Schwartz, R. J. and Olson, E. N. (1999) Building the heart piece by piece: modularity of cis-elements regulating Nkx2-5 transcription. *Development* **126,** 4187–4192.

22. Yu, Y. T., Breitbart, R. E., Smoot, L. B., Lee, Y., Mahdavi, V., and Nadal-Ginard, B. (1992) Human myocyte-specific enhancer factor 2 comprises a group of tissue-restricted MADS box transcription factors. *Genes Dev.* **6,** 1783–1798.

23. Ausoni, S., Campione, M., Picard, A., et al. 1994. Structure and regulation of the mouse cardiac troponin I gene. *J. Biol. Chem.* **269,** 339–346.

24. Potter, J. D., Sheng, Z., Pan, B. S., and Zhao, J. (1995) A direct regulatory role for troponin T and a dual role for troponin C in the Ca2+ regulation of muscle contraction. *J. Biol. Chem.* **270,** 2557–2562.

25. Linhares, V. L., Almeida, N. A., Menezes, D. C., et al. (2004) Transcriptional regulation of the murine Connexin40 promoter by cardiac factors Nkx2-5, GATA4 and Tbx5. *Cardiovasc. Res.* **64,** 402–411.

26. Verheule, S., van Batenburg, C. A., Coenjaerts, F. E., Kirchhoff, S., Willecke, K., and Jongsma, H. J. (1999) Cardiac conduction abnormalities in mice lacking the gap junction protein connexin40. *J. Cardiovasc. Electrophysiol.* **10,** 1380–1389.

27. Verheule, S., van Batenburg, C. A., Coenjaerts, F. E., Kirchhoff, S., Willecke, K., and Jongsma, H. J. (1999) Cardiac conduction abnormalities in mice lacking the gap junction protein connexin40. *J. Cardiovasc. Electrophysiol.* **10,** 1380–1389.

28. Askari, A. T., Unzek, S., Popovic, Z. B., et al. (2003) Effect of stromal-cell-derived factor 1 on stem-cell homing and tissue regeneration in ischaemic cardiomyopathy. *Lancet* **362,** 697–703.

29. Mangi, A. A., Noiseux, N., Kong, D., et al. (2003) Mesenchymal stem cells modified with Akt prevent remodeling and restore performance of infarcted hearts. *Nat. Med.* **9,** 1195–1201.

30. Baschong, W., Suetterlin, R., and Laeng, R. H. (2001) Control of autofluorescence of archival formaldehyde-fixed, paraffin-embedded tissue in confocal laser scanning microscopy (CLSM). *J. Histochem. Cytochem.* **49,** 1565–1572.

31. Hardeman, E. C., Chiu, C. P., Minty, A., and Blau, H. M. (1986) The pattern of actin expression in human fibroblast x mouse muscle heterokaryons suggests that human muscle regulatory factors are produced. *Cell* **47,** 123–130.

32. Yoon, Y. S., Park, J. S., Tkebuchava, T., Luedeman, C., and Losordo, D. W. (2004) Unexpected severe calcification after transplantation of bone marrow cells in acute myocardial infarction. *Circulation* **109,** 3154–3157.

Index